HEALING WITH DEATH IMAGERY

Anees A. Sheikh
and
Katharina S. Sheikh
Editors

Imagery and Human Development Series
Series Editor: Anees A. Sheikh

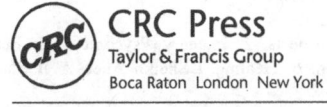

CRC Press is an imprint of the
Taylor & Francis Group, an **informa** business

First published 2007 by Baywood Publishing Company, Inc.

Published 2018 by CRC Press
Taylor & Francis Group
6000 Broken Sound Parkway NW, Suite 300
Boca Raton, FL 33487-2742

First issued in paperback 2018

© 2007 by Taylor & Francis Group, LLC
CRC Press is an imprint of Taylor & Francis Group, an Informa business

No claim to original U.S. Government works

ISBN 13: 978-0-415-78375-0 (pbk)
ISBN 13: 978-0-89503-317-8 (hbk)

This book contains information obtained from authentic and highly regarded sources. Reasonable efforts have been made to publish reliable data and information, but the author and publisher cannot assume responsibility for the validity of all materials or the consequences of their use. The authors and publishers have attempted to trace the copyright holders of all material reproduced in this publication and apologize to copyright holders if permission to publish in this form has not been obtained. If any copyright material has not been acknowledged please write and let us know so we may rectify in any future reprint.

Except as permitted under U.S. Copyright Law, no part of this book may be reprinted, reproduced, transmitted, or utilized in any form by any electronic, mechanical, or other means, now known or hereafter invented, including photocopying, microfilming, and recording, or in any information storage or retrieval system, without written permission from the publishers.

For permission to photocopy or use material electronically from this work, please access www.copyright.com (http://www.copyright.com/) or contact the Copyright Clearance Center, Inc.(CCC), 222 Rosewood Drive, Danvers, MA 01923, 978-750-8400. CCC is a not-for-profit organization that provides licenses and registration for a variety of users. For organizations that have been granted a photocopy license by the CCC, a separate system of payment has been arranged.

Trademark Notice: Product or corporate names may be trademarks or registered trademarks, and are used only for identification and explanation without intent to infringe.

Visit the Taylor & Francis Web site at
http://www.taylorandfrancis.com

and the CRC Press Web site at
http://www.crcpress.com

Library of Congress Catalog Number: 2006050149

Library of Congress Cataloging-in-Publication Data

Healing with death imagery / edited by Anees A. Sheikh and Katharina S. Sheikh.
    p. cm. -- (Imagery and human development series)
Includes bibliographical references and index.
ISBN-13: 978-0-89503-317-8 (cloth)
ISBN-10: 0-89503-317-8 (cloth)
    1. Death--Psychological aspects. 2. Imagery (Psychology) 3. Fear of death. 4. Imagination. 5. Visualization. 6. Healing. I. Sheikh, Anees A. II. Sheikh, Katharina S.

BF789.D4H39 2006
155.9'37--dc22

2006050149

In loving memory of

Dr. Muhammad Ajmal
and
Dr. Gordon H. Turner

*Two extraordinary human beings
who touched our lives deeply*

I died a mineral, and became a plant.
I died a plant, and rose an animal.
I died an animal and I was a man.
Why should I fear? When was I less by dying?

Jalaludin Rumi

(in R. A. Nicholson. *Rumi: Poet and Mystic.*
London: Unwin Paperbacks, 1978)

TITLES IN THE
Imagery and Human Development Series
Series Editor, *Anees A. Sheikh*

HEALING IMAGES
The Role of Imagination in Health
Edited by Anees A. Sheikh

GRENDEL AND HIS MOTHER
Healing the Traumas of Childhood Through Dreams, Imagery, and Hypnosis
Nicholas E. Brink

HANDBOOK OF THERAPEUTIC IMAGERY TECHNIQUES
Edited by Anees A. Sheikh

MEMORIES OF LOSS AND DREAMS OF PERFECTION
Unsuccessful Childhood Grieving and Adult Creativity
Delmont E. Morrison and Shirley Linden Morrison

HEALING WITH DEATH IMAGERY
Edited by Anees A. Sheikh and Katharina S. Sheikh

HYPNOSIS AND IMAGINATION
Edited by Robert G. Kunzendorf, Nicholas P. Spanos, and Benjamin Wallace

THE PSYCHOPHYSIOLOGY OF MENTAL IMAGERY
Theory, Research, and Application
Edited by Robert G. Kunzendorf and Anees A. Sheikh

INDIVIDUAL DIFFERENCES IN IMAGING
Their Measurement, Origins, and Consequences
Alan Richardson

DREAM IMAGES
A Call to Mental Arms
Edited by Jayne Gackenbach and Anees A. Sheikh

IMAGERY IN SPORTS AND PHYSICAL PERFORMANCE
Edited by Anees A. Sheikh and Errol R. Korn

IMAGINATION AND HEALING
Edited by Anees A. Sheikh

Contents

Foreword ix
    Larry Dossey

Preface xiii
    Anees A. Sheikh and Katharina S. Sheikh

CHAPTER 1
    Is There Life Before Death? Healing Potential of Death Imagery . . . 1
    Anees A. Sheikh and Katharina S. Sheikh

CHAPTER 2
    Opening to Loss: Connecting with Life Through the
    Meditations of Stephen Levine 27
    Colleen M. Heinkel and Anees A. Sheikh

CHAPTER 3
    Confronting Death Through Mental and Artistic Imagery 47
    Robert G. Kunzendorf

CHAPTER 4
    Near-Death Experiences: Heading toward Omega? 67
    Anees A. Sheikh, Sundar Ramaswami, and
    Katharina S. Sheikh

CHAPTER 5
    Death Imagery in the Buddhist Tradition 109
    Sundar Ramaswami and Anees A. Sheikh

CHAPTER 6
    The Dynamic, Clinical Use of Imagery to Promote
    Psychotherapeutic Grieving 139
    James K. Morrison

CHAPTER 7
Hypnotic Death and Suicide Rehearsal 165
Alexander A. Levitan

CHAPTER 8
Death Imagery and Death Anxiety 179
Rita T. McDonald and Carolyn J. Salyards

CHAPTER 9
The Use of Guided Imagery in Death Education 203
Thomas A. Droege

CHAPTER 10
Confronting Death: An Experiential Imagery Exercise 223
Anees A. Sheikh

Contributors 229

Index 231

Foreword

The fear of death—its inevitability and finality, its grotesque mysteriousness—is perhaps the source of more misery for more people than anything else. To revise our attitude toward death and modify the immense, dark hold it has on our psychic life must be counted a project of incalculable importance. The accomplishment of this mission is what this book is all about.

Can this be done? Many traditions say yes. A Zen aphorism states, "If you die before you die, then when you die you will not die." What does it mean to die before you die? For one thing it means reassessing the assumptions we habitually and unconsciously make about the meaning of death. Our typical approach is to regard both birth and death as absolutes—the beginning and ending of life. On closer reflection we discover that these images of absolute beginnings and endings depend on deeper assumptions about the nature of reality, specifically about the nature of time. For us, time flows. It is linear, it is stretched from past through the present and into the future; it is one-way. This backdrop is crucial for the finality we attribute to death. It is the reason we "only go around once." It is the reason death for us is the end.

What if we are wrong about the nature of time? It comes as a surprise to many persons to discover that modern physicists, the pundits in our society who tell us about what time "really" is, are not in agreement about its nature. Nobel physicist Richard Feynman, who dominated the physics of his generation, expressed his exasperation about the nature of time. "What is time?" he asked. "We physicists work with it every day, but don't ask me what it is. It's just too difficult to think about" (quoted in Boslough, 1990). Although they cannot assure us what time is, physicists have told us what it is not. It is not, they say, the external, inexorably flowing stuff that is the same for everyone, as Newton intuited. As British physicist Paul Davies puts it, there has never been an experiment in the history of science that shows that time flows.

In the end, however, it seems unwise to base our philosophies of death on the proclamations of physics as to the nature of time. These views change, as history shows. But if physicists are today uncertain about the precise nature of time, and if there is no consensus among them, this suggests that it is perfectly appropriate for the rest of us to reassess our time-contingent meanings of death and to take seriously the life-transforming images of wholeness, unity, completeness, and immortality contained in many of the death images in this book.

Not only may we have it wrong as to the fundamental nature of time, we may also be in error about what we fear will perish at death—the body and the mind—and their relationship to each other. The Swiss psychologist Carl G. Jung once said,

> The psyche's attachment to the brain, i.e., its space-time limitation, is no longer as self-evident and incontrovertible as we have hitherto been led to believe. . . . An objective and critical survey of the available data would establish that perceptions occur as if in part there were no space, in part no time. . . . Anyone who does justice to the facts cannot but admit that their apparent space-timelessness is their most essential quality. The fact that we are totally unable to imagine a form of existence without space and time by no means proves that such an existence is in itself impossible. . . . It is not only permissible to doubt the absolute validity of space-time perception; it is, in view of the available facts, even imperative to do so" (Jung, 1977, pp. 134-136).

Why are Jung's comments relevant to our concerns about the nature of death? One of the most pernicious beliefs of Western man—one on which our morbid ideas of death depend—is the notion that the brain somehow produces "consciousness" or "mind" as a byproduct of its chemical processes. This reasoning has enormously negative psychological consequences for almost everyone because it rules out in *principle* the possibility of any continuation of existence following death. For if all awareness, mind, or consciousness, is dependent on the brain, when the brain dies, that is the end of everything. As Bertrand Russell stoically once put it, "When I die I shall rot, and nothing of my ego shall remain."

What would it take to show that this assumption is false? If we could demonstrate that there are some things that minds can do that brains are incapable of, this would go far in showing that consciousness is not entirely brain dependent. In fact, there is considerable empirical data showing that there is some aspect of the psyche that is *nonlocal*—that is not confined to points in time such as the present moment. It is immensely important to establish a nonlocal model of consciousness because without it much, if not all, of death imagery falls flat; it can always be dismissed as fantasy, wishful thinking, dreamy mysticism, or outright hallucinations—nothing but brain chemistry in action.

In legitimizing death imagery, it is therefore vital, it seems to me, to call attention to the many examples in which the psyche behaves nonlocally; for example, instances in which it escapes its space-time limitation to the brain, the body, and the present. These instances tell us something glorious about our self; that there is some aspect of our psyche that is outside space and time, and that by implication may be unbounded, infinite, and immortal.

One example will make the point. Once Jung experienced a near-fatal heart attack and a subsequent series of "tremendous visions," as he put it. In one of these he foresaw the impending death of the physician who was caring for him at that time. The vision proved correct. On the day the doctor allowed Jung to sit up for the first time, he, the physician, took to bed and died of septicemia a few days later. Here Jung's psyche seemed to break the spatiotemporal limitations we usually assign to the mind; it gained information before the specific events happened, demonstrating a capacity we believe the physical brain is incapable of. Although this might be called a near-death experience today, these events are not confined to the near-death state; they frequently crop up in the voluntary death-imagery experiences described in this book.

When in the past, persons have voiced brighter, less intimidating views of death, they often have been shouted down or derided. Images of death as a transition to another state of being with no ultimate control over us have been dismissed as examples of wish fulfillment, denial, or fantasy, and have been considered amusing fodder for the skeptic. But as this book exemplifies, this harsh attitude may be abating.

Accompanying these experiences frequently is a numinosity that is simply ineffable, as if one has touched absolutes and the deepest meanings. That is why work with death imagery is more than "psychology," "guidance," or "counseling"; and why this book in essence is about a spiritual path and a search for meaning.

There is ample evidence that hopelessness, loss of meaning, and an impending sense of doom are toxic to the body in many ways. These emotions often accompany our attitudes toward death. Today we know they exert a depressant effect on the body's immune function and can set in motion irreversible, sometimes fatal processes in the heart and circulatory system as well. Thus it is no exaggeration to say that our attitude toward death literally can be a matter of life and death.

I can envision no more important task for psychology than a revisioning of death. If death is indeed not the destroyer, avenger, and grim reaper we long have taken it to be in Western culture, the news should be shouted from the rooftops. Finding an alternative to our morbid attitudes toward it justifies an investment of energy that is of Manhattan Project proportions. That is why *Healing with Death Imagery* is a valuable contribution to the enrichment of human life.

Larry Dossey, M.D.
Santa Fe, New Mexico

REFERENCES

Boslough, J. (1990). The enigma of time. *National Geographic, 177,* 109-132
Jung, C. G. (1977). *Psychology and the occult.* Princeton: Princeton University Press.

Preface

> A friend who had been meditating for some time approached a Zen master recently arrived in this country. He asked the roshi if he might study with him. To which the roshi replied, "Are you prepared to die?" My friend shook his head in bewilderment and said, "I didn't come here to die. I came here to learn Zen." The roshi said, "If you are not willing to die, you are not ready to let go into life. Come back when you are ready to enter directly, excluding nothing."
>
> Stephen Levine (1982) *Who Dies?*
> New York: Anchor Books, p. 25

Sages of various traditions and ages have reiterated that we must incorporate the inevitability of death into the fabric of life to experience its breadth and beauty. Imagery is an important tool in dealing fruitfully with death, and this book is devoted to exploring many facets of this fascinating issue.

The first chapter presents an overview of ancient and modern approaches to the use of death imagery for therapeutic purposes, including a discussion of its possible benefits. The second chapter specifically explores Stephen Levine's contributions in this area and shows that it is only by opening to the reality of death that one can make living a conscious process of growth. A number of excellent imagery-based experiential exercises are also discussed in detail. The third chapter demonstrates the significance of confronting death through mental and artistic images and includes a discussion of six examples of death-related religious and existential works of art.

Recently there has been an upsurge of interest in near-death experiences and their salutary effects on the experient's attitudes, beliefs, and values. Of particular interest here are increases in spirituality, concern for others, appreciation of life, and an enhanced sense of meaning and purpose in life. The fourth chapter presents a detailed critical overview of this field of investigation with special emphasis on the transformatory aftereffects of near-death experiences.

Of all the major religions in the world, Buddhism is at the forefront of exploring the topic of death and dying and developing specific meditative exercises for confronting death. Chapter 5 presents an in-depth treatment of death imagery in Buddhist thought.

Chapter 6 continues the theme that confrontation with death can lead to healthful consequences by exploring the use of hypnosis for death rehearsal. A variation of this technique, hypnotic suicide rehearsal, is also discussed: it appears to be effective for use with clients who are ruminating about suicide. Case examples clarify the details of the process.

Over the years, several clinicians have proposed the use of imagery for reconstructing death-related events and thereby facilitating the grieving process in individuals who are experiencing symptoms rooted in unfinished grieving. Chapter 7 gives an exhaustive account of the use of imagery for unresolved grieving and includes a number of case histories.

Researchers have perhaps devoted more time and energy to the investigation of death anxiety than any other death-related topic. Chapter 8 reviews literature on death anxiety and death imagery and demonstrates a core connection between the two phenomena. The authors claim that death imagery has the potential not only to ameliorate death anxiety, but also to lead to a more authentic existence.

Chapter 9 explains how death imagery can be used constructively in death education. The author presents several practical suggestions and specific guided imagery exercises. With Chapter 10, this volume closes with a detailed death-imagery experiential exercise aimed at encountering death to enhance our appreciation of life. The reader will notice that this thread steadily runs through all the chapters in this book.

In conclusion, we thank all contributors for sharing their unique perspectives. Also, we are deeply grateful to the staff of Baywood Publishing Company, especially to its president Stuart Cohen, and Bobbi Olszewski and Julie Krempa. At Marquette University, we are thankful to Stephanie Vainisi and Patricia Johnson for their conscientious help; and last but not least, we are indebted to Rhona Fields for her cheerful and expert assistance throughout the preparation of this volume.

As far as we know, this is the first comprehensive book devoted to the role of death imagery in health and growth. We hope that it will be helpful in changing the rather sinister view of death, prevalent in our culture, to a deeper appreciation of its enhancing potential.

Anees A. Sheikh and Katharina S. Sheikh
Brookfield, Wisconsin

CHAPTER 1

Is There Life Before Death? Healing Potential of Death Imagery

Anees A. Sheikh and Katharina S. Sheikh

> All questions at the public meeting that day were about life beyond the grave. The Master only laughed and did not give a single answer. To his disciples, who demanded to know the reason for his evasiveness, he later said, "Have you observed that it is precisely those who do not know what to do with this life who want another that will last forever?" "But is there life after death or is there not?" persisted a disciple. "Is there life before death?—That is the question!" said the Master enigmatically.
>
> Anthony deMello (1985, p. 74)

> To my question, whether we might not fortify our minds for the approach of death, he answered, in a passion, "No sir, let it alone. It matters not how a man dies, but how he lives. The act of dying is not of importance, it lasts so short a time."
>
> James Boswell (in Straub, 2002, p. 59)

Generally, Western cultures have regarded death as an unpleasant reality, which is not an integral part of life, but exists outside of it or, at least, on its fringes. We try to hide death from view or treat it as a disease to overcome (Aguilar & Wood, 1976; Braga & Braga, 1975; Grof, 2000; Paz, 1961; Straub, 2002). As Kübler-Ross (1975) has stressed,

> It is the denial of death that is partially responsible for people leading empty purposeless lives. For when you live as if you will live forever, it becomes too easy to postpone the things you know that you must do. You live your life in preparation for tomorrow or in remembrance of yesterday, but meanwhile each today is lost. But when you fully understand that each day you awaken may be the last you have, you take the time that day, to grow, to become more of who you really are, to reach out to other human beings (p. 164).

ACCEPTING DEATH BRINGS US TO THE THRESHOLD OF LIFE

It is very surprising that until the late 1960s the subject of death and dying was largely ignored in the West, not only by the general population but also by the scientists and professionals. It is astonishing that even the professionals in health sciences showed a lack of interest in this subject (Blazer, 1978; Grof, 2000). Yet since ancient times, death has been the main source of inspiration of philosophers, writers, artists, and composers. Michelangelo remarked, "No thought exists in me which death has not carved with his chisel," and Thomas Mann felt that "without death there would scarcely have been poets on earth" (Kübler-Ross, 1975, p. 2). Boris Pasternak, in *Doctor Zhivago* (1958), views virtually all human activity as an effort at coming to terms with death.

> Now what is history? It is the centuries of systematic explorations of the riddle of death, with a view to overcoming death. That's why people discover mathematical infinity and electromagnetic waves, that's why they write symphonies. . . . Man does not die in a ditch like a dog—but at home in history, while the work toward the conquest of death is in full swing; he dies sharing in this work (p. 10).

There is general agreement among world religions that a meaningful life is possible only after death has been accepted as a basic condition of life (Long, 1975). The goal is not simply to view death as the final act in life, but to welcome it as a persistent ingredient in the entire process of life. By recognizing the finiteness of one's existence, one is permeated by the urgency to cast off those extrinsic roles and to devote every day to growing as fully as possible (Grof, 2000; Levitan, 1985; Sheikh, Twente, & Turner, 1979; Yalom, 1980, 2002).

Thus the acceptance of death brings one to the threshold of living authentically. This thought is a cornerstone of existential philosophy. Herman Feifel (1961, p. 71) says, "Life is not genuinely our own until we renounce it." Rollo May maintains, "With the confronting of non-being, existence takes on vitality and immediacy, and the individual experiences a heightened consciousness of himself and his world, and others around him" (May, 1958, p. 47). Irvin Yalom (1980, p. 163) feels that "by keeping death in mind one passes into a state of gratitude for the countless givens of existence." Santayana (see Yalom, 1980, p. 163) remarks, "The dark background which death supplies, brings out the tender colors of life in all their purity," and Nietzsche (1974, p. 37) states, "Out of such abysses, from such severe sicknesses, one returns newborn . . . with a more delicate taste for joy, with a more tender tongue for all good things, with merrier senses, with a second dangerous innocence in joy."

Literature is replete with examples of individuals who underwent extensive personal transformation due to their close brush with death. Thomas Mann's (1969) Hans Castorp in *The Magic Mountain*, Max Frisch's (1957) Faber in *Homo Faber*, Tolstoy's (1931) Pierre in *War and Peace*, and Ivan Ilyich in the

Death of Ivan Ilyich (Tolstoy, 1960) are obvious examples. Another striking and well-known illustration is the repentant Ebenezer Scrooge. We may forget that his cold heart was not melted simply by the warmth of the Christmas Spirit—to that it had proven itself totally impervious. What transformed Scrooge was the encounter with his own death. The Ghost of Christmas Yet to Come used a potent form of death-imagery therapy: Scrooge had the opportunity to witness his own death, to overhear acquaintances dismiss lightly his passing, and to observe strangers quarreling over his worldly possessions. Then Scrooge attended his own funeral, and finally, in the last scene preceding his transformation, he examined the inscription on his tombstone (Yalom, 1980).

DEATH IMAGERY: AN OVERVIEW OF ANCIENT AND MODERN APPROACHES

It has become apparent that many thinkers agree that learning to die is a prerequisite to living meaningfully. While the time when death is imminent can be a fertile period of personal growth, we should not and must not wait until then to learn the lessons of death. For centuries, and in several cultures, variations of the experience of death in imagination have been used effectively. These death-imagery techniques provide the opportunity to confront death and to come to terms with it. This section reviews a number of such approaches.

Death Imagery in Ancient Initiatory Experiences

As Metzner (1986) points out, death/rebirth fantasy and associated ritual practices have been an essential component of initiatory experiences in several traditional cultures. For example, the training of shamans/healers involved sloughing off all old attachments and old ways of living. "Sometimes the older shaman, while instructing the apprentice, would symbolically 'kill' the apprentice. This was then followed by a restoration or reconstitution . . . into a new more power-filled form, endowed with healing and magical abilities" (Metzner, 1986, p. 146). This aspect of shamanic training is very similar to the process of *mortificatio* in alchemy, which has a literal meaning of "killing" or "dead making." *Mortificatio* involved conscious and intentional attempts to reduce ego attachments through symbolic meditations and visualizations that stressed "darkness, defeat, torture, mutilation, death and rotting," followed by positive images of "growth, rejuvenation, fruiting, ripening, and rebirth" (Metzner, 1986, p. 146).

Death/rebirth imagery and rituals are also very common in the initiation rites or *rites of passage*, as Arnold van Gennep (1960) calls them, of numerous tribes around the world. Their common denominator is profound confrontation with death and subsequent transcendence (Grof, 2000). Neale (1969, pp. 169-170) describes one such initiation ritual:

After the older men have prepared a sacred place in the bush, the mother brings her son to the edge of the village. She does not know the content of the rites. She has heard only rumors about death and manhood. She does know that occasionally a child fails to return. The little boy knows the same. Both are filled with excitement and pride, but also with great anxiety. The men rush forward and force the boy away from his mother. She weeps and wails over the forthcoming death of her son. He is taken to a hut where he lies down on his back with his arms crossed over his chest. He is covered with a rug and told not to utter a sound. During the coming days, he may be symbolically burned by a fire, buried in a shallow pit, be ritually dismembered, or have a tooth knocked out. All these things—the separation from his mother, the darkness, and the physical dangers—are symbolic experiences of death. The boy is told that the gods are killing him. He does not know for sure whether he will literally survive or not. By means of this first half of the puberty ritual, the world of the child and his personality are destroyed. The second half of the ritual takes place over an extended period of time. The boy meets his god and receives his name. After this he may have to be fed by a guardian for as much as six months, for newborn infants cannot feed themselves without help. During this time he is instructed and trained to meditate on his experiences. By story, dance, and pantomime, he is introduced to the gods, the history of the tribe, and to the way he is to live. Finally, the boy is returned to the community to take his place as a new person in a new world. The boy and his mother may not acknowledge each other for some time to come. After all, her son has died, it is a strange adult who returned to the village. In the spiritual sense, the boy does not know his mother. His old world and old self have been destroyed. Death has led to rebirth and a new creation.

Buddhist Meditation on Death

This type of meditation is very commonly used by Buddhist monks. The monk sits down in the graveyard or crematorium and reflects upon the corpses or ashes, and he even imagines his own body to be among these remains. This exercise renders him more profoundly aware of the brevity and uncertainty of life and the inevitability of death. He realizes that human beings and their objects of pleasure do not endure for long. This insight prompts him to abandon all ambition to shape the world in accordance with his wishes. "And, with the passing of the habit of living a life of willfulness (and its offspring, anxiety and fear) will come automatically a peace of mind and tranquility which will abide unaltered in all conditions of life and all states of mind" (Long, 1975, p. 69).

Many Buddhist teachings concerning death are contained in *The Tibetan Book of the Dead*. It presents not only the most effective method of "living toward death," but also contains instructions on how to die well (Evans-Wentz, 1960). The dying person is advised to remain calm and alert in the face of death and to shun distraction and confusion. He/she is reminded too that his/her life forces are about to disengage themselves from the body and that he/she should focus upon this event. He/she is then prepared for the meeting with death by its description:

death is the "brilliant light of Ultimate Reality" or "the luminous splendor of the colorless light of Emptiness." The moribund should immerse himself/herself in that supernatural brilliance, sloughing off all belief in an individual self and realizing that the "boundless light of this true Reality" is his/her own true self (Evans-Wentz, 1960; Long, 1975; Rahula, 1959; Robinson, 1970).

In a technique involving mindfulness of one's death, Buddhaghosa (1976) encourages the subjects to imagine people who are already dead but who had enjoyed the good things of life, and to repeat, "Death will take place." After a degree of mindfulness has been achieved, the practitioner is advised to remember death in eight ways. These are summarized here from Ramaswami and Sheikh (1991, pp. 182-183):

> 1) One should reflect on the fact that death is inevitable for that which is born and imagine death appearing like a murderer with poised sword. 2) Death should be imagined as the ruin of success—health ending in sickness, prosperity turning to loss, youth yielding to age. 3) One should imagine the death of others and thus infer one's mortality. 4) One should remember that one shares this body with numerous families of worms that live in and depend on our body. They are born, grow old, excrete, and die within one's body. 5) One should reflect on the frailty of one's body. 6) One should reflect that death often attacks without providing prior warning. 7) One should reflect on the limited span of life. 8) One should remember that in the last analysis our life is limited to a single conscious moment: we are constantly dying and being reborn anew every moment.

Benefits of the successful practice of mindfulness of death include conquering attachment to life, avarice, and lust; realizing the impermanence of life and developing serenity; and developing the ability to face death in a composed and fearless manner (Ramaswami & Sheikh, 1991).

Sufi Contemplation Upon Death

The Sufis, in keeping with the Prophet Mohammed's advice, "Die before you are dead," have given great importance to the contemplation of death. They reflect upon the inevitable future decay and disintegration of all living beings and upon the fact that their own bodies soon will be nothing but rotten flesh and dry bones upon which worms will feed. Thus they achieve the awareness of the impermanence of temporal life. For the Sufis, this meditation on death is a vital step toward beatitude—the ultimate goal of all spiritual striving. Death represents the dismemberment of the present imperfect state, which then renders possible the rebirth of a personality with spiritually healthy and stable traits.

The devastation of winter makes way for the renewal of spring. Similarly, the old self must die before it can be reborn. After longings for material riches and bodily pleasures, ambivalence toward others, and above all, egoism are seen in the correct light and abandoned, rebirth is bound to occur (Ajmal, 1979, 1989).

As Andrew Harvey (1994) writes, "Our life is constantly tempting us to identify ourselves with it. Every time we identify ourselves with it, we fall prey to the illusion of separation from other people, we fall prey to the illusion of time and the illusion that we are dying. It is only by dying to that illusion that we can enter reality" (p. 291). He urges, "Transfigure this life into a slaughterhouse of the ego. Burn away the false self and radiate . . . love, knowledge, bliss, and joy to everyone. When you *are*, you will never die, because there is only *Being*" (p. 295).

As it is evident from the preceding passages, according to the Sufis, loss of self is essential for continued integration and growth. "The only Universal Reality is experienced by giving up the 'I,' the 'me,' the 'mine.'" In Sufism this process is called *fana*,[1] or freedom from the self (Shafii, 1985, p. 143). *Fana* ultimately leads to *Baqa*,[2] the ultimate state of existence, "the union and oneness with all beings and God."

Attar, a twelfth-century Sufi, in his book of mystical poetry, *The Conference of Birds*, wrote:

> As long as you are preoccupied with self
>   How can the True Being reach you?
> Unless you become annihilated in humbleness
>   and nonbeing,
> How can ultimate knowing be received
>   from the Great Being (in Shafii, 1985, p. 148).

As Shafii (1985) points out, *fana* or freedom from the self is a universal experience and is not specific to the Sufis only. There are frequent references to the "loss of self" in all major spiritual traditions. The Sufis and other mystical traditions have developed numerous meditative exercises and other procedures to facilitate the process of *fana* (Arasteh, 1980; Shafii, 1985).

Practicing Death

In *The Republic*, Plato maintains that there are four stages of cognitive development: during the first stage one perceives only shadows and other superficial or insubstantial things; the second stage is marked by the perception of the reality of physical objects; the third stage is characterized by the capacity for abstract mathematics and deductive reasoning; the fourth stage involves the experience of the Forms, the eternal archetypes or potentials, that structure all thought and perception. Plato argues that these forms are truly known only by the experience of the highest level of reality, after all physical and mental activity ceases. In the dialogues, such as *Phaedo, Meno, Theaetetus*, and *Phaedrus*, he equates "true knowledge, knowledge of the Forms, with knowledge of the world experienceable

---

[1] *Fana* is an Arabic word meaning passing away, vanishing, annihilation, and nothingness (Shafii, 1985, p. 144).

[2] *Baqa* is an Arabic word meaning permanency, living, life, and eternity (Shafii, 1985, p. 148).

'after death'" (Shear, 1978). In *Phaedo,* he states unequivocally that the philosopher's true method, the method of gaining knowledge of the Forms, consists of practicing death, that is, giving the soul the opportunity to become accustomed "to withdraw from all contact with the body and concentrate itself by itself . . . alone by itself" (*Collected Dialogues of Plato*, edited by Hamilton & Cairns, 1973). How important practicing death was to Plato is evident in an old story. "Plato on his death bed was asked by a friend if he would summarize his great life work, the *Dialogues,* in one statement. Plato, coming out of a reverie, looked at his friend and said, practice dying" (Keleman, 1974, p. 1).

Koestenbaum's Exercises

Koestenbaum (1976) describes several death and immortality exercises that he feels are very effective. Some he has developed and others he has taken from Herman Feifel and Robert Kastenbaum. One exercise consists of composing your own obituary. This act leads you to face the crucial question of what it means to be a human being, what is involved in passing the time on earth well, and most importantly, what it means to be *you.* Other exercises described by Koestenbaum are (1) imaging that you are attending your own funeral and overhearing a friend speak frankly about the significance of your life; (2) experiencing a rebirth fantasy; (3) writing a script for your own death, describing *how, when,* and *where* it took place; (4) reading a vivid and moving account of the death of a 6-year-old abandoned child and, subsequently, completing seven sentences. Koestenbaum maintains that these exercises help to courageously face the reality of your own death and thus to make crucial discoveries.

Koestenbaum (1976) also presents an immortality exercise that has the form of a guided daydream or fantasy. First, he asks the subject to imagine that he/she is a dying patient in the hospital. Then he presents a sequence of thoughts that occur immediately before death. He tells the individual that all worldly things are receding into a meaningless distance, and that he/she now feels more "like a god in outer space observing life than a human being participating in the affairs of the world" (p. 189). Suggestions of this nature are followed by induced images in which the person accepts death, feels at peace, experiences himself/herself as a part of the universal scheme, and has a sense of the eternal nature of consciousness. Koestenbaum claims that this exercise can lead to a premonition of the experience of immortality. "The key dynamism bringing about this realization is relinquishing the sense of being an individual" (p. 189).

Straub's *Death 101*

Sandra Straub's *Death 101: A Workbook for Educating and Healing* (2002) is an excellent resource that includes numerous valuable imagery exercises that will help individuals navigating through death-related issues. According to

Straub, "when you discuss death or acknowledge death, you do not invite death, but rather invite life" (p. 1). These exercises also are extremely helpful for the health professionals who plan to help others resolve death-related complications. It seems obvious that unless we confront our own issues regarding death, we will be of little help to others (Winokuer, 2002).

Stephen Levine's Work on Conscious Living and Conscious Dying

Levine's work (1972, 1979, 1984, 1989, 1991, 1997, 2002) shows that it is only by opening to the reality of death that one can make living a conscious process of growth. His books "demonstrate a remarkable ability to articulate for Western audiences the value of meditation practice in confronting and accepting death. From the point of view of Eastern psychology, particularly Buddhist psychology, real acceptance and understanding of death, illness, and suffering must move beyond mere intellectual speculation and abstraction. Experience is the only teacher. Openness to the fullness of experience is developed through the consistent practice of meditation" (Kruck & Sheikh, 1991, p. 46). Levine offers a series of excellent imagery-based meditational/experiential exercises toward this end. These include *letting the mind float in the heart, losing self-image, self-forgiveness and forgiving others, loving kindness, grief meditation, pain and healing meditation, meditation on heavy emotions, meditation on death and dying, moment of death meditation*, and *after-death meditation*. "Regardless of an individual's theoretical or theological background, Levine provides an outline for rethinking the presuppositions upon which our attitudes toward death and dying are based" (Kruck & Sheikh, 1991, p. 66). He presents an alternative approach that rests on the idea that life and death are complementary dimensions of a single integrated process. For a detailed discussion of his techniques, the reader is referred to other sources (Kruck & Sheikh, 1991; Levine, 1972, 1979, 1984, 1989, 1991, 1997, 2002; Levine & Levine, 1999).

Grieving Through Imagery

In our society, the grief stricken often are discouraged from facing the reality of death by relatives and friends who take over for them and invite them to be mere observers. Consequently, it becomes difficult for the bereaved to come to grips with the death of their loved ones (Nichols & Nichols, 1975). Several clinicians have suggested imagery techniques that, in combination with other therapeutic interventions, reconstruct death-related events, and thus, facilitate the grieving process (Aguilar & Wood, 1976; Droege, 1987; Levine & Levine, 1999; Melges, 1982; Melges & DeMaso, 1980; Morrison, 1978; Ramsay & Noorbergen, 1981; Straub, 2002; Volkan, 1975; Williamson, 1978). Melges and DeMaso (1980), for example, believe that unresolved grief reactions generally persist due to the obstacles that inhibited the grieving process at the time of the loss. When the bereaved is given an opportunity to relive, revise, and revisit scenes of the loss in present-time imagery, and thus remove these obstacles, grief resolution is facilitated. Following is a case history provided by Melges and DeMaso (1980, p. 58).

> A 27-year-old, married mother of two children, became acutely incapacitated with an uncanny fear of death when, shortly after her husband's grandmother died, she revisited the same cemetery where her stepfather was buried three years previously. She had idealized her stepfather as being a "perfect man." During the re-grief therapy, when she was reliving seeing her stepfather's body in the funeral home, she became aware of her anger toward him for having sexually played with her as a girl but she could not express this anger in the relived-remembered scene because her mother, from whom they had kept the secret, was there at the funeral home. The therapist asked her to revise the scene, removing the mother along with all other people, and encouraged her to express her anger and feelings. With the scene thus revised, she gave full vent to her anger and her guilt for having to carry this secret for so long. After that, she felt free to express her love for him, which she had refused to do during his terminal illness. She also acknowledged her complicity in the sexual activities, and then forgave him and subsequently felt he understood and forgave her for not caring for him during his terminal illness. With her guilt and anger dismantled, she felt immediately relieved, no longer "haunted" by the death phobia.

Although techniques such as those described by Melges and DeMaso are not concerned directly with the issue of one's own death, they nevertheless are bound to lead one to confront it. Morrison (1991) offers a note of caution that "imagery techniques may not be appropriate for those therapists who have not carefully analyzed their own imagery" and that therapists "should be aware that directed imagery can occasionally provoke traumatic emotional reactions in clients, and they must be ready for them (pp. 90-91).

Death Imagery Technique

In an article published in 1979, Sheikh et al. report death-imagery techniques that they developed. One can use these procedures to attain mere relaxation, or relaxation may be considered as only the first step in therapy. For relaxation purposes, the subject is asked to take a few deep breaths and lie down. Then he/she is given the following instructions:

> Imagine that you are dead. You have lost all your ability to counter the force of gravity and are completely immobilized and inactive. All your muscles, even all your body cells are pulled down by gravity. You no longer have to struggle, be tense, and spend energy to stay alive. You no longer have to direct your thinking or censor your thoughts. The thoughts come and go as they like. As your "dead" body is pulled more and more by the force of gravity, you have a feeling that you are shedding off your body. Your

thoughts scatter and all the verbal chatter and commotion vanish into thin air. As you shed your body, you become a weightless, bodiless, pure consciousness. There is stillness and quiet and a benign indifference of nature (Sheikh et al., 1979, p. 154).

Often the subject initially experiences some anxiety; however, this soon gives way to feelings of deep relaxation and a sense of being at peace with the world. During this relaxed state, long-forgotten memories, particularly of unfinished issues pertaining to parents, often surface spontaneously. They provide significant material for meaningful therapy. For continuing therapy, specific imagery procedures have been developed. These include (1) visualizing, confronting, and finally saying farewell to all those individuals, alive or dead, with whom the subject had significant emotional contact; (2) visualizing himself/herself as an infant, as a child, as an adolescent, and as he/she is now, and saying goodbye to all these aspects of development; (3) finishing in imagery, the unfinished tasks that arise in associated memories. After the completion of the unfinished business and the farewell process, the subject is directed to experience a departure from his/her body.

Hypnotic Death and Suicide Rehearsal

Levitan (1985) developed a hypnotic death-rehearsal technique initially to help patients faced with imminent death. However, since then he has been using it to assist clients with concerns about the death and dying process. It is very similar to the death-imagery technique discussed above but differs in the sense that "the therapist is continually involved in reframing and interpreting the visualized images reported by the subject. The principal objective of this hypnotic death rehearsal is to demystify the death experience and allow the patient to approach it with familiarity and confidence" (Levitan, 1991, p. 96). A variation of this, the hypnotic death rehearsal, aims at focusing "subjects to critically evaluate the consequences of death by suicide and hopefully eliminate magical thinking in this regard" (p. 96). For further details of these techniques, the reader is referred to other sources (Levitan, 1985, 1991).

Perinatal Experiences and Holotropic Therapy

Grof and Halifax (1977) provide a description of experiences related to the events immediately preceding, accompanying, and following birth that their subjects had during psychotherapy under the influence of LSD. They term these as perinatal experiences. These experiences largely pertain to the problems of biological birth, physical pain, suffering, disease, agony, aging, and death. The encounter with suffering and agony, Grof and Halifax state, ends in an experience of complete annihilation on all levels, including physical, emotional, intellectual, moral, and transcendental.

This is usually referred to as an "ego death": it seems to involve instantaneous destruction of all the previous reference points of the individual. The experience of total annihilation is often followed by a vision of blinding white or golden light and a sense of liberating decompression and expansion. The universe is perceived as indescribably beautiful and radiant; individuals feel cleansed and purged, and talk about redemption, salvation, or union with God (Grof & Halifax, 1977, p. 51).

Grof and Halifax (1977) claim that people return from the perinatal experience with the confidence that they have "confronted the ultimate crisis" and achieved deep understanding into the nature of death and dying. They "discover the importance of accepting, surrendering and relinquishing" (p. 52). Despite its intimate connection with the experience of biological birth, Grof (1985) emphasizes that "the perinatal process transcends biology and has important psychological and spiritual dimensions. It should not therefore be interpreted in a concretistic and reductionistic fashion" (p. 100).

Recently Stanislav Grof and Christina Grof have developed a procedure called holotropic therapy or holomonic integration that they claim achieves the same goals without the use of drugs. Holotropic therapy consists of a combination of intense breathing, music, and focused body work and appears to lead to a variety of salutary consequences including lifting of chronic depression, overcoming phobias and irrational feelings, improvement of self-confidence and self-esteem, disappearance of psychosomatic pain, and in many cases dramatic improvement in the so-called organic diseases such as clearing of chronic infection or solidification of the bones in women with osteoporosis (Grof, 2000). Further details of this procedure are available elsewhere (Grof, 1985, 2000; Grof & Bennett, 1992).

Grof coined the term *holotropic* from the Greek *holos* (whole) and *trepein* (moving toward or in the direction of something) (Grof, 2000; Grof & Bennett, 1992). In holotropic states, he explains,

> Consciousness is changed qualitatively in a very profound and fundamental way . . . characterized by dramatic perceptual changes in all sensory areas. . . . The emotions associated with holotropic states cover a very broad spectrum that typically extends far beyond the limits of our everyday experience, both in their nature and intensity. . . . The intellect is not impaired, but functions in a way that is significantly different from its everyday mode of operation. While we might not be able to rely on our judgment in ordinary practical matters, we can be literally flooded with remarkable valid information on a variety of subjects . . . by far the most interesting insights that become available in holotropic states revolve around philosophical, metaphysical, and spiritual issues (Grof, 2000, pp. 2-3).

Holotropic states, as Grof (2000) points out, were held in high esteem in all indigenous cultures, and effective procedures of induction were very carefully devised by them. They used these procedures in pursuit of a variety of goals, including to diagnose and heal a variety of disorders; to develop intuition, extrasensory perception, and artistic inspiration; and to have direct contact with deities and forces of nature. For an overview of ancient and aboriginal techniques for inducing holotropic states, the reader is referred to Grof (2000).

Other Related Techniques

Yalom (1980) reviews a number of what he calls "artificial aids" to counteract the individual's persistent denial of death.

(a) *The Line of Life*. In this simple yet profound exercise, the subject is asked to draw a straight line on a blank sheet of paper. One end of this straight line represents his/her birth and the other his/her death. Then the subject is asked to draw a cross on the line to indicate the point where he/she is now and then to meditate upon this for brief period.

(b) *Calling Out*. This technique is employed with large groups who are then divided into smaller groups. "Each individual's name is written on a slip of paper, placed in a bowl, and then randomly chosen and called aloud. An individual whose name is called stops talking and turns his back to the others" (Yalom, 1980, p. 174). Yalom reports that this exercise has helped many individuals enhance their awareness of the precarious nature of existence.

(c) *Life Cycle Group*. This procedure was used by Elliot Aronson and Ann Dreyfus, at the National Training Laboratory summer program at Bethel, Maine. In this program, the participants focused on main issues in each developmental stage.

> In the time devoted to old age and death, these participants spent days living like old people. They were instructed to walk old, to dress old, to powder their hair and attempt to play elderly people they have known well. They visited a local cemetery. They walked alone in a forest, imagined passing out, dying, being discovered by friends, and being buried (Yalom, 1980, p. 175).

(d) *Death Awareness Workshops*. A number of workshops have focused on the issue of encountering one's death. Yalom reports one that was conducted by W.M. Whelan. It consisted of one 8-hour eight-member group session in which

> (1) Members complete a death anxiety questionnaire and discuss anxiety-provoking items, (2) Members, in a state of deep relaxation, fantasize in great detail, with awareness of all five senses, their own (comfortable) death, (3) Members are asked to construct a list of their values and then asked to imagine a situation in which a life-saving nuclear fallout shelter is able to save only a limited number of people: each member has to make an argument, on the basis of his or her value

hierarchy, why he or she should be saved, (4) Again in a state of deep muscle relaxation, the members are asked to fantasize their own terminal illness, their inability to communicate, and, finally, their own funerals (Yalom, 1980, p. 175).

(e) *Interaction With the Dying.* Yalom (1980) reports that in group sessions, patients suffering from catastrophic illness often display much affect and wisdom. In order to expose the everyday psychotherapy clients to the wisdom of the dying, Yalom, at times, invited the former to observe group sessions of the latter; or he introduced a seriously ill patient into the group psychotherapy sessions of regular patients. Yalom describes several salutary effects of these interventions.

Yalom suggests that if we as psychotherapists accept the notion that the awareness of our death can be the catalyst for personal change, then we should attempt to use all opportunities to facilitate this process. In addition to providing the structured exercises, we should help clients recognize the reminders of the fragility of life that surround us; for instance, birthdays, anniversaries, children leaving for college, serious illness, and the death of loved ones. Since most of these experiences are painful, we as therapists can easily make the mistake of focusing primarily on the alleviation of pain and miss this opportunity to nudge the patient along on the quest for wisdom and peace (Yalom, 1980).

(f) *The House of Life.* Here is another imagery exercise that can be fruitfully used to explore life/death-related issues (Sheikh & Sheikh, 2002, pp. 348-349). Relax and imagine that you are at the seashore. It is a balmy, sunny day. The sky is blue and the water is a deeper blue with bobbing white caps. The music of the waves, a gentle breeze, and the cool sand under your feet caress and sooth your senses. It feels so good to be alive.

Rising behind the beach are beautiful mountains. As you look up, you see a house perched on top of one of the peaks. What a delightful spot for a house! You are drawn to this house as if it were a magnet, and before you realize what you are doing, you are on your way toward it. Finally, you stand before it and are aching to step inside. You knock on the door, and it is opened by a very kind person who does not hesitate to invite you in. You have never seen or even imagined a house so exquisite in every respect, and the view from the large windows is breathtaking.

As you are drinking in the delights of this place, the owner tells you, "I have to go on an important mission, which may take a week, a month, a year, ten years, fifty years, or even longer. You may live in the house during my absence, but you must vacate it upon my return." Take note of your reaction to this offer.

You accept the terms and the owner leaves. The house is now your home and time flies by. A few months . . . a few years have passed. Assess the quality of your life during this time.

Just as you are in the midst of doing something very important—at least it seems important to you—you hear a knock at the door. You open the door and see the owner. Notice how you react to his/her return.

Now let these images fade away. Take a deep breath and open your eyes.

We can consider this house as a metaphor for life. It has been given to us on uncertain terms. Are we enjoying our stay in this exquisite house—or is uncertainty in the way of fully living our life? When the time comes for that knock at the door, will we feel angry and tell the owner, "Why didn't you drop dead someplace, I was just beginning to enjoy my stay"? Or will we welcome him/her back with a sense of gratitude for letting us be in this heavenly place?

When death beckons, some of us may be resentful, others may feel like the Indian Nobel laureate Rabindranath Tagore (1962, p. 88):

> When I go from hence let this be my parting word, that what I have seen is unsurpassable.
> I have tasted of the hidden honey of this lotus that expands on the ocean of light, and thus am I blessed—let this be my parting word.
> In this playhouse of infinite forms I have had my play and here have I caught sight of him that is formless.
> My whole body and my limbs have thrilled with his touch; and if the end comes here, let it come—let this be my parting word.

POSSIBLE BENEFITS OF DEATH IMAGERY WORK

Whether one examines the death-imagery experiences of the shamans; the near-death experiences reported by Moody (1975), Ring (1980, 1984), Ring and Valarino (1998), and others (Metzner, 1986); the perinatal experiences under the influence of LSD (Grof, 2000; Grof & Halifax, 1977); or the recent death-imagery work by clinicians, they all appear to be overwhelmingly health giving and life transforming. The benefits mentioned in the literature range anywhere from deep relaxation to metaphysical awakening. This section briefly surveys a number of beneficial effects of death imagery.

Deep Relaxation

It has been reported that in the imagination, dying often turns out to be a deeply relaxing experience (Grof, 2000; Metzner, 1986; Ring & Valarino, 1998; Sheikh & Sheikh, 1991; Sheikh et al., 1979). In the beginning, subjects might experience increased anxiety, particularly those who find even the mention of death threatening. This reaction, however, tends to give way to a feeling of deep relaxation: a fully conscious, dreamlike state, which is profoundly soothing at both the physical and mental level. Preliminary laboratory work indicates a slowing down of the heartbeat, flattening of the galvanic skin response, and escaping of trapped air from the body. During death imagery, spontaneous remission of some minor psychosomatic symptoms has been noted, and George Twente (1979) has encountered cases of defecation and sexual orgasm. All of these changes can be considered as objective indicators of a deeply relaxed state of mind and body. At times, the relaxed state produced by death imagery verges on the religious. Koestenbaum (1976) describes it thus:

> I felt suddenly and inexplicably that the burden and weight of living had been lifted. I felt supported. The burden of living was no longer mine alone. I sensed a current stronger than me and one in which I am only a part and which supports me as the sea supports a ship. . . . At that brief moment it became intuitively clear to me that the religious position that there is a God, that I can participate in His life, and that I am not really different from God but a part of Him, made sense. I felt that my body was supported by nature, so my individual awareness was supported by a cosmic consciousness. . . . Did I at that moment lose my freedom? No, but I did lose the sense that I was a capillary cut off from the universal bloodstream. I had a sense of continuity with all of Being, rather than the sense of separation and alienation (pp. 117-118).

Finishing the Unfinished Business

As one gives in to death imagery and enters a relaxed state, unresolved situations from the past as well as from the current scene often make their appearance spontaneously and almost beg to be reexperienced and resolved. This unfinished emotional business more often than not relates to one's parents and potentially can be resolved through continued image therapy. One kind of unfinished situation that often emerges during death imagery is unresolved grief. At times spontaneous regrieving in imagery clears the air. In other cases, the therapist may have to intervene and manipulate certain images (Sheikh, 2001, 2003; also see Morrison's chapter in this book).

Out-of-Body Experience

Some subjects experience a pleasurable and profoundly relaxing feeling of shedding their body. The reports include feelings of well-being, of vitality, of the freedom that perhaps a bird experiences when it is let out of its cage, and feelings of ecstasy. For example, one subject reported that she became lighter and lighter and finally floated away from her body. Suddenly she was adrift in a quiet world of blue-white light. Initially, her body tugged at her and tried to bring her back, but she did not want to come back, for she sensed that out there lay peace. In the beginning, as she floated, she had the shape of a ball, but as she traveled she began to expand and assume new shapes. Suddenly, she separated into a million little particles, mixing with the light and energy and feeling very exhilarated. As she moved farther and farther away from earthly existence, time became meaningless, and a feeling of peace engulfed her. The aftereffects of this experience were very positive. The subject reported that all her senses became very acute, that she felt spiritually revived and totally at peace with her life (Sheikh et al., 1979).

It should be noted that we have no reason to believe that these out-of-body experiences are an indication of *actual* projection of the psychic self, which enables the person to perceive events in a far-off location; but subjects do feel that they are doing so.

Ehrenfeld (1974) speculates that out-of-body feelings occur because of the need to believe that consciousness survives death. Palmer (1978) remarks, "Because of our religious upbringing, (whether we accept it intellectually or not) death means possibility, or at least the hope that our soul is real and will leave the body to carry on in another state. Therefore, a psychological set favoring out-of-body experiences is present in this 'real-life' situation" (see Neher, 1980, p. 194).

Literature on the out-of-body experiences (OBEs), particularly the ones occurring within the context of near-death experiences, has mushroomed within the last decade. A number of cases have been recorded wherein subjects supposedly reported *accurate* observations of events around them about which they had no other way of gaining knowledge. Consequently, several investigators have seriously entertained the possibility of actual separation of a part of us from our body during these experiences (see Ring & Valarino, 1998).

Arguments and speculations aside, the fact remains that a large number of people are capable of having profound experiences of this type, and that they find them exhilarating and deeply therapeutic. It would be worthwhile to conduct systematic research aimed at mapping the various parameters of such experiences and discovering their correlates, antecedents, and consequences. Some of that is already on its way (Alvarado, 2000).

Here and Now: Importance of the Moment

As someone once remarked, "If the stars came out only once in a lifetime, all of us would be out to see them and would be left speechless by the grandeur of that sight. However, when they appear nightly, we often go for long intervals without even noticing them (Adams, Otto, & Cowley, 1984, p. 130).

We often live in anticipation of tomorrow or in reminiscence of yesterday, and meanwhile each day is lost. Martin Buber spoke about "infusing the routines of everyday life with the breath of eternity." He conveyed a sense of the breadth and depth that could be ours if we would give up the preoccupation with the past and develop the skill of sensing fully all that is available to us at any moment (Adams et al., 1984, p. 131).

Alan Watts (1968, 1972) remarked that people who constantly are searching for health, beauty, and fulfillment fail to grasp that they already exist on an intriguing globe floating in a fascinating universe. We have been told by numerous traditions that facing the inevitability of death can lead to the realization that the meaning of life is close at hand. It can foster a new appreciation for the value of time and the beauty and sanctity of life (Barrett, 1988; Butler, 1963; Cumming & Henry, 1961; Sheikh et al., 1979). Dostoyevsky writes in *The Idiot:*

> This man had once been led out with the others to the scaffold and a sentence of death was read over him. . . . Twenty minutes later a reprieve was read to them, and they were condemned to another punishment instead. Yet the interval between those two sentences, twenty minutes or at least a quarter of an hour, he passed in fullest conviction that he would die in a few minutes. . . . The priest went to each in turn with a cross. He had only five minutes more to live. He told that those five minutes seemed to him an infinite time, a vast wealth. . . . "What if I were not to die? What if I could go back to life—what eternity! And it would all be mine! I would turn every minute into an age; I would lose nothing, I would count every minute as it passed. I would not waste one" (quoted in Barrett, 1962, p. 140).

Death and Creativity

Being aware and open to the reality of death appears to be linked to all that we value in human experience, including love and creativity. With regard to creativity, Rollo May wrote,

> Creativity is a yearning for immortality. We know that each of us must develop the courage to confront death. Yet we also must rebel and struggle against it. Creativity comes from this struggle—out of the rebellion the creative act is born (May, 1975, pp. 31-32).

Studies by Goodman (1975) suggest that creativity and the fear of death are significantly related. Creative individuals appear to be able to overcome their fear of death by viewing life in terms of 100-to-1000-year perspectives. On the other hand, those who see life in terms of 2-to-10-year perspectives demonstrate greater concern about death.

The intricate connection between death and creativity is also confirmed by the frequent manifestation of previously dormant creative talents in individuals who narrowly escaped death. Such people undergo the profound experience of rebirth: they now reassess the meaning of life and often struggle to express creative energies that lay buried. The patient who gained a reprieve from death may channel all energy into writing some wonderful verses or working out a new scientific theory (Garai, 1988).

Death and Love

The close relationship between death and love is clear on many levels. Perhaps the most dramatic illustrations are found in the reproductive cycle of some animals. The male bee dies after he has inseminated the queen. The female praying mantis bites off the male's head as he copulates, and as soon as she is inseminated, she eats the male to provide nourishment for the young.

In literature, death and love always have been inseparable. Italian writers commonly play upon the words *amore* (love) and *morte* (death). Mythologies of various cultures portray the sex act as death and rebirth; the ability to surrender one's self must precede the spontaneity of orgasm (May, 1968).

On the psychological plane, passionate love is inevitably accompanied by the specter of death. The lover must grapple with the painful possibilities of the death of the relationship, the death of the beloved, his/her own death, and the death of the offspring. Love heightens the lover's vulnerability and sense of mortality, but the realization of the precarious nature of life also leads to increased reverence for life and more genuine living. As Stephen Levine (1982, p. 99) observes,

> If our only spiritual practice were to live as though we were already dead, relating to all we meet, to all we do, as though it were our own final moments in the world, what time would there be for false games or falsehoods or posturing . . . Only love would be appropriate, only the truth.

Death, Meaning, and Spirituality

As Morgan (1993, p. 5) points out, "human gust is a gust for meaning. . . . We are the only animal that has to decide from moment to moment, who am I? What do I have to do?" What am I here for? What is it all about? These questions about the "meaning" of life are also "spiritual" questions. So when we are talking about spirituality, we also are talking about the meaning of life and vice versa. It has been pointed out over and over again in the existential and spiritual literature that confrontation with death turns our attention in the direction of these crucial questions and motivates us to figure out the purpose and meaning of life.

In one of the death-imagery exercises, participants were instructed to imagine that the Supreme Being confronts them with this ultimatum: "Give me three *good* reasons why I should allow you to continue living. Otherwise your life will end now. Provide three reasons that *you* regard as good, not reasons which you feel *I* might view as valid" (Sheikh, 2005).

Of the hundreds of responses offered by the participants from different cultures, the overwhelming majority fell into three categories. One set fell under the rubric *Love* (e.g., my children are still small and need me; my parents love me and would be devastated if I died; my friends and relatives would be sad). The second category of responses can be put under *Achieving One's Potential*. Respondents spoke about their talents, their purpose in life, and the feeling that they have not yet achieved their potential (e.g., I have not yet sung my best song or danced my own dance; I have great potential for helping the needy; I have just started my medical training, and I feel I can be a great healer). The last category can be labeled *Appreciation of Beauty* (e.g., there is so much to see and enjoy in the world, and I have explored little of it; I want to travel and experience different cultures).

The pattern of the responses is fairly uniform from one culture to the next. It seems that no matter whether we are men or women or in what culture we live, when we are confronted with our demise, our thoughts turn to the same topics; the same values suddenly assume supreme importance. Can we assume that these values describe authentic living? That loving, nurturing our potential, and appreciating beauty make life meaningful for all people? Could it be that the meaning of life is not *created* but *discovered,* that one does not need to dig too deeply or look too far to discover it, that it is just around the corner?

Essence versus Accessory Attributes

Perls visualized the accessory attributes as an edifice constructed of four layers. The first two layers consist of the role playing that we have found useful in everyday life—to please others and to motivate them to support us. Many live out their lives without ever penetrating beyond these outer layers. The third layer envelops the sense of emptiness—the very feeling most people like to keep at a distance with frantic everyday routines. The fourth layer is one that is most difficult to penetrate: it consists of our terror of dying, which is an inescapable and ever-present undercurrent. Only after we have grappled with this condition can we proceed to the center of this edifice and recognize our authentic self (Becker, 1973).

Awareness of death through imagery can spontaneously lead us to sift our essence from accessory attributes. This process has been termed *disidentification*. Assagioli (1965) attempted to help his clients reach their core of pure consciousness by encouraging them to imagine shedding their bodies, emotions, desires, and eventually their intellect.

Yalom employs a structured disidentification exercise that takes only about 30 to 45 minutes. In a quiet setting, Yalom asks the participants to list, on separate cards, eight important responses to the question "Who am I?" He then asks them to arrange the cards in order of importance, placing the cards that come closest to expressing their essence at the bottom. Next, Yalom asks the participants to meditate on what it would be like to give up the attribute described on the top card. After 2 to 3 minutes, he asks them to proceed to the next card and so forth, until they have shed all eight attributes (Yalom, 1980). Yalom feels that disidentification is an effective mechanism of change. The awareness of death brings about a shift in perspective from which the person can easily distinguish between core and accessory attributes.

Along the same vein, Metzner (1986) has found that self-knowledge is the ultimate reward bestowed on those who confront their own death. The self that the individual had thought he/she was, dies; and the true self emerges into prominence. All ego concerns and petty interests dissolve into insignificance in the light of the real self, which is nothing less than a spark from the eternal source of life.

Other Possible Effects

Several other beneficial effects of confrontation with death have been reported in the literature. These include (1) a change of attitude toward dying, including a loss of fear; (2) belief in the survival of consciousness after biological death; (3) diminished earthly ambitions; (4) increased reverence for life; (5) stimulated interest in philosophy, religion, and mysticism; and (6) an altered perception of time.

In the Sufi literature, the experience of *fana*, or annihilation of the ego, is considered to lead to some or all of the following: "1. A feeling of being light as though all burdens of the world had been lifted; 2. Absence of thoughts—quiescence of the mind; 3. Quiet elation and profound joy; 4. Increased sensitivity; 5. Receptivity to internal and external clues; 6. Increased perceptiveness; 7. Awareness of invisible rhythms within and around; 8. Perception of future events; 9. Awareness of the whole as well as the parts; 10. Decreased internal conflicts; 11. Increased feelings of security, certainty, integration, and oneness with all" (Shafii, 1985, p. 159).

CONCLUDING REMARKS

Throughout the ages, all major spiritual and philosophic traditions have stressed the importance of dealing with death; and, as the preceding pages indicate, recently a number of other lines of inquiry have reaffirmed this view. There appears to be general agreement across subjects and across approaches concerning the consequences of a confrontation with death. They are reported to be overwhelmingly positive and can even be self-transcending and life transforming. This emerging consensus invites us to speculate that perhaps "we all harbor functional matrices in our unconscious mind that contain an authentic encounter with death . . . human beings not only know intellectually that they will die, they also possess subliminal knowledge of what it feels like to experience death" (Grof & Halifax, 1977, p. 9).

Recent attempts to induce the experience of death and rebirth through imagery-related approaches under relatively controlled conditions are expected to lead to a deeper understanding of the process of death and the consequences of confronting it. Without a doubt, the study of the death experience is of crucial importance in the understanding of psychological processes. No genuine comprehension of religion, mysticism, or mythology is possible without intimate knowledge of the death experience (Grof, 1985; Grof & Halifax, 1977). A profound symbolic confrontation with death can contribute to better emotional and psychological functioning and a satisfying adjustment to life. Feifel maintains that "only by integrating the concept of death into the self does an authentic and genuine existence become possible" (1961, p. 65).

Those who undergo death-imagery work often end up with an enhanced belief in the survival of consciousness after death in some form, and many even have glimpses of what life after death is going to be like. However, we feel that the true value of this work is not in what it indicates about life after this life, but what it tells us about how to live in the here and now and how to wake up to the countless blessings that come our way. As the Indian poet/mystic Kabir (see Bly, 1977, pp. 24-25) says,

> Friend, hope for the Guest while your are alive.
> Jump into experience while you are alive!
> Think... and think... while you are alive.
> What you call "salvation" belongs to the time before death.
>
> If you don't break your ropes while you're alive,
> do you think
> ghosts will do it after?
>
> The idea that the soul will join with the ecstatic
> just because the body is rotten—
> that is all fantasy.
>
> What is found now is found then.
> If you find nothing now,
> you will simply end up with an apartment
> in the City of Death.
>
> If you make love with the divine now, in the next life
> you will have the face of satisfied desire.
> So plunge into the truth, find out who the Teacher is,
> Believe in the Great Sound!
>
> Kabir says this: When the Guest is being searched for,
> it is the intensity of the longing that does all the work.
> Look at me, and you will see a slave of that intensity.

REFERENCES

Adams, R. S., Otto, H. A., & Cowley, A. S. (1984). *Letting go: Uncomplicating your life*. New York: Science and Behavior Books.

Aguilar, I., & Wood, V. N. (1976, January). Therapy through death ritual. *Social Work*, 49-54.

Ajmal, M. (1979). *Sufi contemplation upon death*. Unpublished paper. National Institute of Psychology, Islamabad, Pakistan.

Ajmal, M. (1989). *Death imagery in Sufism.* Unpublished manuscript. National Institute of Psychology, Islamabad, Pakistan.

Alvarado, C. (2000). Out-of-body experiences. In E. Cardena, S. J. Lynn, & S. Krippner (Eds.), *Varieties of anamolous experiences: Examining the scientific evidence.* Washington, DC: American Psychological Association.

Arasteh, A. R. (1980). *Growth to selfhood: The Sufi contribution to Islam.* New York: Penguin Books.

Assagioli, R. (1965). *Psychosynthesis: A collection of basic writings.* New York: Viking.

Barrett, W. (1962). *Irrational man.* New York: Anchor Books.

Barrett, D. (1988). Dreams of death. *Omega, 19*(2), 95-101.

Becker, E. (1973). *The denial of death.* New York: Free Press, A Division of Macmillan.

Blazer, J. A. (1978). The concept of death as a factor in mental health. *Psychology, 15*(1), 68-77.

Bly, R. (1977). *The Kabir book.* Boston, MA: Beacon.

Braga, J. L., & Braga, L. D. (1975). Foreword. In E. Kübler-Ross (Ed.), *Death: The final stage of growth.* New Jersey: Prentice Hall.

Buddhaghosa, B. (1976). *The path of purification (Visuddhimagga)* (2 Vols.) (B. Nyana Noli, Trans). Berkeley, CA: Shambhala.

Butler, R. N. (1963). The life review: An interpretation of reminiscence in the aged. *Psychiatry, 119,* 721-728.

Cumming, E., & Henry, W. E. (1961). *Growing old.* Illinois: Free Press.

deMello, A. (1985). *One minute wisdom.* New York: Doubleday.

Droege, T. (1987). *Guided grief imagery: A resource for grief ministry and death education.* New York: Paulist Press.

Ehrenfeld, J. (1974). Out-of-the-body experience and the denial of death. *Journal of Nervous and Mental Disease, 159,* 227-233.

Evans-Wentz, W. Y. (1960). *The Tibetan book of the dead.* New York: Oxford University Press.

Feifel, H. (1961). Attitudes toward death: A psychological perspective. In R. May (Ed.), *Existential psychology.* New York: Random House.

Frisch, V. M. (1957). *Homo Faber.* Frankfurt: Suhrkamp Verlag.

Garai, J. (1988). *Birth, death, and rebirth as archetypes of the creative experience.* Unpublished manuscript.

Goodman, L. (1975). *Winning the race with death.* Paper presented as part of a symposium on "Fear, Death, and Creativity." American Psychological Association, Chicago.

Grof, S. (1985). *Beyond the brain: Birth, death, and transcendence in psychotherapy.* Albany, NY: State University of New York Press.

Grof, S. (2000). *Psychology of the future.* Albany, NY: State University of New York Press.

Grof, S., & Bennett, H. Z. (1992). *The holotropic mind.* San Francisco, CA: Harper.

Grof, S., & Halifax, J. (1977). *The human encounter with death.* New York: Dutton.

Hamilton, E., & Cairns, H. (Eds.). (1973). *Collected dialogues of Plato.* New Jersey: Princeton University Press.

Harvey, A. (1994). *The way of passion: A celebration of Rumi.* New York: Tarcher/Putnam.

Keleman, S. (1974). *Living your dying.* New York: Random House.

Koestenbaum P. (1976). *Is there an answer to death?* New Jersey: Prentice-Hall.

Kruck, J. S., & Sheikh, A. A. (1991). Images of life and death: An overview of Stephen Levine's work on conscious living and conscious dying. In A. A. Sheikh & K. S. Sheikh (Eds.), *Death imagery: Comforting death brings us to the threshold of life*. Milwaukee, WI: American Imagery Institute.

Kübler-Ross, E. (Ed.). (1975). *Death: The final stage of growth*. New Jersey: Prentice-Hall.

Levitan, A. A. (1985). Hypnotic death rehearsal. *American Journal of Clinical Hypnosis*, 27(4): 211-215.

Levitan, A. A. (1991). Hypnotic death rehearsal. In A. A. Sheikh & K. S. Sheikh (Eds.), *Death imagery: Comforting death brings us to the threshold of life*. Milwaukee, WI: American Imagery Institute.

Levine, S. (1972). *Death row: An affirmation of life*. San Francisco, CA: Glide Publications.

Levine, S. (1979). *A gradual awakening*. New York: Anchor Press/Doubleday.

Levine, S. (1982). *Who dies? An investigation of conscious living and conscious dying*. New York: Anchor Books/Doubleday.

Levine, S. (1984). *Meetings at the edge*. New York: Anchor Press/Doubleday.

Levine, S. (1989). *Healing into life and death*. New York: Doubleday.

Levine, S. (1991). *Guided meditation, explorations, and healings*. New York: Doubleday.

Levine, S. (1997). *A year to live: How to live this year if it was your last*. New York: Belltower.

Levine, S. (2002). *Turning toward the mystery: A seeker's journey*. New York: HarperCollins.

Levine, S., & Levine, O. (1999). *The grief process: Meditation for healing*. Boulder, CO: Sounds True.

Long, J. B. (1975). The death that ends death in Hinduism and Buddhism. In E. Kübler-Ross (Ed.), *Death: The final stage of growth*. New Jersey: Prentice Hall.

Mann, T. (1969). *The magic mountain*. New York: Vintage.

May, R. (1958). The origins and significance of the existential movement in psychology. In R. May, E. Angel, & H. F. Ellenberger (Eds.), *Existence: A new dimension in psychiatry and psychology*. New York: Simon & Schuster.

May, R. (1968, February). The daemonic: Love and death. *Psychology Today*, 1(9), 16-25.

May, R. (1975) *The courage to create*. New York: W. W. Norton.

Melges, F. T. (1982). *Time and the inner future: A temporal approach to psychiatric disorder*. New York: Wiley.

Melges, F. T., & DeMaso, D. R. (1980). Grief resolution therapy: Reliving, revising, and revisiting. *American Journal of Psychotherapy, xxxiv*, 51-61.

Metzner, R. (1986). *Opening to inner light*. Los Angeles, CA: Jeremy P. Tarcher.

Moody, R. A. (1975). *Life after life*. New York: Bantam.

Morgan, J. D. (1993). The existential gust for meaning. In K. Doka & J. Morgan (Eds.), *Death and spirituality*. Amityville, NY: Baywood.

Morrison, J. K. (1978). Successful grieving: Changing personal constructs through mental imagery. *Journal of Mental Imagery, 2*, 63-68.

Morrison, J. K. (1991). The clinical use of imagery to induce psychotherapeutic grieving. In A. A. Sheikh & K. S. Sheikh (Eds.), *Death imagery: Confronting death brings us to this threshold of life*. Milwaukee, WI: American Imagery Institute.

Neale, R. E. (1969). *In praise of play*. New York: Harper & Row.

Neher, A. (1980). *The psychology of transcendence.* New York: Prentice-Hall.
Nichols, R., & Nichols, J. (1975). Funerals: A time for grief and growth. In E. Kübler-Ross (Ed.), *Death: The final stage of growth.* New Jersey: Prentice-Hall.
Nietzsche, F. (1974). *The gay science.* New York: Random House.
Palmer, J. (1978). ESP and out-of-body experiences: An experiential approach. In D. S. Rogo (Ed.), *Mind beyond the body.* New York: Penguin.
Pasternak, B. (1958). *Doctor Zhivago.* New York: Pantheon.
Paz, O. (1961). *The labyrinth of solitude.* New York: Grove.
Rahula, W. (1959). *What the Buddha taught.* New York: Grove.
Ramaswami, S., & Sheikh, A. A. (1991). Death imagery in Buddhism. In A. A. Sheikh & K. S. Sheikh (Eds.), *Death imagery: Confronting death brings us to the threshold of life.* Amityville, NY: Baywood.
Ramsay, R. W., & Noorbergen, R. (1981). *Living with loss.* New York: William Morrow.
Ring, K. (1980). *Life at death.* New York: Coward, McCann & Geoghegan.
Ring, K. (1984). *Heading toward omega.* New York: William Morrow.
Ring, K., & Valarino E. (1998). *Lessons from the light.* Needham, MA: Moment Point Press.
Robinson, R. H. (1970). *The Buddhist religion: A historical introduction.* Belmont, CA: Dickenson.
Shafii, M. (1985). *Freedom from the self: Sufism, meditation, and psychotherapy.* New York: Human Services Press.
Shear, J. (1978, September). *Plato, Piaget, and Mararishi on cognitive development.* Paper presented at the American Psychological Association Convention, Toronto.
Sheikh, A. A. (2001). Eidetic psychotherapy. In R. J. Corsini (Ed.), *Handbook of innovative therapy.* New York: Wiley.
Sheikh, A. A. (Ed.). (2003). *Healing images: The role of imagination in health.* Amityville, NY: Baywood.
Sheikh, A. A. (2005). *Is the meaning of life discovered or created.* Paper presented at the International Conference for Social Sciences, Honolulu, June 2005.
Sheikh, A. A., Twente, G. E., & Turner, D. (1979). Death imagery: Therapeutic uses. In A. A. Sheikh & J. T. Shaffer (Eds.), *The potential of fantasy and imagination.* New York: Brandon House.
Sheikh, A. A., & Sheikh, K. S. (Eds.). (1991). *Death imagery: Confronting death brings us to the threshold of life.* Milwaukee, WI: American Imagery Institute.
Sheikh, A. A., & Sheikh, K. S. (2002). Good health imaging. In A. Sheikh, *Handbook of therapeutic imagery techniques.* Amityville, NY: Baywood.
Straub, S. H. (2002). *Death 101: A workbook for educating and healing.* Amityville, NY: Baywood.
Tagore, R. (1962). *Gitanjali.* New York: Macmillan.
Tolstoy, L. (1931). *War and peace.* New York: Mudern Library.
Tolstoy, L. (1960). *The death of Ivan Ilych and other stories.* New York: Signet Classics.
Twente, G. E. (1979). Personal Communication.
van Gennep, A. (1960). *The rites of passage.* Chicago: Chicago University Press.
Volkan, V. D. (1975). "Regrief" therapy. In B. Schoenberg (Ed.), *Bereavement: Its psychological aspects.* New York: Columbia University Press.
Watts, A. (1968). *The meaning of happiness.* New York: Harper & Row.

Watts, A. (1972). *The book on the taboo against knowing who you are.* New York: Random House.
Williamson, D. S. (1978, January). New life at the graveyard: A method of therapy for individuation from a dead former parent. *Journal of Marriage and Family Counseling,* 93-101.
Winokuer, H. R. (2002). Foreword. In S. H. Straub (Ed.), *Death 101: A workbook for educating and healing.* Amityville, NY: Baywood.
Yalom, I. D. (1980). *Existential psychotherapy.* New York: Basic Books.
Yalom, I. D. (2002). *The gift of therapy.* New York: Harper.

CHAPTER 2

Opening To Loss: Connecting with Life Through the Meditations of Stephen Levine

Colleen M. Heinkel and Anees A. Sheikh

> Your pain is the breaking of the shell that encloses your understanding.
> Kahlil Gibran (1966, p. 52)
>
> Let your life lightly dance on the edges of time like dew on the tip of a leaf.
> Rabindranath Tagore (in Boerstler, 1982, p. 27)

In his introduction to *A Year to Live* (1997), Stephen Levine writes:

> Preparing for death is one of the most profoundly healing acts of a lifetime . . . a healing process that allows a gradual completion of all that lies behind and a clear-eyed entrance into whatever may lie ahead. A process of clarity, insight, and closure (p. 7).

Levine has worked for decades with the terminally ill, has facilitated workshops for the grieving, and has taught countless others how to heal from a life unlived. His meditations and death imagery focus on a response to grief, rather than on a reaction to it. He demonstrates that it is possible to open one's heart in hell and to heal one's pain from grief.

In this chapter, the foundations for healing in the meditations and imagery of Levine are explored. He has developed an experiential approach that, when practiced regularly, can lead to acceptance of loss and death, to a fuller awareness of life, and ultimately, to deep healing from suffering. His techniques and meditations transform theory into practice, illuminating a path from the mind into the heart.

Levine's imagery has emerged from the fertile ground of his lifelong spiritual seeking, nurtured and defined by the direct experience of those facing death, pain, and loss. Levine's work demonstrates that by opening to loss, living can become a conscious process of growth. His meditations and techniques focus on the source of all healing: the heart's boundless compassion, cultivated by the practice of loving kindness and mercy. He has studied and collaborated with great teachers, among them spiritualist Ram Dass and psychiatrist Elisabeth Kübler-Ross. With Ram Dass, he helped found New York City's first hospice center in 1972 and also coauthored a book entitled *Grist for the Mill* (1976), which explores issues of spirituality and self-growth. He played a key role in the development of the Hanuman Dying Project on the West Coast, and he has served as a consultant to hospitals and hospices worldwide. With his wife, Ondrea, he has operated a telephone counseling service for those facing serious illness. Several publications evolved from this work, including *Who Dies? An Investigation of Conscious Living and Conscious Dying* (1982), *Meetings at the Edge* (1984), and *Healing into Life and Death* (1987).

As his understanding matured, he developed more focused forms of meditation and new meditations, which addressed the suffering of victims of sexual abuse. These evolutions are reflected in his later works that include *Guided Meditations, Exploration, and Healing* (1991), *A Year to Live: How to Live This Year as if it Were Your Last* (1997), and in two audio recordings of his workshops: *In the Heart Lies the Deathless* (1990) and *The Grief Process: Meditations for Healing* (Levine & Levine, 1999). He also reveals his own journey through suffering in his "autobiography of the heart," *Turning Toward the Mystery: A Seeker's Journey* (2002).

The lessons of compassion and of death have spanned the teachings of many spiritual traditions, and Levine has embraced them in his writings. Yet it was Eastern philosophy that provided the impetus and the foundation for Levine's practice. In his autobiography, *Turning toward the Mystery*, he describes his serendipitous introduction to Buddhism:

> At twenty, with already so much done and undone, with time clearly waiting in ambush, I met Buddha in a bus station. From a rack of loosely browsed paperbacks, the Buddha's countenance emerged luminous from A. E. Burt's *The Compassionate Buddha*. In his Four Noble Truths the Buddha told me I wasn't the only one suffering. He said the pain came from the emotional exhaustion of grasping at the ever changing, even illusory, nature of things. He said there was a way out. He offered a path toward clarity and kindness (2002, p. 17).

After this tenuous beginning, Levine found other spiritual teachers who helped him discover his own path through his personal experience of pain and suffering. He found in Buddhist psychology, and specifically in the writings of Eastern spiritual masters Vivekananda, Pantanjali, and Sivananda, a way to reframe his understanding of pain and death. From Vivekananda and Pantanjali, he learned the yogic principles of connecting with the breath and reframing pain by understanding what lies beyond it. He learned that letting go and opening to the fullness of compassion united one with the absolute, the divine, the essence of being. From Sivananda, he learned the blessing of an intense practice of meditation. When grief overwhelmed him during his study with the Buddhist monk Sujata, mercy became his path through it.

Fundamental to Buddhist philosophy is the Doctrine of Impermanence, the belief that the reality one perceives is impermanent and that all things are in continual flux and transformation. Suffering arises as a consequence of attachment, of clinging to things in an ever-changing, kaleidoscopic world. Levine describes the grief process as learning to live with the consequences of love; the pain of grief is the rope burn left when what one has held is wrenched away (1991).

In the tradition of Eastern psychology, all reactions to loss are suffering—the Buddhist word for suffering is *dukha*. Grief, disappointment, anger, doubt, guilt, or resentment are all forms of suffering. They all share the same essence, which is loss. Whether momentary or overwhelming, Buddhism considers them all dukha. The dukha of anger, for instance, arises because things are not the way one wants them to be: anger is a reaction to one's loss of control. Fear is dukha, a reaction to one's loss of feeling safe and comfortable in the world. Doubt is suffering, a loss of not feeling whole and complete. The ultimate loss is the loss of a loved one: the fear, loneliness, pain, and anger experienced during loss of a loved one have been felt before in varying intensities.

It is often the intense feeling of loss from the death of a loved one or from the diagnosis of a serious or terminal illness that awakens one to the suffering one has always felt. The feelings are not new, but the volume is turned up.

> It is not the enormity of our grief we experience that is the problem. It's our everyday grief, our resistance to the unpleasant, our "hard belly," our separation from God and ourselves. It is our common, everyday, ordinary grief, focused on an individual (1990, Tape 1).

The intensified pain from loss awakens one to seek a deeper truth, to find a more accurate picture of what life is. One seeks a reality where suffering makes sense and where it can be integrated. Loss startles one with the realization that one's perceptions just do not make sense, that there are cracks in one's ideas about reality. "We take birth to meet ourselves again in a world so ripped with pain we cannot miss the lesson" (Levine, 1991, p. 328). Yet, it is in this time of deepest despair that one begins to look deeply.

A search for a deeper truth often leads to spiritual seeking. Levine describes this longing for deeper spiritual knowledge as the universal will toward mystery, "our homesickness for God" (2002, p. 10). Suffering, in all its forms, is universal, and regardless of worldview, spiritual traditions seek to alleviate suffering, often by imparting a greater understanding of one's true nature. It may be called "Big Self" in Hinduism, or "living in Christ" in Christianity, or "no-self" in

Buddhism. Many spiritual traditions try to raise one's awareness of a more expansive reality existing beyond the senses, an existence that is one's origin or ground of true being, a reality that by its very essence alleviates suffering.

By looking deeply, one becomes more conscious of a greater sense of being. The renowned Buddhist teacher Thich Nhat Hanh illustrates this sense in *The Heart of the Buddha's Teaching*. He describes a wave on the surface of the ocean having a beginning and an end, like an individual life, and at the same time, the wave is grounded in the ocean. "It is important that a wave knows that she is water, and not just a wave" (1998, p. 211). This understanding of the individual life within a ground of being is at the core of Eastern philosophy about life, about death; and it forms the foundation for Levine's meditations and imagery.

Levine's work builds upon the Eastern spiritual tradition that one's true nature is a formless and vast spaciousness, an endless, nameless being of pure joy and compassion. It does not exist in abstraction but exists here and now, in every moment. Joy and compassion are at the heart of human beingness; yet, the mind cannot perceive it. The limited perception of the mind creates distress, like a child who cries when he loses sight of his parents around a corner of a building. The young child's perceptual skills are too underdeveloped to retain the image of his parents in his mind. Like the corner, the limited perceptual capacity of the mind essentially blocks the view of the ocean of being that is part of every moment and creates the illusion that it does not exist, or that one is separated from it.

Suffering ultimately arises from this illusion of separation from one's true nature. Awareness, on the other hand, corrects the perceptual deficit and teaches one to look *through* the corner imposed by the mind: awareness reveals that joy and compassion exist right now, at this moment, despite the opaque view. It reassures one that there is so much more to life than meets the eye.

The way to decrease suffering, then, is to increase the awareness that one's true nature exists and to expose the illusion imposed by the mind. Healing begins from this search for truth, from the moment one begins to cultivate the awareness of something more. Loss is unparalled for its healing properties.

One cannot think one's way through the illusion, because the mind creates the illusion. Only the heart is capable of revealing the tricks of the mirrored mind. Levine defines "heart" as the very deep, spacious, and universal level of mind. It is found in the farthest reaches of mind: as one penetrates deeply into the mind through the practice of meditation, one encounters more and more heart. One enters into this ground of compassion and joy through the cultivation of loving kindness and mercy.

Fostering awareness of one's compassionate nature through the use of mercy and meditation offers "the way out" promised by the Buddha and removes the shackles of suffering. Awareness unfolds from mercy and loving kindness, unveiling the heart from the mind's illusion, and unleashing the exuberant vibrato of true aliveness. Awareness connects one with the life force itself, opening the direct link to the ground of one's being, to the vast ocean of compassion.

> Investigating our old ways of seeing, we go beyond clinging to the content of old mind and enter directly the energy which effortlessly continues the unfolding, recognizing that what moves thought through the mind moves the stars across the sky. . . . And we go beyond old or new, beyond birth or death, to the timeless, formless, boundaryless nature of awareness itself. We experience the light which produces consciousness on the screen and discover creation itself, our true nature (Levine, 1987, p. 246).

It is the mercy with which one responds to grief that deepens awareness and heals the sense of separation. The healing that emerges from Levine's meditations comes from reconnecting with mercy to the joy and compassion in oneself; but he cautions that this does not always ensure a physical cure. Hearts are healed—unfinished relationships are completed, new joy and intensity in life is found, pain is decreased, fears of death and dying are relieved, forgiveness is rendered and received—but the physical body may not necessarily be cured of its illness. Healing lies in understanding grief, in understanding what hardens the heart and obscures the path to joy in life. To Levine, "healing uncovers the heart" (1991, p. 226).

Levine's meditations challenge one to uncover one's heart by exploring the nature of one's suffering. Descriptions of the nature of fear, for example, might include what one is afraid of, how fear feels in the body, what precedes the feeling, or what thoughts come and go around fear. However, none of these fully describe what the experience of fear *is*. The same is true when one tries to describe anger, doubt, resentment, or all dukka, all the everyday grief.

Being attentive to these feelings or thoughts is the way to most effectively enter into one's experience of grief. Being mindful of how one's fear feels, exploring where one's anger arises, experiencing where doubt resides, or being aware of the origins of suffering make one aware of what creates perception and ultimately of how one's perceptions are limited by the mind.

Reactions to loss with pain, anger, resentment, etc. are conditioned: they occur over and over again. One's *re-actions* to loss block one's ability to access awareness, essentially "armoring the heart" against any form of help (1990). Rather than re-acting to grief by hardening against it, Levine teaches that one must *respond* mindfully to grief with softness and mercy. Healing enters into the hard shell of pain only when it is touched with mercy and loving kindness. Mindfulness and awareness heal by integrating the experience of suffering into the understanding of compassion.

To remain mindful, one of Levine's techniques includes an effective physical reminder: learning how to "soften the belly." Levine suggests that we are a society of the hard bellied, conditioned to re-act, to suffer (1991). When the belly is hard, one is hardening to the moment and holding on to pain. This conditioning may be interrupted by becoming very aware of what one is feeling or thinking and being mindfully present to the experience of one's dukka. Softening the belly helps to soften the armor that surrounds the heart. It softens one to the life that suffuses every moment, to the light that shines through the opening door of one's heart.

As one grows in the practice of awareness and the heart opens to broader vistas, a clearer perception of life and death emerges, revealing a deeper understanding of what lives and what dies. The body may die, but the life force, that compassionate beingness from which life originates, does not. One becomes more conscious that everything in one's life has been impermanent, except for the continual sense of one's being. Awareness reveals what the heart knows: "We go beyond the limited comprehension of the mind, to the enormous intuition of the heart. Being never dies, only the forms it temporarily inhabits. All survive death. Death is just a change in lifestyles" (1991, p. 308).

Death, then, is also understood as an illusion of the mind. By knowing what Death is not, what can die and what cannot, one comes to know what Life is. Each day of riding the wave, yet knowing the ocean, can be treasured. Each moment can be relished without fear, without suffering, because one *is* the ocean just out for a ride.

After his year-long preparation for an imaginary death chronicled in his book, *A Year to Live*, Levine found that he had renewed energy, deeper relationships with friends, more access to love, and fewer troubling emotions. "Ironically, after I have spent a year practicing dying, the quality most noticeably enhanced is a new joy in life" (1997, p. 167).

His feelings mirror those of persons who have been resuscitated from clinical death. They also report an increased appreciation of life, a diminished fear of death, and a new sense of purpose (1997). Beyond an understanding of suffering and a cultivation of mindfulness, meditation practice fosters a deeper understanding of life, exercises one's ability to be fully conscious of our compassionate nature in every moment, and renews one's sense of presence and timelessness in the impermanent flow of time. Of the rewards of meditation, Levine writes: "And yet more important than preparing us for death is their capacity to focus us on life. To let go of the last moment and to open to the next is to die consciously, moment to moment" (1991, p. 308).

By learning to open to his own pain and spacious heart through meditation practice, Levine discovered how to transcend suffering and to find a more conscious life. After his introduction to the Buddha early in life, it took Levine years of painful searching to discover ways to integrate compassion and mercy into his own pain and suffering. "Angels train in hell for the ineffable compassion of heaven," Levine wrote in his autobiography, *Turning Toward the Mystery: A Seeker's Journey* (p. 31). Eastern spirituality had opened his mind to the possibility of healing; yet, it was his meditation practice that revealed *how*.

Levine's meditations, reflections, and visualizations nurture the awareness that all have the capacity to heal to the Infinite, when they open to their suffering with kindness and mercy. Levine developed exercises of imagery and meditation

OPENING TO LOSS / 33

as a way to help others discover their ability to let go of dukha, to soften into the moment.

PRACTICE

"Meditation is a means to an endlessness. It allows us to directly experience our true nature—the ever-healed, the unconditioned, the deathless" (1991, p. 8). Meditation develops the concentration necessary to remain focused on the moment and to liberate consciousness. Concentration intensifies the sense of being: the more concentrated the mind, the deeper the sense of calm. Levine muses that the "open-heartedness and easy-mindedness" of those who have had near-death experiences may come from the fact that, at the time of death, concentration becomes many times increased (1991).

The meditations found in his compilation *Guided Meditations, Explorations and Healings*, and also in *The Grief Process*, have evolved over his many years of practice and have been organized to lead one on a graduated path for cultivating mercy and awareness. The meditations reflected from these works are representative of Levine's work and are most relevant to understanding the therapeutic potential of death imagery. They are being presented in the order recommended by Levine in *Guided Meditations, Explorations and Healings*: Loving Kindness, Soft Belly, Forgiveness, Mindfulness, Grief, Pain, Dying and Guided Death Transition Meditations.

To choose the meditations best suited for one's own healing, Levine recommends trusting one's heart and listening to its suggestions. Frequency of practice is best left to evolve on its own. Some of the meditations build foundations for future work, like the Loving Kindness Meditation, and are recommended for consistent practice. Other meditations will speak to one's heart and recommend themselves as essential to one's own healing, and these should be practiced consistently as well. Although Levine recognizes the value of daily meditation, it is regular practice that is the goal. Also it is the quality of awareness one brings to the practice that provides the healing, not the quantity of time spent practicing.

The following meditations are paraphrased and summarized from Levine's compilation of meditations and from the study guide of *The Grief Process*, but the reader is encouraged to read them in their original form. The poetry of his words breathes life into his imagery; its beauty is a glimpse of what one seeks in the heart and what draws one inward toward its light.

LOVING KINDNESS

For Levine, the meditation practice of Loving Kindness opens one to "the power of the heart to take us beyond the separativeness of the mind" (1991, p. 27). It builds a foundation for further practice, because it leads to the awareness that one's heart is not the seat of emotions but the very essence of mind: It is one's true nature. The meditation achieves this by addressing one's conditioning to suffer. During his workshop, recorded *In the Heart Lies the Deathless*, Levine uses the example of what happens when one stubs one's toe: one is conditioned to send grief into one's pain. A stubbed toe immediately evokes anger or hatred. He asks, "What, then, do we send in when it's a tumor? Anger? Aversion?" (1990, Tape 2).

Judgment, in any form, armors the heart against healing. The meditation imagery of loving kindness, on the other hand, reconditions one to *respond* without judgment, to respond, instead, with mercy. The act of touching pain with love defines mercy, a mercy for one's own grief is the key to healing.

Knowing how merciless one can be with oneself, Levine quotes Buddha, who said, "You could look the whole world over and not find another being more deserving of love than yourself" (1991, p. 25). It is essential to learn to touch one's own pain with love; for Levine, the Guided Loving Kindness Meditation is the first step in learning how to respond to pain with love and mercy.

This meditation was first published in *A Gradual Awakening* (1979) and has evolved into its most recent form in *Guided Meditation, Explorations, and Healings* (1991). The intent of this exercise is to become more fully aware of the loving energies of the universe; the experience of this love lays the groundwork for responding to one's own suffering as well as to the suffering of others. This exercise uses both imaginal and cognitive techniques: Levine demonstrates how both capacities may be used to open the pathway to the heart.

A Guided Loving Kindness Meditation

Begin the exercise by focusing on breathing. Become aware of the rhythm of breathing, and allow yourself to become one with the cycle of inhalation and exhalation. As relaxation begins to occur, send care for your own well-being directly toward yourself.

"Allow the heart, silently, to whisper the words of mercy that heal, that open. 'May I be free from suffering. May I be at peace'" (1991, p. 29). Send loving phrases like these to yourself with every breath, repeat them with every inhalation and every exhalation. Meditate on sending well-being and mercy into your own mind and body.

Expand this healing by sending this same warmth and kindness to someone else—a loved one, a teacher, or a friend. Concentrate on the image of that person and the love you want them to feel. Share with them the feelings of love that you are experiencing; ask also that they be free from suffering. Generate an internal dialogue that reflects the love you have for that person. Continue to connect these loving thoughts with your breath. Let this love grow in your heart; let it fill your heart, then overflow and expand.

Allow loving kindness to expand to the whole world. Open your heart to all and wish all sentient beings happiness and wholeness and freedom from suffering. Imagine enveloping the entire planet in your loving kindness and mercy. Repeat your wishes for love and mercy several times, as you immerse yourself in love for all things. End the meditation by wishing that all beings may dwell in the heart of healing.

SOFT BELLY

This meditation begins to teach mindfulness by noting the feeling of the belly. Is it hard, like stone, or soft? Is it tight, like a closed fist, or loose? For Levine, a hard belly is a sign of hardening to experience (1991, 1999), of judgment, resentment, steeling one's self to pain, and being closed off to the present moment. The softer one's belly remains, the easier it is to remain aware and open to compassion.

Softening one's belly opens one to an exploration of pain and grief in whatever form grief takes. Levine regards the Soft Belly Meditation as key to learning to let go of suffering. Softening to our experience is really a softening of that which separates one from the wisdom of the heart. "Watch breath, soften belly, open heart" (1991, p. 85). This is the path Levine recommends to awareness.

Soft Belly Meditation

Begin this practice by allowing your attention to come into the body. Feel the physical sensation of being in the body, the sensation of the breath, the breath in the chest, the breath as it travels down the neck. Let your attention follow the breath into the belly and allow your belly to soften.

Soften the belly to receive the breath, and notice the sensations of the belly rising and falling with the breath. Let go with each breath. Send mercy into each breath and soften the belly. Let go of grief, of holding on to the old. Breathe out hardness; just let pain dissolve into the softness.

Continue to focus on your breathing, and notice its sensations as it moves in and out of a soft belly. It is important to let go and just trust this process, to allow your mercy to soften the hardness of your belly.

When you have finished meditating and open your eyes, notice where the belly hardens as you finish. When you feel this place harden, you will begin to recognize the conditioning of the body to close off experience, and then you will be able to rebalance it by remembering to soften the belly.

FORGIVENESS

Forgiveness expands on the lessons of softening and loving kindness. It is the completion of business left undone, the resolution of conflict, both internal and external. Through forgiveness, one opens to the pain of hurt and resentment, anger and fear, so that it eventually can be released. Forgiveness exemplifies the process of letting go.

Forgiving others is essential to mindfulness, because forgiveness exemplifies the process of releasing ourselves from suffering. Levine teaches that it is done as a means of self-healing, that "you are forgiving them to make room in your heart for you" (1990). When grief is released, one's load is lightened. By freeing one's mind of grief, one is able to enter into the heart more freely.

In order to forgive others, to accept forgiveness from others, or to assist others in this process, one also must be able to forgive oneself. One's own feelings of unworthiness and mercilessness block the road to forgiveness. Forgiveness also aids the process of healing by sending loving kindness into one's suffering. As forgiveness is experienced, the capacity to share fully with another expands, and the feeling of separation between persons dissolves into an awareness of the inseparable. Levine writes in *Healing into Life and Death*:

> In the deepest stages of forgiveness, one finds there is no "other" to send forgiveness toward, but just a "sense of being" shared. The one mind, the one heart in which we all float. Then, as in unconditional love, there is not forgiveness for another, but forgiveness with another (p. 91).

Forgiveness Meditation

Begin this meditation by asking yourself to reflect on what forgiveness means to you. Slowly, create an image in your mind of someone, alive or dead, who brings forth resentment. Then invite them into your heart. Let the person rest in the spaciousness of the receptive heart center. Holding this image, repeat a statement of forgiveness: "I forgive you for whatever pain you may have caused me in the past, either intentionally or unintentionally, through your words, your thoughts, your actions. However you may have caused me pain. I forgive you" (1991, p. 52).

Focus on awareness of the individual from the heart, and repeat the phrase of forgiveness once more. Try to feel the pain, anger, resentment that still resides inside. Feel the suffering that has been held inside for so long, that has kept you separated from the person you imagine. Recognize that this feeling has prevented you from real contact. Let the openness of your heart surround the hurt, the pain, and the person imagined. Let the separation between you dissolve in mercy and compassion. Allow the image to remain there in your heart, giving yourself whatever time you need. Then, allow it to leave, and notice any feelings that arise as it departs.

Invite an image of a person that perhaps needs to forgive you for past transgressions. Ask that person, now imagined, for forgiveness of any unkind word or action.

"I ask your forgiveness for however I may have caused you pain in the past—through my anger, through my lust, through my fear, my ignorance, my forgetfulness, my blindness, my doubt, my confusion. However I may have caused you pain, I ask that you let me back into your heart. I ask your forgiveness" (1991, p. 54).

Ask yourself to forgive yourself, and allow yourself to be forgiven. If you feel some resistance in the form of resentment, just let it be; let the feeling come and go; just observe the feelings. Let go of any feelings that might block the forgiveness that is being given to you, that is just an unmerciful mind. Once again repeat your request for forgiveness; recall any thoughts, words, deeds, conscious or unconscious, that may have hurt that person; ask for release through forgiveness. Accept the forgiving, letting go of all past feelings of hurt, anger, or resentment. Then allow that image to go, noticing any feelings as it departs.

Now forgive yourself; feel the sense of separateness that comes from pain, fear, and hurt. Allow your heart to open with compassion for yourself; have mercy on yourself; forgive yourself for all imperfections or feelings of unworthiness. Repeat your own first name; let it resonate down in your chest, the center of your heart. Say your name and then state, "I forgive you." Again open your heart to your own anger, resentment, and pain, and repeat the phrase of self-forgiveness. Just as we can hurt others, we also can be hurtful toward ourselves. Allow this realization to occur; surround this hurt with the openness of your heart.

Allow the critical judgments of self to pass. As you do this, feel the compassion in your heart; accept yourself and your imperfections. If resistance emerges in the form of self-criticism, again just observe; do not evaluate; let the unworthy feelings and thoughts go as you open your heart to self-forgiveness. It is so simple, yet so difficult to love ourselves, to truly feel caring deep down within the heart, to accept ourselves and forgive ourselves. As you allow yourself forgiveness, feel the freedom that emerges, the healing of separation and alienation from self. Experience the fullness of caring for yourself; once again, forgive yourself and loved ones who now occupy your heart.

MINDFULNESS

Just as loving kindness and mercy are the foundations for connecting with the compassionate heart, mindfulness is the foundation for developing an attentive, nonjudging mind. Being mindful is the way to most effectively enter grief. If one is mindful of how fear feels, if one explores where anger arises, and if one experiences where doubt resides, one learns what composes our experience, how perceptions arise and what conditions them. When mindfulness is well developed, one is aware of the compassion that is always present, the aliveness in the moment, and mind sinks into heart, becoming inseparable (1991, 1999). Mindfulness heals through its integration of experience.

Mindfulness and the grasping that leads to frustration, to one's dukka, cannot exist in the mind at the same time (1979). If one is present, the other cannot be.

One cannot be mindful and unaware at the same time. During his workshop recorded as *In the Heart Lies the Deathless,* Levine illustrates this with the story of a man who was allowed to emigrate from Korea into Japan during a time of war, although he had been previously denied admittance. After handing the immigration officer the statement, "Drinking my tea, I stopped the war," he was allowed to enter. The same mindfulness one brings to the simple act of drinking tea is the same mindfulness that prevents pain and anger to escalate. When one is mindful of one's drinking, one is mindful of the taste, of how it quenches one's thirst, of what thirst is, of what makes one thirsty, or makes one angry, of what makes others angry, or of what quenches the thirst of others. Being mindful of others' pain and thirst nurtures compassion and mercy, and war cannot continue. The foundation for living fully, mercifully aware of joy and compassion, lies in mindfulness. Levine's Guided Mindfulness Meditation teaches how to cultivate this awareness. "Wherever our attention is, wherever awareness is, that is where our aliveness is" (1991, p. 308).

Guided Mindfulness Meditation

Begin this meditation by closing your eyes and bringing your attention into the body. Let yourself experience the sensations arising there. Notice the sensations created by your breathing, and experience the sensations associated with each breath.

Allowing the body to breathe naturally, focus your attention on the nostrils, and become aware of the sensations produced there by the passing breath. If other thoughts arise during this time, gently acknowledge them, and let them go, always returning to the sensations of breath at the nostrils.

If awareness wanders, return gently, without judgment, to the breath. Awareness simply observes the process, the momentary changes. If feelings arise, simply acknowledge them as such, then gently return to the sensations of breath on the nostrils. Observe the process of arising and passing away of the breath, without holding or controlling.

Notice everything about the breath, the space between inhalations, its texture, its temperature as it passes the nostrils. Allow your awareness to be with the breath, and then let it go within the breath. Notice the span of each breath, its beginning, middle, and end, and begin to enter directly into the experience of breathing.

As your awareness deepens, you sense the impermanence of all experience. Note every thought or feeling or sensation, then allowed them to dissolve, returning with mercy, to the breath. When thoughts or feelings arise, note any tension for things to be different, then return to the breath. Anything that takes you away from the experience of the breath, just note it, then let it go. With mercy, allow yourself to go beyond breath and to enter into the experience of consciousness directly and to be fully present in the moment.

GRIEF

Another step on the path is opening our heart to grief through meditation. Grief offers an opportunity for healing, because it awakens one from the numbness of unconscious living. For Levine, grief is mental activity suppressed, *compressed* into an armor around the heart (1999). Although physical healing may or may not occur, hearts may be healed from grief: true healing removes the sense of separation and connects one with the deathlessness of one's true nature. Compassion eases compression.

Meditation reconditions one to soften into grief, to send loving kindness into pain, to become mindful of it, and to touch one's pain with mercy. Meditation practice enlarges the room in one's heart for one's pain, letting it just be there in mercy. Grief is given a place to exist in the heart, where it is not *removed*, but *integrated*, restoring a sense of wholeness. But Levine cautions one to enter grief work slowly. He compares the denial of one's pain to picking fruit in the midst of a burning orchard, and he advises that "we must not dash into the fire, but take one mindful step at a time" (1987, p. 277).

Levine suggests that before beginning this meditation, one find what he describes as the *griefpoint* in one's own body, the "mind/body convergence point where long-accumulated mental pain (grief) has solidified in the body, thick as armoring" (1991, p. 238). It is the physical locus of unexplored grief. To find it, one presses along the sternum, searching just above the heart for a sensitive spot. This tender area is the *griefpoint*, the point where unexpressed grief accumulates, and the *touchpoint*, the point at which one can touch, or enter, the heart.

The Griefpoint Meditation begins a process of admitting the point of grief to enter the heart, of converting the *griefpoint* into the *touchpoint*. This is the process of laying one's grief onto the ground of compassion, allowing the awareness of compassion to envelop it and to integrate it into a greater understanding of life, of beingness:

> Grief begins to sink from the mind of separation and fear, resistance and dread, into the heart of mercy and loving kindness and pure awareness. In the integration of our pain into our heart, there is no separation to be found, just a unity of being shared in all our lives (1991, p. 239).

Griefpoint Meditation

Sit or lie and relax. With your hands, locate the center of your chest near the base of the sternum; press with your hands against this area in the chest, searching for the point of maximum pressure. Try to feel the place beneath the sternum; notice the feeling of pressure, ache, and pain. This sensation is the feeling of loss, of the grief that we have felt in the past and of the grief that we will inevitably meet in the future. Notice the heavy sense of sadness as you contemplate the loss of your partner, spouse, parent, child, or other loved ones; this feeling is also grief for all the loss and suffering that your neighbors, here and around the world, are experiencing at this instant. It is the feeling of loss and grief that all humankind shares.

Imagine how these deep aches are protected inside your heart. Again take your thumbs and probe for the pressure emanating from the center of the sternum. Feel the painful sensations where the pain and grief are held. Breathe slowly, a little more deeply. Feel the pain in this center as you inhale and exhale. Keep your attention on the feelings, as you allow the feelings of grief and pain to emerge through the layers of protection. Open to the pain as you push into this griefpoint. Keep the pressure constant with your thumbs. Stay with the feeling. Let awareness enter. Allow yourself a vulnerability to all the fear, pain, and anguish of unexpressed grief.

Draw the pain into the immensity of the heart, where it can be accepted and experienced and eventually released. In the process of feeling the pain in the heart, you are accepting that pain and ending the suffering and fear that surround your grief. Allow yourself to breathe deeply into the heart, and let yourself just be in mercy and loving kindness. Breathe in the pain, from past hurts, loss, anger, judgment, the hidden grief, the fear. Let it come into the mercy of the heart that is able to heal all this pain. "Let the mind of grief sink into the heart of healing" (1999, Study Guide, p. 11).

Have mercy on yourself and continue to breathe in the pain. Let the pain flow in, filling the vast spaciousness of your deathless nature, your true nature. It is only in accepting and experiencing grief that we can move beyond it.

If you are grieving for someone, breathe them into your heart through this griefpoint. Little by little, with each exhalation of breath, let them go. Allow the pain of grief to dissolve in the spaciousness of your heart's mercy.

Now let your hand drop gently from your chest, and notice the point where your hand used to be. Continue to breathe from here, breathing in and out of this point. Allow the heart's mercy to expand to all beings, that they may be free of suffering, and know the joy of their deathless nature.

PAIN

Opening to pain is not unlike opening to grief. Often the automatic reaction to pain is to resist it. Psychological techniques to control pain often aim to move awareness away from the sensation of pain. Yet pain, like grief, may become an opportunity for healing.

Opening up to pain is similar to unarmoring the heart or softening the belly. It is not simply an enduring of pain. Instead, pain may be understood in a wider context of meaning and awareness. Levine reminds one that, "there is nothing noble about suffering except the love and forgiveness with which we meet it" (2002, p. 124). Instead of reacting to the pain, he teaches one to respond to it with merciful awareness.

A Guided Meditation on Softening to Pain

Begin this meditation by finding a relaxed position for your body; then slowly bring your attention to the area of your pain. Focus all of your attention on that place, allowing yourself, as fully as possible, to experience the feelings and sensations that emerge. At that point, begin to let the body soften around the pain. Relax the tension there. Let go of the fist of resistance. Let it open to receive mercy and loving kindness. Notice the feelings of pain, allow them to dissolve into softness, and have mercy on them as you let them go.

Feel the resistance changing to a greater openness and acceptance of the sensations at that very moment. As the tension diminishes, feel the softness in the area around the sensations of discomfort, feel the softening of the muscles, of the body. Feel the tension loosening; Levine suggests that now sensations may be easier to accept, to bring into fuller awareness, and to let go.

Continue to send mercy and loving kindness into that area, allowing it to soften further, opening into merciful awareness.

DYING AND DEATH

Levine tells the story of a dying woman who confided in him that two types of people came to visit her during this time (1990). The first group, and by far the largest, could not stand that she was dying or in pain: they wanted her to be different, to be well. As a result, she felt like a failure. Her pain intensified due to their discomfort. A second group would come in to her room with gentleness, and seemed comfortable just being there with her. It was they who made her feel so cared for.

Opening to healing and preparing to die are the same thing (1982). Awareness dissolves one's sense of separateness from one another and from being itself. It reveals that the person is not the body, that the body may die but the essence of being does not. As the illusion of separate bodies and separate minds crumbles, a common ground of being emerges, a place where one is inseparable from another. To be of comfort to the dying, one simply needs to be mindfully present, to silently bear witness to the reality of the inseparable. Levine reminds those who work with the terminally ill that it is important to see the dying person not as their body nor as their pain (1997). For the aforementioned woman, feeling the comfort others had with the dying process became her comfort, and she could relax and trust the process.

The importance of practicing one's dying lies in its capacity for honing the skills necessary for conscious living. As Levine rehearsed his own preparation for death, he reflected that

> the clarity necessary to navigate through death is cultivated in the midst of life. By investigating what is directly ahead we live so thoroughly in the

present that we come to trust the ground beneath our feet and our capacity to stand erect and make our choices from the heart (1997, p. 132).

Levine has used the following Guided Meditation on Dying to help one move beyond the conditioned illusion of separateness. His extensive work with the dying and his own depth meditations have revealed the experience of the death process in its earliest hours. He describes it as one of expansion, an experience of going from solidity to spaciousness (1991). He uses imagery to simulate this experience. The meditation also is designed to help one practice letting go of the last moment and opening to the next—to practice living, and dying, moment to moment, in mindful rebirth.

Guided Meditation on Dying

For this meditation, Levine recommends choosing a place in your home where you would choose to die. As the meditation becomes more familiar, it can be done anywhere.

Assume a relaxed position, and gently close your eyes to enhance concentration. Shift your awareness to the sensations of being in your body; try to feel these sensations as clearly as you can; now do an internal scan of your body. First, focus on your neck and head; notice how it balances on your torso; feel the muscle sensations in your neck; let them loose. Move your attention from your neck down into the musculature of your shoulders; feel the sensation of the muscles of the shoulders. Now move your awareness down into your arms and hands; note the feelings. Keeping your breathing easy and natural, notice your weight, the body. Where does it meet the chair, bed, or floor? Feel where your body meets its support; feel your back, legs, head, feet, and arms. Feel the sensations of your body with full awareness. Just let the sensations coming from your body come into awareness moment to moment. Keep the focus on body sensation. Notice that they appear to be received by an entity much subtler than the body: by awareness.

Focus on breathing now, and try to feel the movement of breathing from the heavy body of sensation to the more subtle body of awareness itself. Visualize the light body balancing inside. Come back to the breathing; follow the breathing with your awareness; feel the inhalation; follow it through to the exhalation. Feel the sensations in the heavy body; now shift attention to the light body of awareness. Feel how the light body is connected to the heavy body with each breath. Each breath is all that exists—just the breathing of the breath. You are now breathing; this is all; each breath is your first and last breath. Do not think of your next breath. This is the only breath. The final breath. Imagine and visualize the light body and the heavy solid body as separate bodies: the light body of awareness is separate from the physical body of sensation. Imagine that this is the end. This is the last breath. Let your breathing go. Let each thought dissolve. Do not cling to life; that is past now. Open to death, and let yourself die.

As the exercise continues, imagine yourself floating away from the heavy body. The awareness body moves away from the heavy body. Open your heart. Let go of your body; let go of your name, your identity, your thoughts; let them go. Float freely in space and awareness. Have mercy on you.

You are one with space; you slowly become aware that something is approaching from far away. Imagine that what is approaching slowly, gently is your breathing. Observe; become aware of the breathing as if you were watching the breathing from a distance. Slowly the breathing becomes more recognizable; it comes closer. Slowly the breathing comes to your body; experience it reentering the body. Focus on the breath. Each breath is the first breath; do not think of your next breath.

Allow yourself to feel the return of conscious awareness to your body; imagine this experience as a rebirth, a new birth to heal, a rebirth to bring kindness, to bring mercy. Simply be aware of breath, of light body reanimating the heavy body. Born again to the world, meditate on the reason for your birth: to learn, to bring mercy, kindness, healing. Be one with your breathing, one with the moment. As this meditation comes to a close, wish all beings the peace of their true nature and freedom from suffering.

DEATH

Levine (1997, pp. 132-133) candidly describes what he has learned during his caregiving and hospice work:

> I know from numerous personal and direct experiences that death has a life of its own. My understanding that awareness survives the body is not a belief system, it's just the way it is. It is not the result of some restless philosophy but the product of numerous experiences of, and with, death that coincided from several different directions, including those that accompanied the dying to the threshold and experienced them cross over. . . . It was from these extraordinary moments that I first experienced the "point of remembrance" and was allowed repeated observation of the dissolution of the elements as they lost sway over a lightening spirit.

His familiarity with the death process ends a few hours after clinical death, and he readily admits that he does not know what comes next. Yet, to help others through the death process, he sought inspiration from the various translations of the *Tibetan Book of the Dead*. He developed the meditation presented here from those texts in collaboration with Lama Yeshe, a Tibetan Lama. It is meant to be only a guide for an exploration of dying and death, one possible scenario among infinite possibilities.

As one grows in mindful practice of this meditation, one must learn to trust one's own intuition, to linger where the heart wants to, or to alter the meditation in any way that feels appropriate. The renewal of death, as in life, relies on the readiness of one's connection to compassion and joy. Gentle practice in life creates a well-worn path to the heart. When death ultimately arrives, the scenery might be different, but the path will be familiar. Knowing the way, one can relax and trust the process.

Death Transition Meditation

Although this meditation is often repeated by a guide to a dying or dead person, one also can meditate on these words to practice living with an engaged heart.

The guide's main task is to assist the dying person to let go of the body. The guide begins by asking the dying to imagine that his/her body no longer has the energy to remain connected to the life force and to experience it dissolving out of the body. The guide asks the dying to leave the solid, heavy body behind for a flowing one. The guide tells the dying person that death has arrived and encourages him/her to gently let go.

The dying person is asked to recognize the clear light as it emerges into awareness. This clear light is identified by the guide as the dying person's true nature. He/she is prompted to open, without holding or clenching, to the clear, white light. The dying person is asked to feel the love and compassion emanating from the light, as he/she opens to the reality and experience of the light. He/she is encouraged to let go of any fear or confusion. He/she is gently encouraged to let go of his/her separations and to become one with the clear light.

If the dying person becomes attached to memories, he/she is gently brought back to the experience of the light. He/she is encouraged to experience the wholeness and unity in the light. If projections arise, he/she is asked to simply note these moments and let them go: to let the mind and body separate. He/she is reminded that the physical body has been shed and that he/she now has a light body, a body of light, one of pure being.

Even though the body has separated and died, the dead person can still be capable of projecting a world of thought. The person is encouraged to recognize the fact that the body is gone. Projections of fear and desire may continue, but this is just the rising and falling of thought. The person is encouraged once again to let go of present and past fears, to accept the light of true essence and being. He/she is encouraged to recognize that he/she is beyond death; there is no death. As projections continue to emerge based on the past idea of who he/she was, they are neutralized and purified in the presence of the white light.

From an Eastern spiritual perspective, the dead one may not fully accept his/her oneness with the clear light and as such be pulled away from the light toward greater separateness. As this happens, the dead person may be moving toward a new birth, a new incarnation. If this occurs, the guide reminds the dead one to recall the essence of his/her being and to remain aware in the new birth, to go beyond the conditioned in the unconditioned heart, to merge with the light of his/her own great heart. As the meditation moves toward closure, the dead one is reminded that he/she is Awareness itself, and that as Awareness, he/she does not depend on life or death for existence. He/she is the essence of all things, the light.

CONCLUDING REMARKS

Levine challenges the perceptions upon which the pain of loss, death, and dying are based, and offers instead, a new way of responding. Opening to loss heals ultimately by revealing a deeper awareness of life. Healing comes not from the intellectual mind but from connection with the vast compassion of the heart. It lies in the merciful awareness that joy and compassion always have been there and will always be there in every moment.

His meditations speak to the deathlessness of one's being and to one's timeless essence found in the intimate awareness of the present moment. Here, in this moment, one discovers that conscious dying is the same as conscious living, and that one dies the way one lives. "As we pass through this 'point of remembrance,' it becomes clear, as it is said, that we were not human beings having a spiritual experience, but spiritual beings having a human experience" (2002, p. 212).

REFERENCES

Boerstler, R. (1982). *Letting go.* Watertown, MA: Associates in Thanatology.
Dass. R., & Levine, S. (1976). *Grist for the mill.* Santa Cruz, CA: Unity Press.
Gibran, K. (1966). *The prophet.* New York: Alfred A. Knopf.
Levine, S. (1979). *A gradual awakening.* New York: Anchor Press/Doubleday.
Levine, S. (1982). *Who dies? An investigation of conscious living and conscious dying.* New York: Anchor Press/Doubleday.
Levine, S. (1984). *Meetings at the edge.* New York: Anchor Press/Doubleday.
Levine, S. (1987). *Healing into life and death.* New York: Doubleday.
Levine, S. (1990). *In the heart lies the deathless: Facing personal loss through spiritual contemplation* (audiocassettes). Boulder, CO: Sounds True Recordings.
Levine, S. (1991). *Guided meditations, explorations and healings.* New York: Doubleday.
Levine, S. (1997). *A year to live: How to live this year as if it were your last.* New York: Belltower.
Levine, S. (2002). *Turning toward the mystery: A seeker's journey.* New York: HarperCollins.
Levine, S., & Levine, O. (1999). *The grief process: Meditations for healing* (audiocassettes and study guide). Boulder, CO: Sounds True.
Nhat Hanh, T. (1998). *The heart of the Buddha's teaching: Transforming suffering into peace, joy, and liberation.* New York: Broadway Books.

CHAPTER 3

Confronting Death Through Mental and Artistic Imagery

Robert G. Kunzendorf

> Well! we are all *condamnés*, as Victor Hugo says: we are all under sentence of death but with a sort of indefinite reprieve—*les hommes sont tous condamnés à mort avec des suris indéfinis*: we have an interval, and then our place knows us no more. Some spend this interval in listlessness, some in high passions, the wisest, at least among "the children of this world," in art and song.
> Walter Pater, *The Renaissance*, 1919, p. 198

This chapter advances the thesis that the psychologically most basic image of death is the image of personal annihilation. As discussion of this thesis will show, certain mental images directly *express* self-annihilation. Other images, both mental and artistic, serve to *repress* this basic image of death. Many religious images of death do both, and thereby *sublimate* the basic image of personal annihilation. Through the different sections of this chapter, these various types of death imagery and their psychological implications will be explored.

The first section of the chapter examines the subjectively experienced image of personal annihilation and its depressing connotations. The second section reviews evidence that less depressing images of death, particularly images of an afterlife, serve to repress self-annihilative imagery. In the third section, the debilitating consequences of repressing the subjective image of annihilation are contrasted with the debilitating consequences of not repressing this depressing image. The final section shows how, by contemplating either religious or existential artworks that objectify the subjective image of personal annihilation, people can sublimate the possibility of such annihilation, instead of succumbing to depression or denying the very possibility.

PHENOMENOLOGICAL DESCRIPTION OF DEATH IMAGERY

To mentally to confront death as directly as one can is to imagine the possibility of personal annihilation, as phenomenologically described by Koestenbaum (1964-1965):

> If I think of my death as the end of everything, then, in a manner of speaking, I must think as well of the termination of the universe itself. After all what mental image is present when I think of the real meaning of the death of myself? Honest analysis will disclose that there is then no image of the world left. Thus, my image of the death of myself is tantamount to asserting the end of the world.
>
> There is a fundamental phenomenological error in the thought that the death of myself means the cessation of heartbeats, burial, and yet assures the continuation of the world. That is *not* how the threat of my own death presents itself to me. That threat is the death of the observer, and if I should think of my own burial, the settling of my estate, the cessation of my breathing, etc., then I tacitly—and erroneously—also think of myself as some eternal observer contemplating the tragic scene of his own death! What the observer has done here, in effect, is not to have considered candidly enough the reality of his own death. The understanding of what it means for him to be dead cannot include the presence of himself as an observer at his own death. He has, in fact, slipped back surreptitiously into the picture of his own death as some sort of eternal observer. But we must remember that his death is supposed to be the death of the observer itself. And with extinction of that observer, the entire scene vanishes as well.[1]

According to Koestenbaum's phenomenological description, the basic image of subjective annihilation is an image of forever losing the ability to experience this world or any other world.

Inasmuch as this "end of the universe" image constitutes the foundation for the remaining discussion, it is necessary to rebut arguments that such an image is (a) too subjective, (b) too intellectual, (c) impossible to generate. The first argument—that the universe, as an object of knowledge, does not cease to exist when the knowing subjects dies—is certainly true from the standpoint of a surviving observer. But this same argument is meaningless (neither true nor false) from the standpoint of an annihilated observer whose subjective experience of that universe has forever ended. Moreover, it is psychologically significant that the possibility of self-annihilation can be experienced only as a mental image of the "subjective" universe, not as a mental image or an artistic image of the "objective" universe. Accordingly, as the final section of this chapter will show, artistic images cannot *directly* recreate Koestenbaum's subjective image of the end of the

---

[1] From "The Vitality of Death" (pp. 142-143) by P. Koestenbaum, 1964-1965, *Journal of Existentialism, 5*. Copyright by Libra Press. Reprinted by permission.

universe, because artistic images of annihilation are experienced as *objects in the universe.*

The second objection to Koestenbaum's image of annihilation is that such an image is too intellectual to be biologically instinctual or otherwise universal. In so denying the universality of self-annihilative image, Michael Chapman (personal communication, 1986) argues that "there was a stage in human development historically, as well as a stage of ontogenesis, in which the concept of personal annihilation does not yet exist" (pp. 1-2). However, Chapman's objection is rejoined by Heilbrunn's (1955) argument that "in the newborn [and] in every human being [is an] inherited fear of annihilation . . . the dread of annihilation by being eaten . . . ordinarily dormant within the organism but easily activated by relatively innocuous external and internal stimuli" (pp. 448, 462, 464). Indeed, James (1905) compares both normal death-anxiety and abnormal depression to the instinctive fear of being eaten.

> Here on our very hearths and in our gardens the infernal cat plays with the panting mouse, or holds the hot bird fluttering in her jaws. Crocodiles and rattlesnakes and pythons are at this moment vessels of life as real as we are; their loathsome existence fills every minute of the day that drags its length along; and whenever they or other wild beasts clutch their living prey, the deadly horror which an agitated melancholiac feels is the literally right reaction on the situation (p. 164).

The subjective image of being eaten, which arises in the fairy tales and religious myths of many cultures, is a concrete and compelling image of the end of one's existence and one's universe. As such, it appears to be the instinctual, if not primal, version of the generic "end of the universe" image described by Koestenbaum (1964-1965).

The third objection to Koestenbaum's image of death stems from Freud's (1963/1915) arguments against the possibility of consciously imaging annihilation or of fearing it per se.

> Our own death is indeed unimaginable, and whenever we make the attempt to imagine it we can perceive that we really survive as spectators (pp. 222-223).

> The dread of death, which dominates us oftener than we know, is on the other hand something secondary (p. 231). . . . merely a fear of libidinous deprivation (p. 137).

Freud's first argument—that total unconsciousness cannot be consciously imaged— rightly recognizes that a person imaging the annihilation of conscious experience must meanwhile be self-conscious *that he or she is imaging* (Kunzendorf, 1987-1988, 2000). Otherwise such a person would be totally unconscious. However, Freud's second argument—that death imagery and death anxiety are, therefore, secondary or derivative phenomena—fails to recognize that Koestenbaum's "end of the universe" image is, but for the self-consciousness which accompanies it, a veridical image of personal annihilation: an image that brings living persons as close as they can *consciously* come to the annihilation of consciousness.

Indeed, contrary to Freud's second argument, fear of death is a primary fear: a *direct and immediate urge to escape* the "end of the universe" image, which cannot be reconciled with one's desire to continue living indefinitely or one's pursuit of long-term goals. The inability to escape this image of personal annihilation can be a cause of debilitating depression and hopelessness, as later discussion will demonstrate. However, the repression of death imagery can also be psychologically debilitating, as the next two sections of this chapter will show.

PSYCHOLOGICAL REPRESSION OF DEATH IMAGERY

Several empirical studies indicate that, whereas the fear of personal annihilation is expressed in the subconscious behavior of all adults, it is sometimes repressed from the conscious experience of those who fantasize religious salvation as an alternative to annihilation. For example, Williams and Coe (1968) found that, although conscious expressions of death anxiety are less severe in religious persons than in unbelievers, the degree to which galvanic skin response is elevated by death-related words is the same in both groups. Similarly, Lester (1970) found that, although conscious death anxiety is lower in believers than in unbelievers, the degree to which associative response latencies are increased by death-related stimuli is equivalent in both groups. To the extent that increases in GSR and response latency are valid measures of subconscious fear, these results suggest that death-denying images of religious salvation may serve to repress the more instinctual and more depressing image of personal annihilation.

The validity of the response latencies is confirmed by two sets of findings. First, subjects who are repressers exhibit longer identification times for death-related words than subjects who are sensitizers exhibit (Magni, 1972). At the same time, repressers express less overt death anxiety than sensitizers express (Jaervinen, 1975; Magni, 1972; Toler & Reznikoff, 1967). Still, Kastenbaum and Costa (1977) have criticized the assumption that increases in response latency and in GSR reflect repressed fears, rather than unconscious physiological factors.

In response to Kastenbaum and Costa's criticism of these nonverbal measures of subconscious fear, Kunzendorf (1985) examined a more direct verbal measure: the degree of death-related fear expressed subconsciously through "automatic writing." When the religious subjects in Kunzendorf's study were deeply hypnotized and were automatically writing their subconscious answers to death-related questions, their fear of personal annihilation rose to the level of fear that was expressed consciously (and subconsciously) by unbelievers. Notably, this hypnotic recovery of subconscious death anxiety was observed only in response to questions about personal annihilation, not in response to other death-related questions.

Finally, Spencer (1976) directly measured the repressed death anxiety of people who, during near-death encounters, experienced "life after life" imagery and lost their conscious fear of death. In their conscious responses to Spencer's death-related questions, subjects with "life after life" images reported less fear than control subjects without near-death encounters reported. However, in their verbal responses on the Thematic Apperception Test, the "life after life" subjects produced more subconscious expression of death anxiety than the control subjects produced. The "life after life" image itself—the image of comfort and light at the end of a tunnel—has been compared to a drug-induced hallucination and to a flashback of the birth experience (Siegel, 1980). In either case, it—like other images of an afterlife—apparently represses and replaces the more basic and more dreadful image of personal annihilation.[2]

A question that emerges from the above studies is whether repressing the instinctual image of personal annihilation fosters an abnormal psyche or a healthy one. As the next section shows, such repression seems to produce certain abnormalities, and the absence of repression seems to produce others.

ABNORMAL MANIFESTATIONS OF DEATH IMAGERY

Becker (1973) suggested that, as people move from total repression of death imagery to no repression thereof, they move from one extreme of psychological debilitation to another—from existential psychosis to existential depression. In depicting the psychotic extreme on this continuum, Becker relied on existential psychoanalysts like Searles (1961), who "touched upon the evidences that schizophrenia is a defense against recognizing the inevitability of death" (p. 640). Accordingly, Becker observed that the schizophrenic's hallucinatory images "of magical omnipotence and immortality are a reaction to the terror of death by a person who is totally incapable of opposing this terror with his own secure powers" (p. 218).

Becker made similar observations about nonpsychotic images that repressively defend against existential angst—images that range from fetishistic fantasies, on one hand, to genocidal fantasies, on the other. In fetishists studied by the existential analyst Boss (1949), and described by Becker (1973), human sexuality

---

[2] My late colleague and friend Michael Chapman argued that, although Western images of an afterlife serve to deny the annihilation of personal consciousness, Eastern images of reincarnation seem to embrace the annihilation of personal memory. This author's counterargument is that believers in reincarnation *deny personal annihilation* by positing both an afterlife and a previous life, and that they *have to deny the survival of personal memory* in order to explain why no previous life can be remembered.

was associatively linked with filthy animal carnality and with animal mortality and, ultimately, with personal annihilation. The perverted fantasies of these fetishists "magic[ally]" "spiritualized" human sexuality and, as a result, served to disinhibit sexual arousal by repressing its linkage with inhibitory images of personal annihilation (p. 236). And just as fetishists' perverted fantasies serve to cleanse sexistential filth, so too, according to Becker (1975), the Nazis' genocidal fantasies served to cleanse existential evil.

> I think it is time for social scientists to catch up with Hitler as a psychologist, and to realize that men will do anything for heroic belonging to a victorious cause if they are persuaded about the legitimacy of . . . identifying evil and moving against it (p. 142).
>
> Burke and Duncan have amply described the religious horror drama of Germany under Hitler, where the dirty and evil Jews were purged from the world of Aryan purity by the Nazi priesthood. Buchenwald and Auschwitz were the result of one of the most massive mystifications of history, a religious use of man's fundamental motives and fears (p. 117).
>
> The logic of killing others in order to affirm our own life unlocks much that puzzles us in history (p. 110).
>
> If you kill your enemy, your life is affirmed because it proves that the gods favor you. . . . As Winston Churchill discovered in one of his first military experiences: "Nothing in life is so exhilarating as to be shot at without result." And as Hitler concluded—after miraculously surviving the bomb blast that was meant to take his life but instead took several others, "Providence has kept me alive to complete my great work" (pp. 105-106).

Upon reading this in a seminar ten years ago, one of this author's students came to the realization that his image of a hellish afterlife for Jews was a genocidal fantasy *in which* the Christian godhead was overseeing the dirty work instead of the Nazis, and *through which* the student himself was aggressively repressing both his doubt about his own religion and his angst over his anticipated annihilation (Kunzendorf, 2002-2003).

At the opposite extreme from the existential hallucinator's psychotic repression of the reality of death is the existential depressive's equally debilitating confrontation with this reality. As recent studies comparing depressives and normals have shown, the depressive person *fails to repress* grim realities such as death. In two studies of dying patients, Kastenbaum and Aisenberg (1972) observed that the "depressed patients were those who openly recognized the prospect of death" (p. 72); and Zung and Gianturco (1971) confirmed that depression among the dying is negatively correlated with repression. Similarly, in two studies of college students, Sackeim (1983) and Roth and Ingram (1985) have confirmed that depression is negatively correlated with self-deception. In an experimental study with college students, Nelson and Craighead (1977) found that normal students underestimate the frequency of punishment in a laboratory task, whereas depressed students accurately recall the amount of punishment. In related experiments, Alloy and Abramson (1979, 1988) found that, when estimating the degree of contingency between responses and reinforcements, normal subjects make low estimates for undesired reinforcements and high estimates for desired reinforcements, whereas depressed subjects make accurate estimates in both cases. In addition, both Powell and Hemsley's (1984) and Kunzendorf and McLaughlin's (1988-1989) studies of *liminal* percepts—brief percepts near the *limen*, the threshold for self-conscious apperception—found that normal subjects perceive death-related words less accurately than congenial words, whereas depressed subjects perceive death-related words just as accurately as congenial words. Experiment 2 by Kunzendorf and McLaughlin revealed that, *unlike depressed subjects, normal subjects attenuate reality testing during the liminal perception of death-related words*, and a subsequent experiment by Kunzendorf, Moran, and Gray (1995-1996) revealed that, *unlike existentially depressed subjects, psychosis-prone subjects attenuate reality testing during the regular perception and imaging of congenial words*. Accordingly, in refuting the Freudian suggestion that normal people are less repressive than depressed people, the above experiments suggest that normality lies in the middle of the continuum between psychotic repression and existential depression.

In order for normal people to maintain this golden mean between repression and depression, they must not repress the image of personal annihilation, but also must not image it too directly. On one extreme, in attempting totally to repress the image of death, schizophrenics and other psychotic hallucinators have lost touch with death's reality and have hallucinated god-like immortality (Becker, 1973; Kunzendorf, 2000; Searles, 1961). On the other extreme, in attempting directly to image death until it loses its "sting," Montaigne, Mozart, and others have been driven into acute depression instead (Choron, 1964). To maintain a normal mental state between these two extremes, a person needs sublimated death imagery that promotes *psychologically safe confrontation* with personal annihilation, rather than repression or depression. Death imagery of this very sort abounds in works of art, both classical and modern, as the next section of this chapter illustrates.

ARTISTIC EXPRESSIONS OF DEATH IMAGERY

For at least 4000 years, people have been confronted with artistic images of death: Egyptian sarcophagi, Greek steles, medieval and Renaissance crucifixes, plus more modern images of death. Focusing on six specific examples of such art, the remaining discussion will show how certain artistic images objectify the subjective termination of the universe and thereby foster psychologically safer confrontations with personal annihilation. Focusing first on crucifixions by Grunewald, Perugino, and Rodin, the discussion will examine how viewers can consciously confront the end of the universe by projecting their own annihilation onto the heroic image of Jesus. Turning then to more modern death imagery in existential works by de Chirico and Munch, the discussion will examine how such works also sublimate the subjective image of annihilation, but objectively portray it as insignificant rather than heroic.

The possibilities for indirect confrontation with personal annihilation are, perhaps, best exemplified in artistic images of Jesus' crucifixion. In Figure 1, for example, *The Small Crucifixion* by Grunewald (c. 1511/1520) confronts the viewer directly with the end of Jesus' universe and indirectly with the end of his or her own universe. Grunewald's artistic image of a night-like void enveloping the dying Jesus is visually similar to the subjective image of the end of the universe. At the same time, neither this artistic image nor any other can directly re-create the subjective image of nothingness, inasmuch as the artistic image itself is perceived to be an object in the universe. Rather, a crucifixion like this one by Grunewald allows the viewer to confront the end of the universe *indirectly* by projecting oneself into the objective image of Jesus' death.[3]

The tendency to project oneself into Grunewald's image of the crucified Jesus is easily appreciated by comparing it to the reproduction in Figure 2 of a radically different crucifixion by Perugino. In *The Crucifixion with the Virgin, Saint John, Saint Jerome, and Saint Mary Magdalene* by Perugino (c. 1482/1484), there is no night-like void. Rather, there is light blue sky surrounding Jesus' body, and there is "business as usual" in the background, suggesting that Jesus' death is not the end of the world. Whereas Grunewald's painting of the crucifixion *objectifies the subjective image of annihilation*, Perugino's artistic image portrays Jesus' crucifixion from a survivor's point of view. Thus, one can project one's own annihilation onto Grunewald's subjectively dying Jesus, but not onto Perugino's objectively dying Jesus.[4]

Another crucifixion with a psychologically significant approach to death is *Christ and the Magdalene*, sculpted by Rodin (c. 1894) and pictured in Figure 3. This piece of sculpture confronts the viewer with a linkage between death and sex. That is, at one level of artistic expression, this crucifixion portrays grief and death on the cross, as Mary Magdalene clutches the lifeless Jesus. At another level, it expresses desire and sexual death, as she passionately embraces him. However, Rodin's artistic linkage between sex and death is psychologically unlike the mental linkage that Becker and Boss observed in fetishists. For such persons,

---

[3] On a psychological level, this projection of the self is paralleled by the Jungian identification of "Christ with the archetype of the self" (Ellenberger, 1970, p. 725). On an artistic level, the identification of the crucifixion with personal annihilation is paralleled by the filmmaker Bergman's *The Seventh Seal* (1956) wherein he identifies the apocalypse, as described in *Revelations*, with the end of the world, as encountered by every individual.

[4] Indeed, Perugino's artistic image might represent a psychological defense against the anxiety-provoking image of subjective death. Perugino "disbelieved in the immortality of the soul" (Walker, 1974, p. 86); and disbelievers tend to avoid death anxiety by entertaining more pleasant thoughts (Alexander & Adlerstein, 1959).

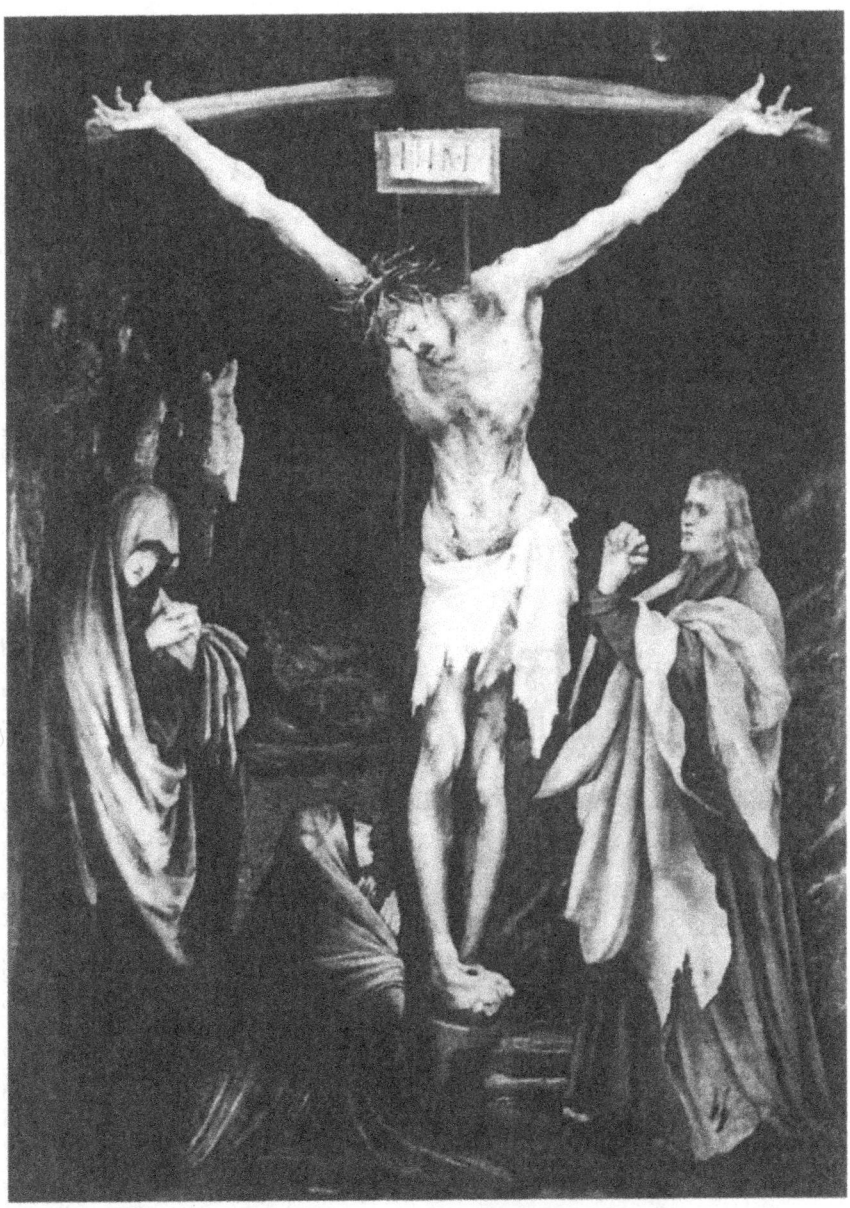

Figure 1. Grunewald, Matthias. *The Small Crucifixion,* c. 1511/1520, Samuel H. Kress Collection, Image © 2005 Board of Trustees, National Gallery of Art, Washington, oil on panel.

56 / HEALING WITH DEATH IMAGERY

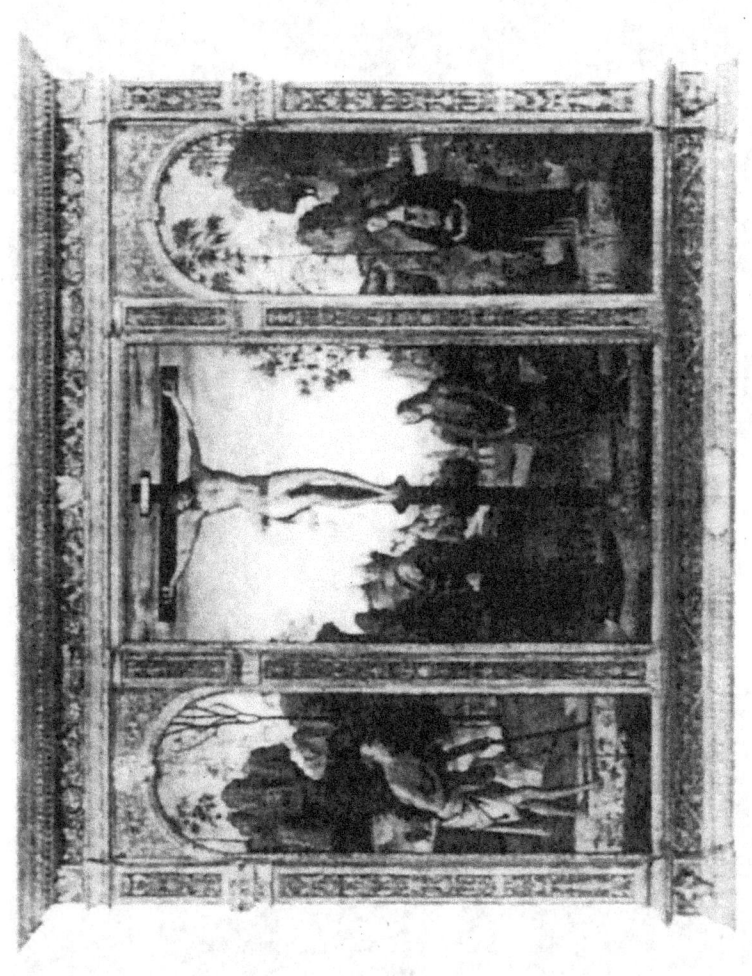

Figure 2. Perugino, Pietro. *The Crucifixion with the Virgin, Saint John, Saint Jerome, and Saint Mary Magdalene,* c. 1482/1484, Andrew W. Mellon Collection, Image © 2005 Board of Trustees, National Gallery of Art, Washington, oil on panel transferred to canvas.

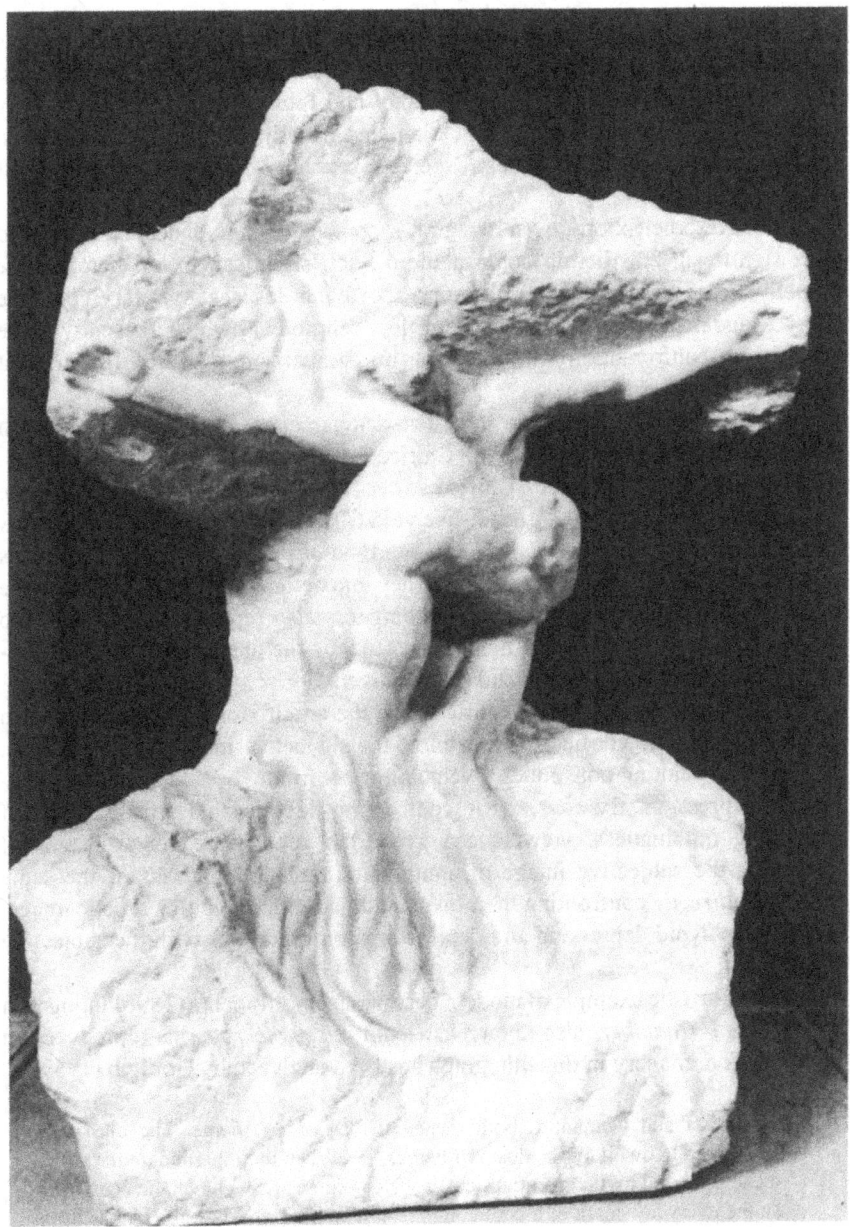

Figure 3. Rodin, Auguste. *Christ and the Magdalene (Le Christ et la Madeleine)*, c. 1894, Gift of Mrs. Alma de Bretteville Spreckels, Fine Arts Museums of San Francisco, plaster, © 2005 Artists Rights Society (ARS), New York/ADAGP, Paris.

sexuality subconsciously implies mortality and creates anxiety, which inhibits the normal sexual response. For Rodin, it is the reverse: it is death—even Jesus' death—that consciously implies materiality and thus, sexuality. By artistically reversing the direction of the implication, and by bringing it to consciousness, Rodin's crucifixion, unlike most, liberates sexuality from the inhibitions of death anxiety.

In all three crucifixions, even Perugino's, confrontation with death is portrayed as a significant and heroic confrontation. Such significance and heroism are visually expressed simply by elevating the dying Jesus above survivors like Mary Magdalene. In the more modern, less religious artworks presently to be considered, confrontation with death is, by comparison, a rather insignificant and pathetic matter.

The pathos and insignificance of modern death imagery are readily discerned in *The Anxious Journey*, painted by de Chirico (1913) and reproduced in Figure 4. In this and other paintings, de Chirico strove "to find artistic expression for the void" (Jaffe, 1964, p. 295). A death-like void fills the very center of *The Anxious Journey*. As the viewer travels into this void, *no one is watching* from the sides of the painting. Thus, a lone person's journey into nothingness is a heroic example to no one. Finally, this journey into nothingness also represents a journey into the mind itself. At the core of mental existence is the dark, sometimes subconscious, image of the subjective end of the universe.

This modern painting by de Chirico (like the crucifixion by Grunewald) can be viewed as an objectified expression of the subjective image of annihilation. As such, the painting constitutes a vehicle for confronting death without repression or depression. By *consciously* confronting de Chirico's artistic image of impending nothingness, viewers can avoid the debilitating consequences of repressing the subjective image of annihilation and nothingness. At the same time, by *indirectly* confronting their own annihilation through this artistic image, viewers can avoid depressing and debilitating confrontations with the subjective image itself.

A second artistic example of modern death imagery, Munch's (1896) lithograph of *The Death Chamber*, also known as *Death in the Sickroom*, is reproduced in Figure 5. The imagery in this lithograph has been analyzed by Gottlieb (1959).

> Classicists and Romantics both treated the *Deathbed* theme. The classic artist liked to dwell on the death of heroes. . . . When the inherited *deathbed* scene is treated by the twentieth-century Norwegian artist Munch, he centers on the everyday death of a common person who has passed away. This is in harmony with the values of nineteenth-century modern art. What is new, and shocking, and twentieth-century in his painting, *Death in the Sick Chamber*, is the fact that the interest focuses on the living instead of the dead. The expressions and stances of the surviving family members are powerful and expressive; and the bed and deceased are shifted into the background. The second shocking fact about Munch's interpretation of death is that the faces

CONFRONTING DEATH / 59

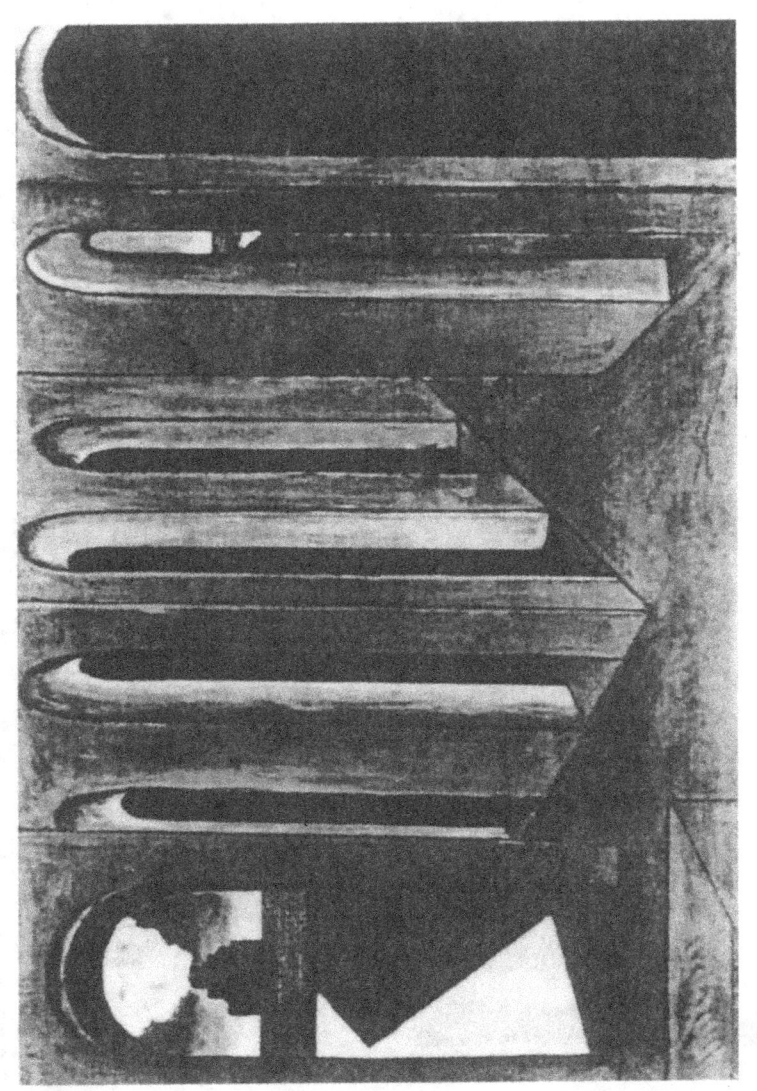

Figure 4. de Chirico, Giorgio. *The Anxious Journey*, 1913, Acquired though the Lillie P. Bliss Bequest, The Museum of Modern Art, New York, Image © The Museum of Modern Art / Licensed by SCALA/Art Resource, New York, oil on canvas, © 2005 Artists Rights Society (ARS), New York / SIAE, Rome.

60 / HEALING WITH DEATH IMAGERY

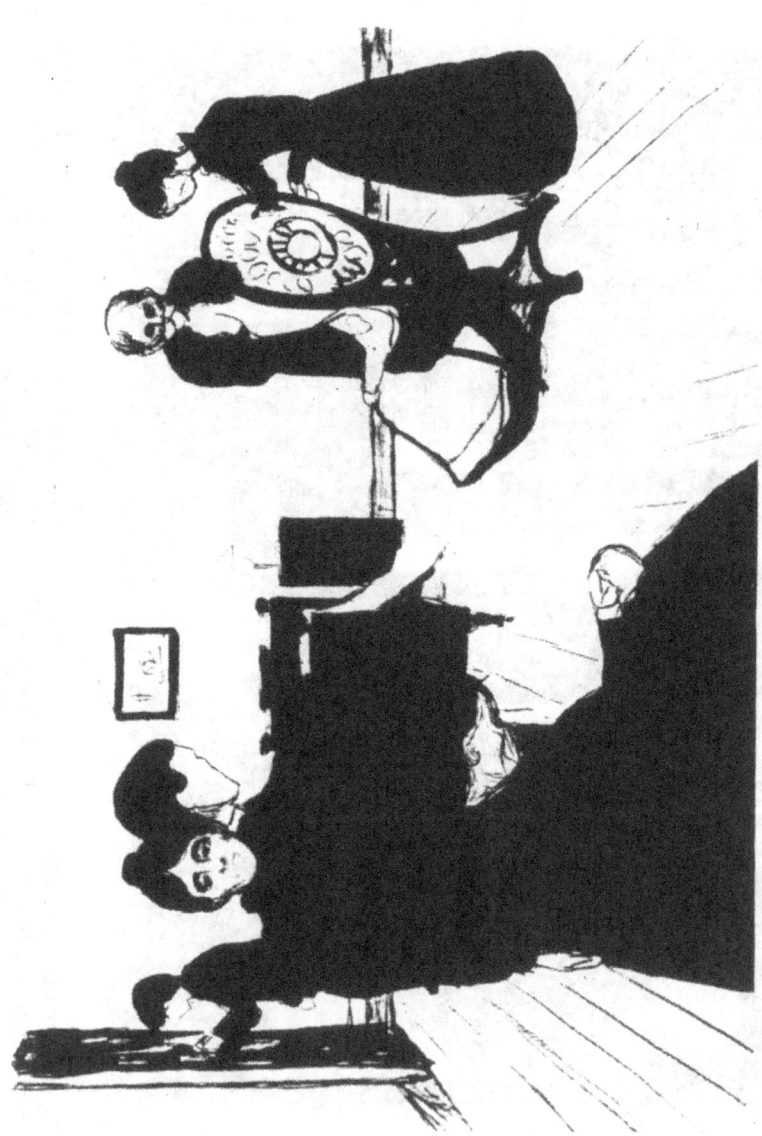

Figure 5. Munch, Edvard. *The Death Chamber (Sterbezimmer)*, 1896, Courtesy of the Fogg Art Museum, Harvard University Art Museums, Gift of Charles Bain Hoyt and John S. Thacher, lithograph, © 2005 The Munch Museum/The Munch-Ellingsen Group/Artists Rights Society (ARS), New York.

are contorted, not in mourning for a beloved lost member, but in fear of the unknown which has just swallowed the deceased, fear for themselves who are eventually to meet the same fate. In this agony, each person is alone; each survivor turns away not only from the dead but also from the other participants in the scene.[5]

In Munch's lithograph, as in de Chirico's painting, death is insignificant, rather than heroic, because *no one is watching*. However, unlike de Chirico's unpeopled image, Munch's image is one of survivors who appear unable to watch death. Accordingly, Munch's lithograph captures the fact that, as a survivor, one can neither perceive nor image the subjective termination of another person's universe, but can subjectively image only the end of one's own universe. At the same time, the survivors in Munch's lithograph appear to sense the insignificance of dying—and living—unwatched. They are like playwright Camus' (1958) protagonist Caligula, who realizes the insignificance of life, not while he is actively grieving for his deceased mistress, but as soon as he is "not watching" and forgets her.

Although *The Death Chamber* effectively expresses the subjectivity of personal annihilation, some of Munch's other artistic images more completely objectify this subjectivity. In *The Scream*, for example, Munch (1895) portrayed not only death, but the rest of the world as well, from a subjective standpoint. As Figure 6 indicates, *The Scream* pictures a skeleton-like person, terrified and transfixed. This contorted person, like the similarly contorted sky behind him, seems to scream with emptiness as two men, oblivious to their mortality, walk toward the sky and out of the picture. Clearly, such an artistic image does not portray objective reality—the world as it is. Rather, this artistic image portrays subjective reality—the world as it is phenomenally experienced. Thus, *The Scream* is similar in its perspective, as well as its content, to the subjective image of personal annihilation. Consistent with this subjective perspective that he introduced into works of visual art, Munch asserted that "we do not die—the world takes leave of us."[6] Such an assertion, like Koestenbaum's phenomenological description at the beginning of this chapter, simply characterizes in words, rather than artistic objects, the subjective image of the end of the universe.

In all of the artistic images described above, the crucifixions as well as the more modern images, viewers are confronted with objectified and sublimated expressions of the subjective image of personal annihilation. By consciously confronting artistic objects like these, viewers can avoid the debilitating consequences of repressing the subjective image of personal annihilation. At the same time, by engaging in such confrontation with artistic images, which can only

---

[5] From "Modern Art and Death" (p. 181) by C. Gottlieb, in *The Meaning of Death*, H. Feifel (ed.), McGraw-Hill, New York, 1959. Copyright by McGraw-Hill. Reprinted by permission.

[6] This assertion by Munch was quoted on a poster at the *Munch: Symbols & Images* Exhibition, National Gallery of Art, Washington, DC, 11 November 1978–19 February 1979.

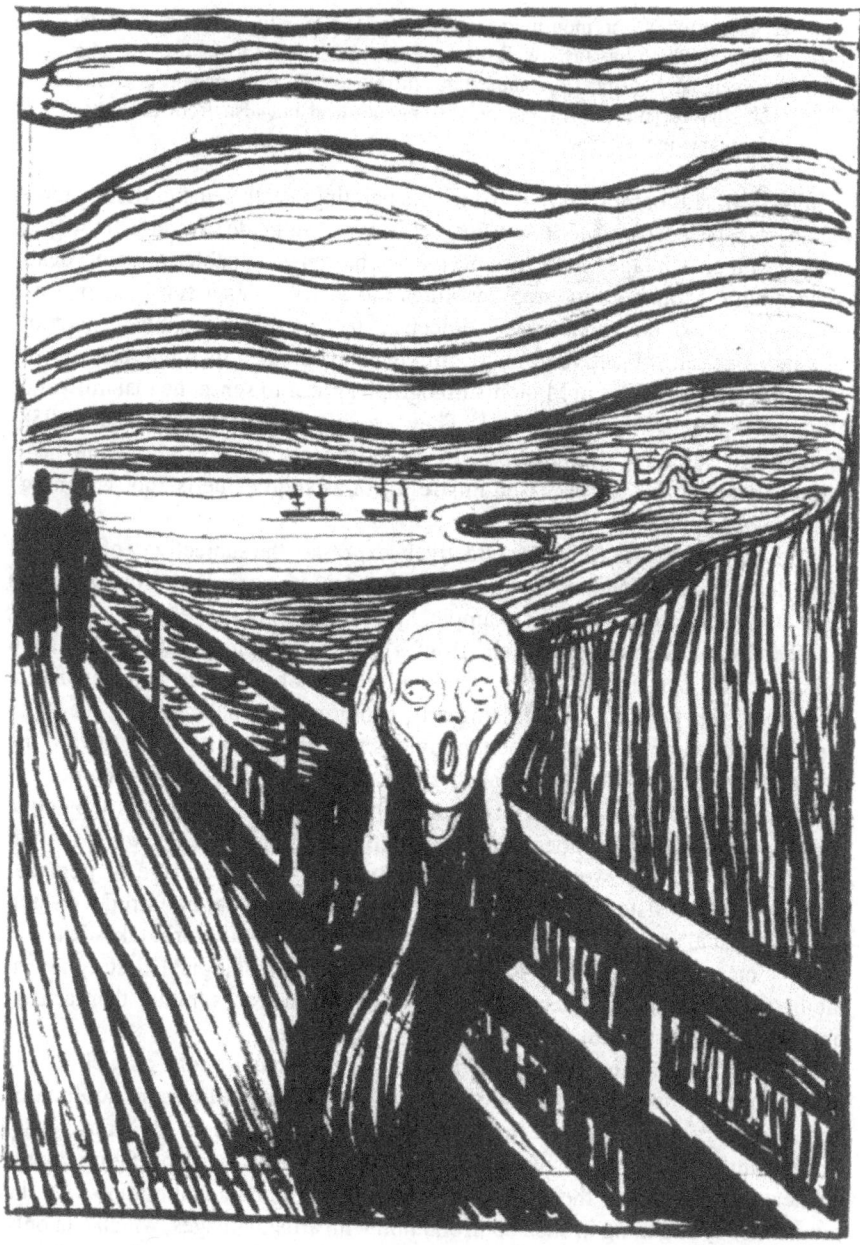

Figure 6. Munch, Edvard. *Geschrei (The Scream),* 1895, Rosenwald Collection, Image © 2005 Board of Trustees, National Gallery of Art, Washington, lithograph, © 2005 The Munch Museum/The Munch-Ellingsen Group/ Artists Rights Society (ARS), New York.

express personal annihilation indirectly, viewers can avoid direct and depressing confrontations with the subjective image itself.

ACKNOWLEDGMENTS

The author gratefully acknowledges helpful and insightful critiques by Elizabeth Ritvo, Anees Sheikh, and the late Michael Chapman.

REFERENCES

Alexander, I., & Adlerstein, A. (1959). Death and religion. In H. Feifel (Ed.), *The meaning of death* (pp. 271-283). New York: McGraw-Hill.
Alloy, L. B., & Abramson, L. (1979). Judgment of contingency in depressed and nondepressed students: Sadder but wiser? *Journal of Experimental Psychology: General, 108*, 441-485.
Alloy, L. B., & Abramson, L. (1988). Depressive realism: Four theoretical perspectives. In L. B. Alloy (Ed.), *Cognitive processes in depression* (pp. 223-265). New York: Guilford.
Becker, E. (1973). *The denial of death*. New York: Free Press.
Becker, E. (1975). *Escape from evil*. New York: Free Press.
Bergman, I. (Director). (1956). *The seventh seal* [film]. New York: Janus Films.
Boss, M. (1949). *The meaning and content of sexual perversions*. New York: Grune and Stratton.
Camus, A. (1958). Caligula. In A. Camus (Ed.), *Caligula and three other plays* (pp. 1-74). New York: Alfred A. Knopf. (Originally published in French, 1944.)
Choron, J. (1964). *Death and modern man*. New York: Collier.
de Chirico, G. (Artist). (1913). *The anxious journey* [painting]. New York: Collection, The Museum of Modern Art, acquired through the Lillie P. Bliss Bequest.
Ellenberger, H. F. (1970). *The discovery of the unconscious*. New York: Basic Books.
Freud, S. (1963). Reflections upon war and death. In P. Rieff (Ed.), *Character and culture* (pp. 107-133). New York: Collier. (Originally published in German, 1915.)
Gottlieb, C. (1959). Modern art and death. In H. Feifel (Ed.), *The meaning of death* (pp. 157-188). New York: McGraw-Hill.
Grunewald, M. (Artist). (c. 1511/1520). *The small crucifixion* [oil on panel]. Washington, DC: Samuel H. Kress Collection, National Gallery of Art.
Heilbrunn, G. (1955). The basic fear. *Journal of the American Psychoanalytic Association, 3*, 447-466.
Jaervinen, L. (1975). Psychodynamics of fear of death. *Psychiatria Fennica, 6*, 139-143.
Jaffe, A. (1964). Symbolism in the visual arts. In C. G. Jung (Ed.), *Man and his symbols* (pp. 255-322). New York: Dell.
James, W. (1905). *The varieties of religious experience*. London: Longmans, Green and Company.
Kastenbaum, R., & Aisenberg, R. (1972). *The psychology of death*. New York: Springer.
Kastenbaum, R., & Costa, P. T. (1977). Psychological perspectives on death. *Annual Review of Psychology, 28*, 225-249.
Koestenbaum, P. (1964-1965). The vitality of death. *Journal of Existentialism, 5*, 139-166.

Kunzendorf, R. G. (1985). Repressed fear of inexistence and its hypnotic recovery in religious subjects. *Omega: Journal of Death and Dying, 16*, 23-33.

Kunzendorf, R. G. (1987-1988). Self-consciousness as the monitoring of cognitive states: A theoretical perspective. *Imagination, Cognition, and Personality, 7*, 3-22.

Kunzendorf, R. G. (2000). Individual differences in self-conscious source monitoring: Theoretical, experimental, and clinical considerations. In R. G. Kunzendorf & B. Wallace (Eds.), *Individual differences in conscious experience* (pp. 375-390). Amsterdam: John Benjamins.

Kunzendorf, R. G. (2002-2003). Book review of "In the wake of 9/11: The psychology of terror by T. Pszczynski, S. Solomon, and J. Greenberg." *Imagination, Cognition and Personality, 22*, 427-431.

Kunzendorf, R. G., & McLaughlin, S. (1988-1989). Depression: A failure to suppress the self-conscious "monitoring" of dismal cognitions. *Imagination, Cognition and Personality, 8*, 3-17.

Kunzendorf, R. G., Moran, C., & Gray, R. (1995-1996). Personality traits and reality-testing abilities, controlling for vividness of imagery. *Imagination, Cognition and Personality, 15*, 113-131.

Lester, D. (1970). Religious behavior and the fear of death. *Omega: Journal of Death and Dying, 1*, 181-188.

Magni, K. G. (1972). The fear of death: An exploratory study of its nature and its correlates. In A. Godin (Ed.), *Death and presence: The psychology of death and the afterlife* (pp. 125-138). Brussels: Lumen Vitae Press.

Munch, E. (Artist). (1896). *Sterbezimmer (The death chamber)* [lithograph]. Cambridge, MA: Fogg Art Museum, Harvard University.

Munch, E. (Artist). (1895). *Geschrei (The scream)* [lithograph]. Washington, DC: Rosenwald Collection, National Gallery of Art.

Nelson, R. E., & Craighead, W. (1977). Selective recall of positive and negative feedback, self-control, and depression. *Journal of Abnormal Psychology, 86*, 379-388.

Pater, W. (1919). *The Renaissance.* New York: Boni & Liveright. (Originally published in 1873 as *Studies in the History of the Renaissance.*)

Perugino, P. (Artist). (c. 1482/1484). *The crucifixion with the Virgin, Saint John, Saint Jerome, and Saint Mary Magdalene* [oil on panel transferred to canvas]. Washington, DC: Andrew W. Mellon Collection, National Gallery of Art.

Powell, M., & Hemsley, D. R. (1984). Depression: A breakdown of perceptual defence. *British Journal of Psychology, 145*, 358-362.

Rodin, A. (Sculptor). (c. 1894). *Le Christ et la Madeleine (Christ and the Magdalene)* [plaster cast]. San Francisco, CA: The Fine Arts Museums of San Francisco, Gift of Mrs. Alma de Bretteville Spreckels.

Roth, D. L., & Ingram, R. E. (1985). Factors in the self-deception questionnaire: Associations with depression. *Journal of Personality and Social Psychology, 48*, 243-251.

Sackeim, H. A. (1983). Self-deception, self-esteem, and depression: The adaptive value of lying to oneself. In J. Masling (Ed.), *Empirical studies of psychoanalytical theories* (Vol. 1, pp. 101-157). Hillsdale, NJ: Erlbaum.

Searles, H. E. (1961). Schizophrenia and the inevitability of death. *Psychiatric Quarterly, 35*, 632-655.

Siegel, R. K. (1980). The psychology of life after death. *American Psychologist, 35*, 911-931.

Spencer, C. S. (1976). The effect of near-death experience on death anxiety. *Journal of Undergraduate Psychology Research, 3*, 21-26.

Tolor, A., & Reznikoff, M. (1967). Relation between insight, repression-sensitization, internal-external control, and death anxiety, *Journal of Abnormal Psychology, 72*, 426-430.

Walker, J. (1974). *National Gallery of Art, Washington, DC.* New York: Harry N. Abrams.

Williams, R. L., & Coe, S. (1968). Religiosity, generalized anxiety, and apprehension concerning death. *Journal of Social Psychology, 75*, 111-117.

Zung, W. W., & Gianturco, J. A. (1971). Personality dimension and the self-rating depression scale. *Journal of Clinical Psychology, 27*, 247-248.

CHAPTER 4

Near-Death Experiences: Heading Toward Omega?

Anees A. Sheikh, Sundar Ramaswami and Katharina S. Sheikh

> I was filled with an ecstasy beyond my wildest dreams. . . . I felt now as if I had been made anew. I saw wondrous meanings everywhere, everything was alive and full of energy and intelligence.
> Ring and Valarino (1998, p. 299)

> It was as if I was "seeing" things from a much greater depth of understanding!!! Needless to say, the absolute joy of learning was incredibly new to me and my mind felt like it was literally starving for new and interesting information. I could not pile it in fast enough.
> Ring and Valarino (1998, p. 42)

> I had the strong urge to hug total strangers with overpowering feelings of care and concern. I didn't understand where all this empathy was coming from, but I just knew it felt beautiful . . .
> Ring and Valarino (1998, p. 43)

The preceding excerpts are considered quite representative of the reports of tens of thousands of near-death experiences (NDEs) of individuals from around the world (Fox, 2003; Morse & Perry, 1992; Ring & Valarino, 1998; Sabom, 1998). It is not surprising that extensive parallels have been drawn between NDEs and mysticism (Cressy, 1996), NDEs and shamanism (Green, 2001), NDEs and perennial wisdom (Lorimer, 1996), and NDEs and Tibetan Buddhism's bardo teachings (Rinpoche, 1996). For example, as Tibetan Buddhist Sogyal Rinpoche states, "The central message that the near-death experiencers bring back from their encounters with death, or the presence or 'being of light', is exactly the same as that of Buddha and the bardo teachings: that the essential and most important qualities in life are love and knowledge, compassion and wisdom" (Rinpoche, 1996, p. 359). First, let us consider in detail what constitutes an NDE.

NDEs are defined as "profound psychological events with transcendental and mystical elements, typically occurring to individuals close to death or in situations of intense physical or emotional danger" (Greyson, 2000, p. 316). Probably NDEs have been occurring in some form for centuries. Valarino (1997) points out that descriptive fragments of NDEs occur both in the Bible and in the classic works of philosophy. Zaleski (1987) notes, "In nearly all cultures, people have told stories of travel to another world, in which a hero, shaman, prophet, king, or ordinary mortal passes through the gates of death and returns with a message for the living" (p. 3). One of the earliest descriptions of such an experience is mentioned in Plato's *The Republic*. Zaleski (1987) summarizes it thus:

> A soldier named Er, slain in battle comes back to life on the funeral pyre and describes his visit to the next world. He tells of leaving his body and journeying with a great throng to the place where souls are judged; the righteous ascend through an opening in heaven, while the wicked travel downward and to the left to meet their punishment.... The moral of the story, which Er has been sent back to proclaim, is that only those who have led an "examined life" will be able to turn fate to their advantage (p. 19).

Accounts of similar occurrences are contained in the folklore and writings of European, Middle Eastern, African, Indian, East Asian, Native American, and Pacific peoples (Greyson, 2000). For example, for early Hawaiians,

> their observations of *apparent* death, or persons who had "left the body prematurely," were interpreted in accordance with beliefs about the ancestor-gods. On each island, there was a special promontory overlooking the sea; this was the *leina*, or leaping place, of the soul or spirit on its journey to the realm of the ancestors. If, on its way to the *leina*, a soul was met by an ancestor-god and sent back, the body would revive. Otherwise, the ancestor-god would lead it safely to and over the *leina*; once beyond that hurdle, the soul was safe with the ancestors. For various reasons ... an ancestor-god might delay a soul's acceptance into eternity. For instance, if a person died before his or her earthly work was done, the ancestor-god conducted the soul back to the body (DeSpelder & Strickland, 2005, pp. 519-520).

Bremmer (2002), Abanes (1996), and Fox (2003) trace in detail the history of near-death experiences from antiquity, through the middle ages, down to modern times. The interested reader is referred to these sources.

Albert Heim, a Swiss geologist and mountain climber, is credited with the first systematic data collection on near-death experience. In 1892, he published a report based on the "subjective experiences of mountain climbers who had fallen in the Alps (as he himself had done), soldiers wounded in the war, workers who had fallen from scaffolds, and individuals who had nearly died in accidents or near-death drownings" (Greyson, 2000, p. 316). Heim reported that his subjects experienced a detachment from their bodies and panoramic memory or life review. Heim's data was later reviewed by Oscar Pfister (1930, 1981), a psychoanalyst, who proposed that these experiences were caused by shock and depersonalization before imminent danger.

The modern concept of NDE was well in place by the 1950s. Numerous prominent people have reported NDEs, including writer Ernest Hemingway, explorer Richard Byrd, and psychologist Carl Jung (Audette, 1982; Morse, 1996). For example, Jung provided an elaborate account of his NDE following a heart attack in 1944, which involved out-of-body travel, removal of earthly obstacles, entry into a rock temple, reluctant return, and other visions. Jung commented, "We shy away from the word 'eternal,' but I can describe the experiences only as that ecstasy of a non-temporal state in which present, past and future are one. . . . Face to face with such wholeness one remains speechless, for it can scarcely be comprehended" (Basford, 1990, p. 17).

Recent interest in NDEs can be clearly traced back to the publication of *Life After Life* by Raymond Moody (1975), a philosophy professor turned psychiatrist. This book caused a stir immediately. Eventually it was translated into more than thirty languages; it led to the foundation of societies for near-death studies in many Western countries; and prompted the birth of two journals devoted to the subject, *Omega* and the *Journal of Near-Death Studies* (formerly named *Anabiosis*); and it inspired numerous books (Bremmer, 2002). Television networks and Hollywood also have played a role in making the term "near-death experiences," coined by Moody, a concept familiar to the general public.

PERCEIVED CHARACTERISTICS OF THE NEAR-DEATH EXPERIENCE

On the basis of 150 anecdotes, collected over an 11-year period, Moody (1975) constructed the following model of a NDE:

> A man is dying and, as he reaches the point of greatest physical distress, he hears himself pronounced dead by his doctor. He begins to hear an uncomfortable noise, a loud ringing or buzzing, and at the same time feels himself moving very rapidly through a long dark tunnel. After this, he suddenly finds himself outside of his own physical body, but still in the immediate physical environment, and he sees his own body from a distance, as though he is a spectator. He watches the resuscitation attempt from this unusual vantage point and is in a state of emotional upheaval.
>
> Others come to meet and to help him. He glimpses the spirits of relatives and friends who have already died, and a loving warm spirit of a kind he has never encountered before—a being of light—appears before him. This being asks him a question, nonverbally, to make him evaluate his life and helps him along by showing him a panoramic, instantaneous playback of the major events of his life. At some point he finds himself approaching some sort of barrier or border, apparently representing the limit between earthly life and the next life. Yet, he finds that he must go back to the earth, that the time for his death has not yet come. At this point he resists . . . and does not want to

return. He is overwhelmed by intense feelings of joy, love, and peace. Despite his attitude, though, he somehow reunites with his physical body and lives.

Later he tries to tell others, but he has trouble doing so. . . . He also finds that others scoff, so he stops telling other people. Still, the experience affects his life profoundly, especially his views about death and its relationship to life (pp. 21-23).

In this model, Moody (1975) identified 15 recurring elements, to which he added four more in his second book (Moody, 1977). These are presented in Table 1. Greyson (2000) has summarized the attempts of a number of investigators to classify the common features of near-death experiences. Noyes and Slymen (1978-1979) classify them into mystical, depersonalization, and hyperalertness elements; and Greyson (1985) groups them into cognitive, affective, paranormal, and transcendental features.

As Greyson (2000) points out, some researchers maintain that the NDE unfolds in a predictable temporal pattern (Noyes, 1972; Ring, 1984), and others believe that there are discrete phenomenological types of experiences (Greyson, 1985; Greyson & Bush, 1992; Sabom, 1982). Since Kenneth Ring is the first major

Table 1. Common Elements Recurring in Adult Near-Death Experiences (Moody, 1975, 1977)

Elements occurring during near-death experiences:
Ineffability
Hearing oneself pronounced dead
Feelings of peace and quiet
Hearing unusual noises
Seeing a dark tunnel
Being "out of the body"
Meeting "spiritual beings"
Experiencing a bright light as a "being of light"
Panoramic life review
Experiencing a realm in which all knowledge exists
Experiencing cities of light
Experiencing a realm of bewildered spirits
Experiencing a "supernatural rescue"
Sensing a border or limit
Coming back "into the body"

Elements occurring as after effects:
Frustration relating the experience to others
Subtle "broadening and deepening" of life
Elimination of fear of death
Corroboration of events witnessed while "out of body"

Based on Greyson (2000).

investigator to systematically examine this phenomenon and thus provided impetus for scientific inquiry, a closer look at his description of the NDE is warranted. Unlike Moody, Ring advanced research in this area by employing structured interview and measurement scales that he had developed.

In his first book, based on his study of 102 individuals who had come close to death, Ring (1982) refines Moody's composite into a fivefold coherent pattern which he terms the basic thanatomimetic narrative—the experience of near-death in its developmental form. This "core experience," which Ring identified, consists of five stages. However, "this series of stages is better described as a trend rather than as an invariant sequence" (Roe, 2001, p. 145). It should be noted that Ring's later work (Ring, 1984, 1992; Ring & Valarino, 1998) and that of others (e.g., Morse & Perry, 1992; Sabom, 1998) largely support his earlier conclusions. Furthermore, Hampe's study (1979),[1] the only significant work clearly uninfluenced by Moody's *Life After Life*, also essentially supports Ring's conclusions.

According to Ring (1982), the first stage, wherein one receives the first intimations of dying, is heralded by feelings of peace and well-being. He (1982) quotes a woman who had attempted suicide by leaping off a cliff overlooking the sea: "This incredible feeling of peace came over me. . . . All of a sudden there was no pain, just peace" (p. 41).

The second stage of the core experience involves a sense of detachment from one's physical body, now commonly known as out-of-body experiences (OBEs).[2] A man injured in an auto accident remembers this:

> At that time I viewed myself from the corner of my hospital room, looking down at my body which was very dark and gray. All the life looked like it was out of it. And my mother was sitting in a chair next to my bed looking very determined and strong in her faith. And my Italian girl friend at the time was crying at the foot of my bed (Ring, 1982, p. 47).

One remarkable feature of the separation stage is the quality of the mind during this sequence: Ring's subjects report an observer-like detachment congruent with the feeling that the experience was perfectly normal. It is interesting to note here that, contrary to reports found in occult literature, few subjects mentioned a second body, and the two who did denied seeing any cord linking the two bodies.

The third stage, a transitional one between this world and beyond, consists of entering the darkness. It was Moody (1975) who first implied that many individuals experience traveling through a dark tunnel. The majority of Ring's

---

[1] At about the same time that Moody's first book was published (Moody, 1977), Hampe (1979), a German Lutheran minister, was conducting his own investigation on this phenomenon. His findings appeared in English in 1979 in his book *To Die is Gain*.

[2] During the last decades, a good deal has been written on OBEs, with or without NDEs. A review of this topic is beyond the scope of the chapter. The reader is referred to other sources (e.g., Alvarado, 2000; Barušs, 2003).

subjects did not describe a tunnel but characterized the space as devoid of specific dimensions but, nevertheless, peaceful.

The next stage of the core experience is characterized by a brilliant golden light. This light is described as restful, never blinding, ineffably beautiful, all embracing, and comforting. It is perceived as the beginning of a new life, the experience of the presence of a Supreme Being or of incredible love.

The fifth and final stage appears to be an extension of the previous one. The difference between the stages is the difference between seeing the sugar cube and tasting the sugar, between seeing the light and entering into the world wherein the light appears to have its origin. According to most descriptions, it is a world of preternatural beauty. The colors are said to be unforgettable. One of Ring's near-death experiencers (NDErs) described it thus:

> I happened to go down this path and it was beautiful. Beautiful flowers and the birds were singing, and I was walking down. . . . I did reprimand my surgeon and my cardiologist. I said, "Why, in heaven's name, did you bring me back? It was so beautiful" (Ring, 1982, p. 61).

Another gave the following description:

> I took a trip to heaven. I saw the most beautiful lakes. Angels—they were floating around like you see seagulls. Everything was white. The most beautiful flowers. Nobody on this earth ever saw the beautiful flowers that I saw there. . . . I don't believe there is a color on this earth that wasn't included in that color situation that I saw. Everything, everything. Of course, I was so impressed with the beauty of everything there that I couldn't pinpoint any one thing. . . . Everything was bright. The lakes were blue, light blue. Everything about the angels was pure white (Ring, 1982, p. 61).

According to Ring, the majority of near-death experiencers reach a point where they are faced with a crucial decision: should they return to life or continue into the beyond? Several phenomenological features appear to be associated with this point: the life review, an encounter with a "presence," an encounter with deceased loved ones, and the making of the decision itself.

The life review seems to take place in the form of images. Either one's entire life or selected aspects are experienced in a matrix of vivid images like a hologram. These images occur either as flashbacks or flash-forwards.

Next, the individual becomes aware of a "presence." This presence is never actually seen but always "sensed, inferred or intuited" (Ring, 1982, p. 67). Ring's experiencers often felt as if there were mutual communication between the presence and themselves.

> Although there is some variation here, the presence usually states or implies that the individual is at a choice-point in his life and that it is up to him to elect whether to return to it (that is, physical life). At this point the individual seems led either to reflect on his life or to reexperience it in the form of the panoramic life review just described, as he attempts to make up his

mind. In some cases, the individual seems to be given information about his future physical existence, should he decide to live (Ring, 1982, p. 67).

Occasionally, the NDErs became aware of the spirits of deceased loved ones, and they both saw and recognized the spirits. Typically, the spirits were warm and friendly toward the NDErs but urged them to go back because it was not yet their time. As a result, a decision was made either by or for the NDErs to return to life.

The subjects of Ring's interviews stated that their decision to return had hinged on the pull of loved ones and on a sense that their life's mission was not yet fulfilled. The nuances of the decision making are described by Ring by means of several illustrative interviews. The following is the testimony of a woman who felt that she was sent back by God:

> I could feel myself just slipping away. I could feel myself in a chamber. I could hear them say I was in shock. I could hear the nurse say, "I can't get a pulse. No respiration. She's gone."... It was all echoey. Meanwhile... I felt very detached and very at ease. I was completely panic stricken before when I was going in, I was terrified, but when I was in there, it was the most peaceful, happy time. I never saw God. No one ever came walking up to me. But I did hear somebody say, "You're needed, Patricia, I'm sending you back now" (Ring, 1982, p. 80).

Ring's subjects overwhelmingly affirmed that their NDE was very real and rejected the suggestion that it was either a dream or a hallucination. They described their cognitive processes as rational and their sensory awareness as lucid and sharp. For most of Ring's respondents, their sense of body, space, and time disappeared. Another common feeling expressed by them is a heightened appreciation of life, of nature, and of other humans. One subject told Ring, " I appreciate things more. And I should tell people I love them more than I do. Life is precious. And it is a gift of God. Everyday I've got is a gift" (Ring, 1982, p. 142). Those who survive a brush with death often report a sense of rebirth. Along with this comes a sense of mission. They believe they have been spared for a reason.

CORRELATES OF NEAR-DEATH EXPERIENCES

Recent estimates indicate that about a third of all individuals who come close to death have NDEs (Fenwick & Fenwick, 1995; Roe, 2001). Several studies have determined a number of correlates of these experiences (Greyson & Stevenson, 1980; Irwin, 1999; Ring, 1982; Sabom, 1982).

Demographic Factors

In general, the occurrence of NDEs is not related to variables such as socio-economic level, race, age, marital status, occupation, and religious affiliation (Irwin, 1999). Even skeptics have been noted to have NDEs (Lansberry, 1994).

However, the content of these experiences may correlate with some factors, such as occupation; for example, professional people experienced fewer encounters with discarnate beings (Sabom, 1982).

Sex Differences

Gender appears to be a factor associated with the incidence of NDEs. A number of studies indicate that these experiences are reported more frequently by women than by men (Greyson & Stevenson, 1980; Noyes & Kletti, 1977; Ring, 1982; Sabom & Kreutziger, 1977; Twemlow & Gabbard, 1984). Gender also seems to influence the characteristics of the experience. Females report encounters with discarnate beings more frequently than males do (Sabom, 1982). Also, an interaction between gender and the situation in which the experience happens has been noted (Ring, 1982; Twemlow & Gabbard, 1984):

> Women were relatively more likely to have their experience during illness whereas men tended to have their NDEs more often in an accident or a suicide attempt (Irwin, 1999, p. 209).

Social Conditioning

Several researchers have investigated the possible effects of social conditioning through cross-cultural studies of the societies of China, India, Australia, the South Pacific, and of Native Americans, among others (e.g., Alcock, 1978; Blackmore, 1993; Counts, 1983; Kellehear, 1996; Pastricha & Stevenson, 1986; Rodabough, 1985). While the majority of descriptions appear to follow the core experience, some significant exceptions have been noted. For example, Pastricha and Stevenson (1986) discovered that NDErs in India "did not have panoramic life review nor an out-of-body impression of their physical body, and that they were taken directly by 'messengers' to a transcendental realm where discarnate beings consulted some records, decided a mistake had been made and ordered their return to terrestrial life" (Irwin, 1999, p. 210). Out-of-body experiences also were absent in the experiences of Melanesians (Counts, 1983). A recent survey of the cross-cultural data by Kellehear (1993, 1996) reveals that panoramic life review and the tunnel effect are perhaps the most culture-specific aspects of the NDE. As Barušs (2003) points out,

> These cultural differences strengthen the argument that NDEs cannot simply be experiential byproducts of the physiological changes taking place in a dying brain. Because people in some cultures have never reported seeing a tunnel, although they may have experienced a period of darkness, it would appear that tunnel imagery during NDEs may not be the result of physiological events but of psychological development in a modern technological culture. Similarly, life reviews have occurred in societies admonishing personal responsibility through Hindu, Buddhist, or Christian religions but

not in traditional native societies, suggesting a role for cultural factors in NDEs (p. 223).

Greyson (2000, p. 321) points out that "cultural influences have led some scholars to interpret NDEs as nothing more than emotional reactions to the threat of imminent death (Ehrenwald, 1974; Lukianowicz, 1958; Noyes, Hoenk, Kuperman, & Slymen, 1977; Noyes & Kletti, 1976), but they may reflect not so much the experience itself as the experient's ability to process and express an event that is largely ineffable."

Circumstances of NDE Occurrence

Twemlow and Gabbard (1984) report a more frequent awareness of golden light when the subjects were under anesthesia and more encounters with discarnate beings when the experient's heart had stopped beating; however, this study has been criticized for methodological flaws, and further research is warranted (Irwin, 1999).

Psychological Profile

Individuals who have had NDEs appear to be psychologically healthy and indistinguishable from others of their age, gender, race, or religion, (Gabbard & Twemlow, 1984; Greyson, 1991; Irwin, 1985; Fox, 2003; Ring, 1982; Ring & Valarino, 1998; Sabom, 1982). They are comparable to others who have not had NDEs in intelligence, neuroticism, extraversion, and anxiety (Greyson, 2000; Locke & Shontz, 1983). Also, NDEs can be easily distinguished from the hallucinations due to schizophrenia or organic brain dysfunction (Bates & Stanley, 1985; Blackmore, 1986).

Although some have speculatively linked NDEs and *dissociating tendencies*, Irwin (1993) failed to find any significant difference in dissociative coping style between NDErs and non-NDErs. However, he did discover that childhood traumas were more prevalent in the lives of NDErs than nonexperients. Irwin suggested that NDErs may tend to dissociate in the face of very stressful unexpected events, but do not adopt a general dissociative style to deal with common stressors (Greyson, 2000). This tendency, according to Ring (1992), enables the child to "tune out" (dissociation) threatening features of the environment and "tune into" (absorption) alternate realities where he or she can feel safe, realities that others may not perceive. This combination of dissociation and absorption is what goes into the making of what Ring calls the *encounter-prone* personality. Thus, for some, the NDE becomes "a kind of compensatory gift in return for the wounds they have incurred in growing up" (Ring, 1992, p. 146). However, Ring (1992) also adds that childhood trauma is only one of the factors that fosters extraordinary encounters such as NDEs. Some individuals have an inborn predisposition for such experiences. In imaginative play, this tendency is nurtured in childhood (Greyson, 2000).

It is interesting to note that childhood abuse and trauma are generally considered to be predictive of *fantasy proneness,* which, according to Wilson and Barber (1981, 1983), is "characterized by strong investment in fantasy life, vivid hallucinatory ability, intense sensory experience and excellent eidetic memory" (Greyson, 2000, p. 324). Wilson and Barber (1981, 1983) suggested that the fantasy-prone individuals may be more disposed to have NDEs. Also, they speculated that this tendency may develop as a result of dealing with traumatic experiences in childhood or due to encouragement by significant adults in childhood.

NEAR-DEATH EXPERIENCES IN CHILDHOOD

The social conditioning theory of NDEs would predict that these experiences in children would have fewer elements of the core experience, because the young have had much less social conditioning than adults (Irwin, 1999). Aside from the many adults who claim to have had NDEs as children, it has been difficult to find children who recently had a NDE. Psychiatrists Gabbard and Twemlow were the first to report an NDE of a young child in their book, *With the Eyes of the Mind* (1984).

> Todd was two years, five months old when he bit into the electrical cord from a vacuum cleaner while playing with his siblings. His mother came upon this some two or three minutes after the accident occurred. He was lying motionless. . . . [S]he realized he was not breathing and called an ambulance." [The paramedics instituted CPR and rushed Todd to the emergency room.]
>
> Medical records from the hospital emergency room indicate that there was a period of approximately twenty-five minutes when the child had no heartbeat or respiration. These records also indicate that Todd's pupils were dilated and that he was completely unresponsive. [Todd remained unresponsive for several days, in fact, and it took four to six months before he gradually regained much of his cortical and neurological functioning again. Remarkably, there was no evidence of any permanent brain damage.]
>
> About three months before his third birthday, he was playing in the living room when his mother asked him, "Could you tell Mommy what you remember when you bit the cord of the vacuum cleaner?" Without even looking up, he told her, "I went in a room with a very nice man and sat with him." His mother asked him what the room looked like. Todd replied, "It had a big bright light in the ceiling," which his mother took to mean some kind of chandelier. Todd's mother then asked him what the man said to him. Todd responded, "He asked me if I wanted to stay there or come back

to you." Looking up at his mother he said, " I wanted to be with you and come home." Then he smiled, and went back to his toys (in Ring & Valarino, 1998, p. 105).

It should be noted that the above incident occurred in 1972, before Moody's *Life after Life* (1975) was published and Todd's mother had not heard of NDEs.

In the 1980s, a number of significant studies began to appear that investigated the incidence of NDEs in children (Bush, 1983; Morse, 1994; Morse, Castillo, Venecia, Milstein, & Tyler, 1986; Morse & Perry, 1990, 1992; Serdahely, 1989, 1990; Sutherland, 1995). Foremost among these is the work of pediatrician Melvin Morse and his colleagues. Morse's involvement in this field was "purely adventitious, not deliberate, and occurred because of a conversation he had with a patient of his named Kristle" (Ring & Valarino, 1998, p. 100). Morse met her in the emergency room, and at this point she had been without a heartbeat for almost 19 minutes. Morse was successful in resuscitating her. "An emergency CAT scan showed massive swelling of her brain; she had no gag reflex; and only an artificial lung machine could keep her breathing. Kristle had a 10 percent chance of survival" (Abanes, 1996, p. 57).

Later, Morse was startled by the information Kristle revealed. Even though she had been profoundly comatose, she accurately described what had gone on in the emergency room. In addition, she talked about a tunnel opening, about bright light and flowers, about meeting her dead grandparents, her maternal aunt, Jesus and the Heavenly Father, and about meeting Heather and Melissa, two souls waiting to be born, and Elizabeth, a guardian angel to her.

Kristle told the whole story in a matter-of-fact way. Morse was amazed, and he and his colleagues began to research NDEs in children. NDEs of children, argued Morse, "might be expected to be particularly interesting, given that they would not have had time to acquire the cultural baggage of adults and therefore might be expected to narrate correspondingly pure experiences of the NDE's core, perhaps permitting researchers to glimpse the NDE in its 'essence'" (Fox, 2003, p. 50).

Morse's book, *Closer to the Light: Learning from Children's Near-Death Experience* (Morse & Perry, 1990) was enthusiastically received and became *The New York Times'* bestseller. Morse and his colleagues concluded that the experiences of the children in their study paralleled those of adults and had similar transformative effects, and that their experiences could not be understood by reliance on conventional neuroscientific knowledge (Fox, 2003). In a review article, Greyson (2000) concludes that "children's NDEs are similar to those of adults, except that they tend not to include a life review or meetings with deceased friends and relatives, two differences that could be expected because of children's brief experience with life" (p. 317). Sutherland's study of NDEs in Australian children, discussed in the book *Children of the Light*, also supports these conclusions.

NEAR-DEATH EXPERIENCES IN THE BLIND

Maria's story is one of the most widely mentioned cases in the NDE literature. In 1984, following a heart attack and subsequent cardiac arrest, she was rushed to a hospital in Seattle. Maria claimed not only to have simply witnessed the resuscitation attempts upon her "but also to have floated during this time *outside* the hospital altogether. Taking full advantage of the sudden freedom which her temporary out-of-body condition afforded her, she continued to float up" and spotted a single tennis shoe sitting on a ledge (Fox, 2003, p. 205). After having been resuscitated, Maria told her story to her critical care social worker, Kimberly Clark, and asked her to check if the shoe was actually there. Clark acted according to the request and later recalled,

> With mixed emotions I went outside and looked up at the ledges but could not see much at all. I went up to the third floor and began going in and out of patients rooms and looking out their window, which were so narrow that I had to press my face to the screen just to see the ledge at all. Finally I found a room where I pressed my face to the glass and saw the tennis shoe! My vantage-point was very different from what Maria's had been for her to notice that the little toe had worn a place in the shoe, and that the lace was stuck under the heel and other details about the side of the shoe not visible to me. The only way she would have had such a perspective was if she had been floating right outside and at very close range to the tennis shoe. I retrieved the shoe and brought it back to Maria; it was very concrete evidence for me (Wilson, 1997, p. 98).

Maria was not blind. If she really saw what we are told, she could not have "seen" with her "eyes of flesh." There was probably some other "mechanism" involved. Hence it would not be farfetched to expect that, during NDEs, the blind also may be able to "see." In a retrospective study of 31 blind individuals, of whom 14 had been blind since birth, Ring and his collaborators discovered that the NDEs of 21 of them were practically indistinguishable from the NDEs of sighted individuals (Ring & Cooper, 1997; Ring & Valarino, 1998). Overall, 80% of the participants claimed to have had visual impressions during their experience. They described "both perceptions of this world as well as other worldly scenes, often in fulsome, fine-grained details, and sometimes with a sense of extremely sharp, even subjectively perfect acuity" (Ring & Cooper, 1997, p. 122). In a few of these cases, Ring and Cooper (1997) were able to collect some corroboration of the veridicality of the out-of-body observations, and they found that the claims of the blind NDErs were "in fact noted in a direct and accurate . . . perception of the situation" (Ring & Valarino, 1998, p. 85). However, skeptical critics may find this evidence insufficient to draw firm conclusions.

It is an established fact that individuals blind from birth or others who lost their sight within the first five years of their life do not experience visual images in their dreams (Kerr, 2000). But in other respects their dreams are very similar to those of sighted persons. Ring and Cooper (1997, 1999) noticed that some of the congenitally blind NDErs mentioned that their NDEs were very different from their dreams because they contained visual imagery. Since the brains of these individuals have not had a chance to develop sufficiently for visual processing, their visual impressions appear especially striking, even apart from the question of "accuracy" of their observations (Barušs, 2003).

Ring and Cooper (see Ring & Valarino, 1998, p. 9) ask the obvious questions concerning the visual perceptions of the blind NDErs: "If the blind do indeed *see* during these NDEs, how is it possible for them, under these extreme conditions, apparently to transcend sensory restrictions that have hitherto imprisoned them in a sightless world? . . . Or, alternatively, is there another form of awareness that comes into play when, *whether one is blind or not*, an individual is thrust into a state of consciousness in which one's sensory system is no longer functional?"

Ring and Cooper (1997) considered numerous alternative answers based on conventional psychology and even esoteric metaphysical systems, and concluded that none of them could provide a satisfactory explanation for their findings.

In the end, Ring and Cooper (1997) concluded that the visual aspects of the NDEs of blind subjects "may not have much to do with seeing as sighted individuals ordinarily do with the eyes, but may be some form of direct knowing that" they have called *transcendental awareness* or *mindsight*, a kind of eyeless vision or "understanding" or "taking in" rather than the usual visual perception (Barušs, 2003, p. 221). This mindsight is not restricted to the blind, but is available to others who experience an NDE or an out-of-body experience (OBE) or perhaps in some other nonordinary states of consciousness.

Ring and Valarino (1998) wonder why it is that when casually read, the NDE reports of the blind generally seem to imply that the blind do see in a way that is similar to physical sight. They conclude, "Our ordinary language is rooted in the experiences of sighted persons and is therefore biased in favor of visual imagery. . . . Because the blind are members of the same linguistic community as sighted people, we can certainly expect that they will tend . . . to phrase their experiences in a *language of vision*, almost regardless of its appropriateness to the qualities of their own personal experience" (p. 93).

DISTRESSING NEAR-DEATH EXPERIENCES

A vast majority of the NDEs that have been reported over the years and across cultures appear to include "profound feelings of peace, bliss, joy, and a sense of cosmic unity" (Greyson & Bush, 1992, p. 95). However, a substantial number of individuals have reported extremely distressing experiences. Estimates range from less than 1% (Ring & Valarino, 1998) to 12% (Grey, 1985). Greyson and Bush (1992) have analyzed a sample of 50 distressing NDEs, and Atwater (1992) came across 105 individuals between 1978 and 1992 who recalled negative NDEs.

Grey (1985) and Rawlings (1979, 1993) have brought a number of "hellish" experiences to light. Here are two examples:

> I found myself in a place surrounded by mist. I felt I was in hell. There was a big pit with vapors coming out and there were arms and hands coming out trying to grab mine. . . . I was terrified that these hands were going to claw hold of me and pull me down into the pit with them (Grey, 1985, p. 63).

> As I got drowsy, I remember going down this black hole round and round. Then I saw a glowing red-hot spot getting bigger and bigger until I was able to stand. It was all red and hot and on fire. The earth was like slimy mud that sank over my feet, and it was hard to move. The heat was awful and made it hard to breathe. I cried "Oh Lord give me another chance" (Rawlings, 1979, p. 96).

Even though there is some variation in the estimates of the percentage of distressing NDEs, most researchers maintain that such occurrences are rare. Also, it seems that in many cases "[t]he experiences themselves are similar to positive ones, but the patients misunderstand the experience. They may see it as psychiatric pathology or interpret various elements of the experience (especially the dark void) to mean that they are in hell or having a negative experience" (Morse, 1996, p. 313).

On the basis of a thorough analysis of 50 cases of negative NDEs, Greyson and Bush (1992) classified these experiences into three categories: "(a) experiences phenomenologically like the blissful type but interpreted as terrifying, (b) experiences of nonexistence or eternal void, and (c) experiences with blatant hellish imagery" as illustrated in the foregoing examples (Greyson, 2000, p. 319). What factors contribute to the occurrences of such experiences? How can these be explained? Do they have any clinical usefulness? What kind of aftereffects do they have? Due to the relative rarity of these experiences, it is difficult to conduct research in this area. Consequently, these questions still await answers.

CONSEQUENCES OF NEAR-DEATH-EXPERIENCES

Ring (1993) suggests that, aside from sexual orgasm, there has been no experience of such brief duration—many NDEs appear to last less than a minute—that has elicited so much reflection and commentary. Perhaps one major reason behind this interest is the belief that NDEs offer proof that there is life after death. Two major sets of theories have been advanced to explain NDEs. One group of investigators see in NDEs a strong proof of survival after death, and this stance resonates deeply with the general public. Another group of investigators are loathe to even entertain this possibility and are bent upon demonstrating that NDEs are nothing but "a response to the threat of death . . . the ego's defensive reaction to a life-threatening situation. . . . Perhaps both of the explanations are valid: There is life after death and there is also a psychological phenomenon involving various defense mechanisms whereby the *personality is radically altered* as the transition from one state to the next is negotiated" (DeSpelder & Strickland, 2005, p. 522).

This radical personality alteration as a result of a NDE is intriguing and in itself would render the NDE worthy of investigation (Greyson, 1996; Irwin, 1999). The literature on the consequences of NDEs reveals an overwhelmingly positive impact, but a number of negative aftereffects also have been noted. Many of the individuals experiencing the latter require expert help to deal with the experience.

Negative Consequences of NDEs

Most of the systematic work in this area has been conducted by Greyson and his associates (Bush, 1991; Flynn, 1986; Greyson, 1997; Greyson & Bush, 1992; Greyson & Harris, 1987; Insinger, 1991). They describe a number of disturbing aftereffects (also see Abanes, 1996):

1. Some NDErs are ostracized by family and friends, who fear that the NDErs have come under the sway of evil forces.
2. Some NDErs have reentry problems and react to the return with anger or depression.
3. Some find it difficult to reconcile the NDE with prior religious convictions or values.
4. Some identify excessively with the experience and think of themselves primarily as an NDEr.
5. Some fear that the NDE is indicative of mental instability.
6. Some encounter interpersonal problems because they feel separated from those who have not had an NDE.
7. Some fear that they may be the object of ridicule.
8. Some struggle to integrate changes in their attitude with the expectations of others.
9. They may have difficulty fulfilling a role that has lost meaning for them after the NDE.
10. Those who have an NDE in childhood or following a suicide attempt have unique difficulties.
11. The feeling of having been used for a higher purpose may lead to problems.
12. Guilt or ambivalence with regard to having returned or wished not to return is a further source of problems.
13. Some find that the timeless quality of the NDE has diminished their ability to deal with the present.
14. Some become obsessed with the past due to the life review part of the NDE. Or they focus on the future due to the visions in the NDE.
15. Some may need counseling to deal with the disintegration of careers and relationships.

As Greyson (2000) points out, most individuals experiencing negative aftereffects slowly manage to adjust without any assistance. However, this adjustment often necessitates altering attitudes, interests, and values; and close relations may find it hard to comprehend these changes. They may avoid the NDEr thinking that he/she has been subjected to some "unwelcomed influence." Or, they "may place the experient on a pedestal and expect unrealistic changes," such as "super human patience and forgiveness" or "miraculous healing and prophetic powers and may become bitter and reject the experient who does not live up to these unrealistic expectations" (Greyson, 2000, p. 328).

As Greyson (2000) warns, although the undesirable consequences of NDEs occur in only a relatively small number of cases, their effect can be disabling. Furthermore, competent help is not easily available, and little has been written on this issue. To compound the problem, the popular media focus on the positive effects of NDEs may stop those facing problems from seeking help.

Greyson (2000) further explains that the "way a psychotherapist responds to a near-death experient can have a tremendous influence on whether the NDE is accepted and becomes a stimulus for psychospiritual growth or whether it is regarded as a bizarre experience that must not be shared for fear of being labeled as mentally ill" (p. 328). A group of 32 clinicians with extensive experience in this field have developed strategies to be employed in therapy with individuals struggling with the negative aftereffects of NDEs. Some major guidelines presented by that group follow. These have been extracted from Greyson (2000, pp. 330-331).

1. It is usually valuable to let these individuals verbalize their confusions and distress. They usually become more frustrated if told not to talk about their experience.
2. Reflections and clarifications of patients' perceptions and emotions are usually more helpful than interpretations.
3. Objective information about the frequency and common effects of NDEs often alleviates concern about their implications and consequences.
4. Regarding the near-death experient as a victim is often counter therapeutic.
5. The induction of controlled alterations in experience through hypnosis or guided imagery and non-verbal media such as art may help patients express conflicts that they deem to be ineffable.
6. Regrets, ambivalences, and frustrations over the "return" should be explored.
7. Changes in values, beliefs, and attitudes may require changes in old careers. Couple or family therapy may be indicated when changes in the experient demand changes in close relationships.
8. Near-death experients rarely want to eliminate intrusive reminders of their experience. More commonly, they request help integrating the experience and its lessons into their daily lives.

9. Exploring problems and solutions with fellow experients can reduce the sense of bizarreness associated with the phenomenon.
10. There is no evidence that psychotropic medications can help with problems following an NDE. Medicating individuals in the midst of spontaneous spiritual awakening may freeze the process in mid-course and prevent any further reparative development.
11. Taking up a contemplative discipline such as meditation or prayer may help the individual in spiritual crisis.

Positive Aftereffects of Near-Death Experiences

Ring's *Heading Toward Omega* (1984) was the first major investigation of the aftereffects of NDEs. However, interest in this topic has steadily increased, and most of the subsequent publications support Ring's observations (e.g., Atwater, 1988, 1994; Brinkley, 1994, 1995; Flynn, 1986; Grey, 1985; Greyson, 1992; Morse & Perry, 1992; Musgrave, 1997; Ring, 1992; Ring & Valarino, 1998; Sutherland, 1992). The majority of investigators assert that the consequences of near-death experiences are overwhelmingly positive in nature. Ring regards NDEs as basically revelatory experiences that convey an intuitive sense of the "transcendent aspect of creation." An NDE is the universe's signal to the individual to wake up. It is a seed experience: the seed may or may not take root. In other words, a core experience is not necessarily transformatory because "much depends on how the experience is interpreted and integrated" (Ring, 1982, p. 256).

Ring (Ring & Valarino, 1998) also documents that learning about NDEs and their transformative consequences possibly can inspire similar changes in others: they can catch the "benign virus" from the NDErs. This claim has received some support from others (Horacek, 1997; Lundahl, 1993; Morris & Knafl, 2003). On the other hand, others have pointed out that perhaps there is nothing special about NDEs: similar changes have occurred in people who encountered death, in reality or in imagination, with or without hypnosis (Blackmore, 1993; Kinnier, Tribensee, Rose, & Vaughan, 2001; Schwenk, 1999; Van Quekeberghe, Goebel, & Hertweck, 1995). While it is generally true that encounters with death tend to bring people to the threshold of life and can result in positive aftereffects (Sheikh & Sheikh, 2003; Yalom, 1980), it seems doubtful that the changes, in general, are of the same breadth and depth (Groth-Marnat & Summers, 1998; Ring & Valarino, 1998).

The Call to Awaken

The NDE may be construed as a brief glimpse of a higher reality. In this sense, it is a call to awaken to higher consciousness. Ring, much like the philosopher Teilhard de Chardin, believes that a new consciousness, the so-called planetary consciousness, is making itself manifest on earth. In this view, the NDE is an evolutionary device, a sort of trigger, that would serve the purpose of awakening the individual to a higher potentiality. Ring (1984) argues that the NDE has at its core a spiritual radiance so overwhelming that it leaves the individual with little alternative but to be thrust forever into a new mode of being.

> The NDE is essentially a spiritual experience that serves as a catalyst for spiritual awakening and development. Moreover, the spiritual development that unfolds following an NDE tends to take a particular form. Finally, as a by-product of this spiritual development, NDErs tend to manifest a variety of psychic abilities afterward that are an inherent part of their transformation (p. 51).

In order to fully understand this spiritual core of the NDE and its sweeping aftereffects, it would be worthwhile to examine an illustrative case. The following is the account of a 40-year-old man who nearly drowned when the car he was driving was caught in a flash flood. He writes:

> I knew I was either dead or going to die. But then something happened. It was so immense, so powerful that I gave up on my life to see what it was. I wanted to venture into this experience, which started as a drifting into what I could only describe as a long tunnel of light. But it wasn't just a light, it was a protective passage of energy with an intense brightness at the end which I wanted to look into, to touch. There were no sounds of any earthly thing. A soothing symphony of indescribable beauty blended with the light I was approaching.
>
> I gave up on life. I left it behind for this new wonderful thing. I did not want to go back to life. For what I knew was that what lay ahead was to be so wondrous and beautiful that nothing should stop me from reaching it.
>
> As I reached the source of the light I could see in. I cannot begin to describe in human terms the feeling I had at what I saw. It was a giant infinite world of calm, and love, and energy and beauty. It was as though human life was unimportant compared to this. And yet it urged the importance of life at the same time it solicited death as a means to a better, different life. It was all being, all beauty, all meaning for existence. It was all the energy of the universe forever in one immeasurable place (Ring, 1984, pp. 54-55).

The preceding account, by no means unrepresentative, illustrates the spiritual energy at the core of the NDE. The light and the brilliance, the love and the acceptance, the peace and the calm, the paradisiacal music, all illustrate the spirituality inherent in the NDE.

Many other accounts illustrate the kind of knowledge that is given to those who have the core experience. The NDErs refer to knowledge of both universal principles (such as the belief that consciousness and life are inextricably linked) and personal knowledge (flashbacks and flash-forwards). Most NDErs come away with the feeling that they have been vouchsafed a glimpse of the Godhead. They believe they have "directly penetrated into the experiential source of humanity's universal belief in a higher religious dimension" (Ring, 1984, p. 84).

Another aspect of the NDE is the "presence" encountered during the core experience. The identity of this presence remains inexact: some NDErs describe a hierarchy of luminous beings and others encounter only one. Whether the being is one or many, the luminosity has an important consequence. Most of Ring's subjects experienced a union with the light, a transfer of energy from the light source into themselves, a blending with the luminosity that enabled them to return to this world with some of that luminous energy. This luminous energy appears to be the source of the evolutionary transformation that seems to follow the core experience. If the NDE is indeed a call to awaken, the luminosity is the catalyst for the awakening. Morse and Perry (1992) emphatically assert that "those who have the experience of light are the ones who have the greatest transformation. And the deeper the experience of light, the greater the transformation. It does not matter who has the experience—Marines, punk rockers, real-estate agents, corporate executives, housewives, ministers, or holy men—they are all transformed by their exposure to light" (Morse & Perry, 1992, p. 68).

The Revolution of the Self

The core experience holds such rapture that many NDErs return reluctantly. It is a return from timelessness, spacelessness, and freedom to the mundane world. The anguish of such a return is first revealed in personal relationships. Primary relationships, such as marriage, are buffeted and often end in divorce. The following account provides some clues:

> "It was at least, at least six months after the incident," reports one NDEr, "that I, that I could even speak to my wife about it. It was such an emotional, beautiful, swelling feeling inside that every time I tried to express it, I think I would just explode, you know; I would break down and cry. And she, for the longest time couldn't figure out what was wrong with me" (Ring, 1984, p. 96).

The turbulence experienced in interpersonal relationships is but a hint of the revolution in the self that is yet to come. Many NDErs report radical changes in their personality, attitudes, beliefs, values, and preferences, such as enhancement of self-esteem, a more tolerant and altruistic outlook, greater compassion, a loving interpersonal orientation, a greater appreciation of life, and a reverence that extends to all life including sensitivity to the health of the planet (Morse & Perry, 1992; Ring, 1984; Ring & Valarino, 1998). One correspondent reported, "I have a fierce desire to live every wonderful moment of as many days as I can manage to be gifted with. My life unquestionably is richer than before for having had the near-death experience" (Ring, 1984, p. 123). These "zestaholics" are solidly in the here and now, "savoring life as it happens, making as much of it as they can" (Morse & Perry, 1992, p. 76). Status and social comparison games, and accumulating the trappings of worldly success are unimportant to them. One NDEr stated, "Before I was living for material things.... Before I was conscious of only me, what I had, what I wanted.... I have gradually sloughed off the desire to have and to hold earthly possessions, material possessions to any great degree" (Ring, 1984, p. 132).

Other common aftereffects of NDEs include heightened spirituality, decreased fear of death, less competitiveness (Flynn, 1986; Grey, 1985; Morse & Perry, 1992; Sabom, 1982), a strengthened belief in the afterlife (Noyes, 1980), an increased interest in understanding the purpose and meaning of life, a tremendous thirst for knowledge, and expanded mental awareness (Bauer, 1985; Morse & Perry, 1992; Ring & Valarino, 1998). Morse and Perry (1992; Morse, 1996) report that NDErs exercise more frequently, consume more fresh fruits and vegetables, ingest fewer medications, and spend more time in quiet contemplation compared to the general population. Also they report more time spent alone and with family members. Consequently, it is not surprising that NDErs have fewer symptoms of depression and anxiety, fewer psychosomatic complaints (Morse & Perry, 1992), stronger objections to suicide, and significantly increased scores on tests of general mental health and spiritual well-being (Greyson, 1992-1993) compared to control samples. Morse and Perry (1992) also report that many of the NDErs believed that they had become more intelligent as a result of their experience. The authors suspect that it actually is true in many cases. They also appear convinced that "the NDE itself subtly changes the electromagnetic forces that surround our bodies and each and every cell in it. This change is so profound that it affects such things as personality, anxiety response, ability to have psychic experiences, and even the ability in some to wear watches" because they simply stop working (p.133). Spontaneous healing of illnesses as a result of NDE also has been reported (Krishnan, 1995; Morse & Perry, 1992).

The Search for Higher Consciousness

The NDE is, above all, a spiritual experience. It is not surprising that Ring's respondents seem to develop in a decidedly spiritual or religious direction. They turn to the church, take up healing or counseling, or increase service to their families or communities. It is noteworthy that NDErs adopt a universalistic spiritual orientation rather than a strictly religious one: the formal trappings of religious life and worship lose importance; they are convinced that there is life after death and believe in the unity of all religions. NDErs are more open to Eastern religions and ideas of reincarnation; they also report feeling close to God. They view their spiritual growth as intrinsic to the shift to a higher mode of consciousness. They have been given a hint of a higher mode of being, and after the return, they strive to realign themselves with this higher plane of consciousness (Morse & Perry, 1992; Ring, 1984; Ring & Valarino, 1998).

NDE and Psychic Development

Ring (1984) reports that NDErs manifest psychic abilities that seem to be an epiphenomenon of their transformation. The development of psychic abilities as an almost inevitable by-product of spiritual practice is well-known among practitioners of Eastern religions. Both Hindus and Buddhists describe the occult powers gained in the course of spiritual practice, but they also warn about their dangers. NDEs and meditational practices used in Eastern religions manifest several similarities. Both thrust the individual into a higher state of consciousness, albeit briefly; both leave similar aftereffects on the personality. Finally, both appear to confer psychic abilities. However, there are also differences between the two: the breakthrough to higher consciousness achieved through meditation involves prolonged, voluntary, and arduous spiritual training under the supervision of a master. The NDE, on the other hand, is an involuntary and sudden push into spiritual illumination. However this spiritual illumination is achieved, the psychic abilities that attend the experience are the same. In other words, NDErs report the same psychic gifts that meditators in Eastern mystical traditions have long described. This is not surprising since the result of both the meditative path and the NDE is the same: a higher, unitive state of consciousness.

The psychic abilities that demonstrate accelerated development after an NDE include clairvoyant and telepathic experiences, precognitive dreams, precognitive flashes, déjà-vu experiences, and synchronistic occurrences. Most NDErs who report these psychic abilities also state that they are more intuitive than before, more in touch with a perennial source of wisdom or with a spiritual guide.

One remarkable NDE phenomenon is what Ring (1984) calls the personal flash-forward. Personal flash-forwards normally occur during the life-review stage of the core experience and typically are described as images or visions of the future. They seem to be the life design of the individual, revealing how his or her life will unfold should he or she choose to return to life. In support of the veracity of personal flash-forwards, Ring (1984) describes another precognitive phenomenon occasionally associated with the NDE: the planetary vision, which seems to be a collective, global flash-forward.

On the basis of interviews with several NDErs, Ring offers an elegant summary of the planetary vision (PV):

> There is, first of all, a sense of having total knowledge, but specifically one is aware of seeing the entirety of the earth's evolutions and history, from the beginning to the end of time. The future scenario, however, is usually of short duration, seldom extending much beyond the beginning of the twenty-first century. The individuals report that in this decade there will be an increasing incidence of earthquakes, volcanic activity, and generally massive geophysical changes. There will be resultant disturbances in weather patterns and food supplies. The world economic system will collapse, and the possibility of nuclear war or accident is very great (respondents are not agreed on whether a nuclear catastrophe will occur) (1984, p. 197).

But this dire forecast has a positive outcome. NDErs report that the aforementioned cataclysms will be followed by an era of universal brotherhood, world peace, and universal love. The planet will survive! Curiously, the NDErs who report these visions not only believe that this scenario is inevitable, but they go on to assert that it is necessary and desirable. A new beginning, it seems, can only happen when the old dies. Omega not only follows Alpha but is necessary for Alpha.

THEORIES OF NEAR-DEATH EXPERIENCES

Near-death experiences have been explained on the basis of perspectives as diverse as psychological, sociological, pharmacological, physiological, parapsychological and religious. Preliminary attempts have also been made to explain NDEs in terms of modern physics (Brumblay, 2003; Crumbaugh, 1999; Lundahl, 2000). Many of these perspectives are not mutually exclusive. Psychological and pharmacological interpretations, for example, may complement each other, for instance when depersonalization is thought to be triggered by release of specific transmitters. Clearly "no theory has yet been proposed that can account satisfactorily for all of the common elements of NDEs. There is no logical reason, however, to demand that one comprehensive theory explain the entire phenomenon" (Greyson, 2000, pp. 336-337). This section presents most of the significant explanations of NDEs. These are grouped into three categories: neuropsychological, psychological, and metaphysical.

Neuropsychological Theories

Anoxia and Hypercarbia

Anoxia refers to a condition during which the brain is deprived of oxygen supply, and hypercarbia refers to elevated levels of carbon dioxide in the brain. It is assumed that the crisis situations of the NDErs lead to anoxia and or hypercarbia, which in turn can trigger altered states of consciousness and visionary experiences often amazingly similar to the one's reported by NDErs. However, it is a fact that individuals have gone through NDE's without being stricken by anoxia or hypercarbia (Bailey & Yates, 1996; Sabom 1998). Fenwick and Fenwick (1995) assert that anoxia would cause confusion and feelings of disorientation that are seldom reported by NDErs. Blackmore (1993) comments that anoxia and hypercarbia perhaps only trigger the NDE event and after that many other factors become involved.

Temporal Lobe Seizures

When the supply of oxygen to the brain is drastically reduced, its temporal lobe is considered to be susceptible to seizure activity. Blackmore (1993) points out that sudden release of endorphins under stressful conditions can also cause seizure activity in the temporal lobe, which is believed by many to be the physiological basis for NDE. Blackmore also adds that temporal lobe dysfunction can be responsible for the sudden emergence of memories resembling the life reviews of NDErs. It is interesting to note that during the 1930s, when Wilder Penfield electrically stimulated the temporal cortex of his epileptic patients, some saw their lives flash before them and experienced long-forgotten events (Zaleski, 1987). But as Abanes points out, "not every NDEr is an epileptic." Furthermore, "some NDErs have their experiences well before hypoxia or anoxia occurs" (Abanes, 1996, p. 102). Similarly, Sabom (1982, 1998) emphatically denies the role of temporal lobe seizures in NDEs. He argues that unlike NDEs, these seizures involve sensory delusions; predominant negative feelings such as fear, sadness, and loneliness; and forced thinking and random ideas beleaguering the mind. Further, Sabom quotes the work of Michael Persinger (1989), which reports that artificial stimulation of the lobe led to changes in mood and consciousness, which remained "fragmented and variable" unlike the "integrated and focused" state in NDEs (Sabom, 1998, p. 179). Sabom cites evidence even questioning the role of endorphins in these experiences and concludes:

> The dying brain hypothesis, which attempts to explain the NDE on the basis of endorphins, hypoxia, and temporal lobe seizures, cannot adequately account for the near-death experience. To do so would be like confusing bronchitis and pneumonia—there may be similarities, but the trained medical observer knows that they are fundamentally different conditions with different symptoms and methods of treatment (Sabom, 1998, p. 181).

Fenwick and Fenwick (1995) further support Sabom's position by pointing out that "if effects and disturbances within the temporal lobe are the basis of the NDE, then the experience would be expected to be forgotten," which is obviously not the case (Fox, 2003, p. 167). Morse and Perry (1990, 1992; also see Morse, 1996) describe NDEs as neurobiological events not as dysfunction of the temporal lobe, but as normal activity of the temporal lobe. The controversy continues.

Endorphins

Several researchers have reported that feelings of peace and calm are frequently experienced by NDErs (Ring, 1982; Sabom, 1982), and this sensation generally occurs before the other elements such as the life review, the tunnel, or the bright light are encountered (Abanes, 1996). Many researchers speculate that these peaceful sensations are caused by the release of endorphins, the brain's natural painkillers, during extreme stress. Endorphins also are responsible for the triggering of seizures in the limbic system, which includes the temporal lobe, that have been associated with mystical experiences (Carr, 1982; Persinger, 1984, 1989; Zaleski, 1987). Morse, Venecia, and Milstein (1989) also speculate along the same lines, but consider serotonin, rather than endorphins, as the initiator of NDEs (Abanes, 1996). Blackmore (1993) is a strong supporter of the role of endorphins in NDEs and believes that life-threatening situations alone may be enough to release endorphins and thereby lead to an NDE. Sabom (1982) points out that in studies where endorphins were injected into the cerebrospinal fluid of cancer patients, those patients were relieved of pain for 22 to 73 hours. However, with NDErs who experienced pain, the pain returned almost immediately upon resuscitation. And although runners experience increased levels of endorphins, "it is rare to observe runners experiencing life-review, tunnel sensation, and meeting with deceased relatives" (Kellehear, 1996, p. 121). Futhermore, most people under stress and near death have higher levels of endorphins, but very few have NDEs (Fenwick & Fenwick, 1995).

Drugs

It is commonly acknowledged that a wide range of drugs can lead to dissociative or visionary experience, and NDEs do occur under their influence. Jansen's Ketamine theory is of special relevance here. Ketamine is an anesthetic that has been used with patients suffering from cardiovascular and respiratory problems, and many NDErs were under the influence of Ketamine. However, Ketamine is no longer commonly used, but NDEs still continue to be reported. Recently Jansen has suggested that under severe stress, the body synthesizes a Ketamine-like chemical with similar NDE-like effects. On the other hand, Ketamine is known to produce feelings of disorientation and horror, which rarely are reported by NDErs (Fox, 2003). As Zaleski points out, "one cannot build a coherent theory of near-death experience on a pharmacological basis; not all near-death subjects were under medication, and in any case, the effects of different drugs vary endlessly" (Zaleski, 1987, p. 165). Also, as Greyson (2000, p. 334) remarks, individuals "who are febrile, anoxic, or given drugs when near death report fewer NDEs and less elaborate experiences than do people who remain drug free and are neither febrile nor anoxic." Several surveys support this conclusion (Osis & Haraldson, 1977; Ring, 1982; Sabom, 1982).

Dimethyltryptamine (DMT):
A Naturally Occurring Psychedelic

DMT is a chemical that is believed to be "released during naturally occurring psychedelic states including childbirth, the dying process, dreams, and a variety of subjective mystical experiences" (Hirshfeld-Flores, 2002, p. 1448). Participants who were administered DMT in a study by Strassman (see Hirshfeld-Flores, 2002) reported experiences similar to typical NDEs; however, they had no long-term positive effects on the subjects.

Massive Cortical Disinhibition:
Multiple Factor Theories of Siegel and Blackmore

Researchers now widely recognize that death is a *process*, not one *event* (Fox, 2003). In light of this recognition, Siegel (1980, 1993) and Blackmore (1993), among others, have proposed that a theory that enlists a number of factors to explain all the elements of the subjective reality of this process is more likely to succeed than a single-factor theory (Audain, 1999; Fox, 2003; Paulson, 1999). Siegel (1993) and Blackmore (1993) both feel that basically NDEs are an artifact of a dying brain. Under unusual circumstances, such as life-threatening events, "control is lost over the random activity of the central nervous system and consciousness reflects the system's efforts to make sense of this endogenous activity" (Irwin, 1999, p. 214). Both Siegel and Blackmore discuss psychological factors along with physical factors to explain the event. For example, Siegel (1993) asserts that during some drug administration or simply during the process of dying, religious and cultural fantasies may come to the surface from *within* the self and seem to appear from *outside* of it to the dying person (Fox, 2003). He illustrates his view by the case of a man looking through a window of a lighted room as night falls.

> He is absorbed by the view of the outside world and does not visualize the interior of the room. As darkness falls outside, however, the images of the objects in the room behind him can be seen reflected dimly in the window. With deepening darkness the fire in the fireplace illuminates the room, and the man now sees a vivid reflection of the room, which appears to be outside the window. As the analogy is applied to the near-death experience, the daylight (sensory input) is reduced while the interior illumination (the general level of arousal in the brain) remains bright, so that images originating within the rooms of the brain may be perceived as though they came from outside the windows of the senses (Siegel, 1993, pp. 254-255).

Along similar lines, Blackmore (1993, p. 161) suggests that our "system takes the most stable of its models and attributes to it the status of 'real'." Ordinarily, this model is "a rich composite which consists of information processing from a range of sources: *inner* (memory, imagination, expectation) and *outer* (the senses of seeing, hearing, and so on). Both are normally combined in ways we are not entirely conscious of, but the result is a livable model of self in the world which we call real" (Fox, 2003, p. 174). However, as the dying process advances, and our senses begin to fail, our model of reality is "powered progressively less and less by outer stimuli and more and more by inner stimuli" (Fox, 2003, p. 175). For Blackmore, this altered model of reality is no less real than the everyday model. To her, they are both "a fiction created to make sense of the world" (Blackmore, 1993, p. 223).

Beyond the above psychological factors, both Siegel and Blackmore do not hesitate to incorporate various physical factors into their theories to explain different aspects of the near-death experience. For example, to explain the tunnel and the light, they both refer to "Kluver's form constants" of tunnels, spirals, lattices, and cobwebs that seem to occur in the hallucinations of experimental subjects. Blackmore thinks that "their origin probably lies in the structure of the visual cortex, the part of the brain that processes visual information" (Bailey & Yates, 1996, p. 291). Blackmore enlists Kluver's constants and disinhibition of brain activity in the visual cortex due to anoxia or drug effect to develop a complex explanation for the experience of tunnels and lights by NDErs. According to her explanation, one would expect these phenomena in all NDEs, which is definitely not the case, according to Kellehear (1996). Although Blackmore's explanation is perhaps the most comprehensive one, it is definitely not problem free (Fox, 2003).

Psychological Theories

Depersonalization

This theory rests on the axiom that the mind will go to great extent to avoid entertaining the possibility of its own annihilation. As Goethe said, "It is entirely impossible for a thinking being to think of its own nonexistence" (see Zaleski, 1987, p. 244). Freud wrote in 1915,

> Our death is indeed unimaginable, and whenever we make the attempt to imagine it we can perceive that we really survive as spectators. Hence the psychoanalytic school could venture on the assertion that at bottom no one believes in his own death, or to put the same thing in another way, in the unconscious everyone is convinced of his own immortality (pp. 304-305).

Oscar Pfister (1930), a close friend of Freud, was the first psychologist to apply Freudian principles to explain NDEs, followed thirty years later by psychiatrist R. C. A. Hunter. Pfister's and Hunter's works provide in essence "the guiding principles for subsequent psychological interpretation of near-death experience; the central idea is that the mind cannot accept its death and therefore imagines itself detached from the body, fantasizes immortality, and regresses to infantile and 'oceanic' consolations" (Zaleski, 1987, p. 172).

Psychiatrist Russell Noyes, who collected over 200 accounts by survivors of life-threatening emergencies, offers a psychoanalytic perspective. He, along with Kletti, advances a depersonalization explanation of the NDE (Noyes, 1979; Noyes & Kletti, 1976). They propose that the sense of peace and well-being, detachment, life-review, and spiritual transcendence are defensive operations to insulate the ego from decompensating in the face of annihilation. A comparable depiction of the NDE also has been proposed by Roberts and Owen (1988) and others.

This explanation has been criticized on several grounds: For one, the depersonalization experience differs significantly from the NDE. The depersonalized individual experiences confusion over the reality of his/her self and feels she/he is not a person; whereas the NDErs report their sense of self to be strong. This explanation is also inadequate in explaining the perception of a deceased individual whom the dying person does not know to be dead. Several of these cases have been reported, and a psychodynamic interpretation is hard put to account fully for these occurrences. Also, the depersonalization theory assumes that the perception of threat to life precedes the NDE. Sabom (1982) mentions instances when the two were reversed. It is worth noting that young children who have not experienced ego differentiation yet and have a different concept of death compared to adults, also experience NDEs (Morse, 1996).

Noyes and Kletti (1977, p. 113) do acknowledge possible transformative effects of the NDE:

> The vastly altered mind may be set to work upon final tasks ... the individual near death may accept the reality before him and, from a transcendent perspective, capture a glimpse of his life in harmony with the universe.

However, Noyes and Kletti leave us wondering "how a hallucinatory condition that is intrinsically regressive and delusionary could come to be the vehicle for such high attainment" (Zaleski, 1987, p. 174).

Motivated Fantasy

This theory drops the concept of depersonalization and emphasizes wishful and defensive fantasy. As Irwin (1999) clearly points out, the motivational bases vary from narcissism (Rank, 1971), to the denial of death (Ehrenwald, 1974; Greyson, 1981; Sagan, 1979), to a basic dread of catastrophe (Gabbard & Twemlow, 1991). The content of this fantasy may come from different sources, including the experient's belief system (Norton & Sahlman, 1995), popular images of an afterlife (Vaisrub, 1977), and media portrayal of the NDE itself (Walker, 1989).

The motivated-fantasy hypothesis fails to explain the consistency of the characteristic features of the core experience across different individuals. It is reasonable to expect individuals to harbor different expectations in regard to an afterlife; yet, the sequence of the NDEs is remarkably similar. Both Moody (1975) and Ring (1982) assert that expectations do not have any relationship to the NDE.

Both depersonalization and motivated-fantasy models suggest that near-death experiences "are products of imagination, constructed from one's personal and cultural expectations, to protect ourselves from facing the threat of death" (Greyson, 2000, p. 332). Greyson clearly summarizes the empirical evidence that contradicts this hypothesis. He cites research indicating that the details of NDEs often conflict with the subjects' religious and personal expectations about death (Abramovitch, 1988; Ring, 1984); the details of NDEs are generally independent of the individual's familiarity or lack thereof with the phenomenon (Greyson, 1991; Greyson & Stevenson, 1980; Ring, 1982; Sabom, 1982); and children who have not undergone much cultural or religious conditioning report NDEs that are similar to those of adults (Bush, 1983; Gabbard & Twemlow, 1984; Herzog & Herrin, 1985; Morse et al., 1986; Serdahely, 1991; Serdahely & Walker, 1990).

NDEs as False Memory Syndromes

Abanes (1996) considers a number of separate facts and proceeds to speculate that an NDE may just be a case of false memory syndrome. What are these facts that might persuade one to draw this conclusion?

It has been established that both imagination and perception activate exactly the same brain centers, and when we generate images through concentration, which then "get recorded in the web of neurons as if they were real, we might actually convince ourselves that confabulations are true" (Neimark, 1995, p. 85). Also, we do not have precise recollections of our dreams and memories, we constantly recreate them (Calvin, 1990; Taylor, 1979), and whenever our brain is faced with gaps in our memory or bits of data that do not fit, it makes its best attempt to create a memory and then believes it (Blackmore, 1993; Morse, 1996). So it is not surprising that about a quarter of all individuals "recollect" events that never occurred (Loftus, 1991). It is also noteworthy that much of our brain's emotional processing occurs unconsciously, and that of all our senses, we lose our hearing sense the last due to unconsciousness (Abanes, 1996).

In light of the above information, Abanes (1996, p. 127) speculates that possibly in a crisis situation, "NDErs perceive the environment around them and, although unconscious, and visualizing what is taking place such visualization might then get confused and combined with added information unconsciously received while in recovery" and with information provided by family and friends after consciousness is regained. All of this together possibly could create a basic NDE that is tantamount to a false memory. Whether one can explain all NDEs and all characteristics of NDEs in this way seems highly implausible at the moment. Future research, hopefully, will shed further light on this issue.

NDEs as Recollections of the Birth Experience

The explanation that NDEs are recollections of the birth experience (Grof, 1975; Grosso, 1983; Sagan, 1979) has been refuted successfully. Extensive evidence supports that mental alertness, visual acuity, spatial stability of visual images, and cortical capacity to register the birth experience are lacking in newborns (Becker, 1982; Greyson, 2000). Also, Blackmore (1983) reports that descriptions of out-of-body experiences provided by those born by cesarean section are not different form those born the normal way. While Grof (1975) and Grosso (1983) also emphasize the birth experience in their explanation, they conceptualize "NDEs as representations of Jungian archetypes of a birth experience rather than as memories of actual birth events" (Greyson, 2000, p. 333).

NDEs as Archetypes

Another way to explain NDEs is to assume that these images are "wired" into the brain. "That is, people of all cultures and all eras are born with an inclination to generate certain mental images or *archetypes* that form the mythological elements of our common humanity" (Irwin, 1999, p. 216). While Jung (1971) first postulated the concept of archetypes, Grof (1975), Grosso (1983), Heaney (1983), and Quimby (1989) have applied it to explain NDEs. How the concept can lead to a testable hypothesis or to therapeutic interventions is not clear (Greyson, 2000). There is no independent evidence that the alleged "near-death archetypes" actually exist. Irwin (1999) points out that, "it does not seem very constructive to attribute the uniformity of NDEs to the uniformity of people's archtypical images: appeal is being made to one unknown in order to explain another" (p. 216).

NDEs as Fear-Death Experiences (FDEs)

Richard Abanes, in his book *Journey Into the Light* (1996) argues that NDEs are perhaps "fear-death experiences." According to him, FDEs occur when subjects believe that they are "going to die soon, although no physical near-death condition is present" (p. 87). Therefore NDEs may just be FDEs intensified by the additional element of physical stimulus. It is not suprising that many FDEs seem remarkably similar to NDEs and that FDErs reported more NDE elements when they held a deeper conviction that they were going to die (Schultz, 2004). This explanation amounts to calling NDEs by another name and does not constitute a satisfactory explanation of the phenomenon.

NDEs as a Sociocultural Phenomenon

In *Experiences Near Death,* Allan Kellehear (1996) proposed that NDEs are a "culturally influenced and socially mediated experience" that are better explained from a sociological perspective (Balk, 1997, p. 314). Kellehear (1996) states that "for too long now, the debate about the NDE by medical and psychological workers has given this area of human experience the appearance of oddity. . . . Far from being abnormal experiences, NDEs are surprisingly common, normal responses to uncommon, unusual circumstances" (p. 42). As discussed earlier, several differences in the descriptions of the NDEs in various cultures have been noted. Hence, Kellehear proposes that NDEs are a product of societal and cultural forces. Kellehear's theory attempts to explain why NDEs take a certain form, but not their cause.

NDEs as Altered States of Consciousness

Ring (1984) reports several case histories from his archives that relate experiences strikingly similar to the NDE, except that the individuals never had an NDE. From the earlier brief discussion of the meditative experience, it is reasonable to assume that the NDE is an altered state of consciousness which also occurs under a variety of other situations. The altered state of consciousness experienced during the NDE seems to have little to do with approaching death, except that the prospect of dying itself seems to be a reliable trigger that sets off the altered state of consciousness.

The NDE, then, appears to belong to the family of mystical experiences, which is as old as humankind. These transcendental experiences are known to induce what has variously been called "cosmic consciousness" or "ultra consciousness." In Eastern meditative lore, the transformation to cosmic consciousness is achieved through the activation of the kundalini. This Sanskrit term means "coiled up."

> The term represents a postulated, subtle form of bioenergy said to lie latent, like a sleeping serpent, at the base of the spine. Under certain circumstances, however, this energy can be activated, and when it is, it is said to travel upward through the spine (in a special channel). As it travels, it affects certain energy centers (called chakras in the yogic tradition) and may induce explosive and destabilizing energy transformations that are experienced both psychologically and physically (Ring, 1984, p. 230).

The arousal of the kundalini catapults the individual into a higher state of consciousness. It throws his/her nervous system into overdrive and transforms the brain cells. It awakens latent potentialities and capacities and permits the individual to experience the world in a rapturous manner and also allows for the flowering of psychic abilities.

Admittedly the kundalini experience has not been scientifically verified, due in part to the lack of instrumentation as well as lack of agreement on what to measure. Nevertheless, there is wide consensus that the kundalini experience does occur, and that it is remarkably similar to the NDE. In fact, NDEs, the kundalini experience, and other transformations of consciousness appear to belong to the same class of transcendental mystical experiences. They seem identical in content and aftereffects, differing only in the ways in which they are precipitated. Krishna's (1970, 1975) account of his kundalini awakening could well be a report of the NDE. The hypothesis that kundalini is the energy released during the NDE and underlies the event deserves further research (Harris, 1994; Kasan, 1994; Kieffer, 1994).

Metaphysical Theories of Near-Death Experiences

While popular interest in NDEs appears to be due primarily to the implication that these events are an introduction to the afterlife, the majority of investigators in the field have ignored this question and have offered explanations in terms of universal processes, psychological or physiological (Greyson, 2000). However, there are a number of findings that do not readily lend themselves to such explanations and point toward the possibility of the survival of consciousness beyond the death of the body. For example, a number of investigators have presented examples of subjects who described with unusual accuracy the events happening around them, or occurrences at a distance beyond the reach of their sense organs, or objects located in spots beyond their access from the period they were ostensibly unconscious (Ebon, 1977; Greyson, 2000; Hampe, 1979; Moody, 1977; Ring & Lawrence, 1993; Sabom, 1982, 1998). Ring and Cooper (1997, 1999) present evidence that in their NDEs, blind persons, some blind from birth, had accurate visual perceptions. Such veridical out-of-body perceptions do not necessarily prove survival after death, because the experients are obviously still alive and their consciousness may still be dependent on the bodies. "However, if minds are capable of functioning outside the body while it is alive, then it is conceivable that they are capable of functioning after the body dies" (Greyson, 2000, p. 341, also see Osis & Mitchell, 1977).

Cobbe (1982) describes "Peak in Darien," a type of near-death vision in which individuals "on their deathbeds see a recently deceased person of whose death they had no knowledge" (Greyson, 2000, p. 341). Such cases, which apparently point toward a survival hypothesis, have been reported by a number of other researchers (Badlaw & Badlaw, 1982; Callahan & Kelley, 1993; Kübler-Ross, 1983; Moody, 1975; Moody & Perry, 1988; Ring, 1982; Sabom, 1982; Spraggett, 1974).

One can perhaps conclude that current theories based on neurophysiological or psychological processes cannot explain the NDE data satisfactorily and have created room for metaphysical speculation (Sabom, 1982). For example, the *Soul Travel Theory* refers to a possible "transitional journey of the soul or spirit to another mode of existence or realm of reality," and the *Psychic Vision Theory* implies "glimpses into another mode of reality, though not necessarily providing proof of soul-survival after death" (DeSpelder & Strickland, 2005, p. 520).

In *Life at Death*, Ring (1982) embraces a metaphysical interpretation that derives from the holographic theory advanced by Karl Pribram and supported by the British physicist David Bohm, among others (Revision 1, 1978, entire issue).

It is Ring's belief that the first two stages of the NDE represent an out-of-body experience involving the actual (as opposed to subjective) separation of personal consciousness from the physical body. Such a split, then, provides a parsimonious explanation for the feelings that are reported by NDErs. After all, a disembodied consciousness, by definition, would be bereft of the cares of a physical body. The feelings of ease, beatitude, worrylessness, and calm that accompany the true NDE may well be the affective concomitants of the out-of-body experience.

Green (1968) and Tart (1974) convincingly present the case for the reality of the out-of-body experience. It is very likely, but by no means definitive, that the out-of-body experience falls squarely within the realm of human experience. At this point it may be worthwhile to consider whether the separation of disembodied consciousness at death also involves the separation of a second body, the so-called double. In both esoteric writings and in the wide-ranging explorations of the British organization, the Society for Psychical Research, there is mention of a "cord," usually of silver, connecting the physical body with the ethereal double. This cord supposedly snaps at death. Both self-reports of the NDE and accounts of witnesses to the separation of the ethereal double need to be examined with extreme caution. These accounts, even if accurate, raise more questions than they purport to answer. For example, what is the precise composition of the cord? What are its functions? What causes the separation? Suffice it to say that the mere separation of consciousness at the stage of death, with or without a second body, would account for all the stages of the core experience if examined in the light of the holographic theory.

Holography, simply put, is photography without a lens. "In holography, the wave field of light scattered by an object—say, an orange—is recorded on a plate as an interference pattern. . . . When the interference pattern is then illuminated by a laser beam, the orange reappears as a three-dimensional image. This image is a hologram" (Ring, 1982, p. 235). An extraordinary property of this pattern is the capacity of any part to contain information about the whole. According to Pribram (1978), the human brain functions holographically by mathematically analyzing the interference wave pattern so that images of objects are seen. Thus the brain functions as a frequency analyzer with different parts and cells responding to different frequencies. Our normal "reality" is constructed out of one set of frequencies. In the construction of reality out of frequencies, ordinary boundaries of space and time collapse.

If space and time collapse within a holographic reality, then, in tapping into that reality (which is behind the world of appearances), which also ushers in a new frequency domain, one may be entering a different state of consciousness with myriad possibilities. Among these possibilities may be access to paranormal phenomena such as telepathy and clairvoyance as well as a transformatory experience, which may represent humankind's next evolutionary step.

Can this holographic theory account for the core experience? Ring has argued that the first two stages of the core experience can be explained to some extent by accepting the evidence for the out-of-body experience. Then he proceeds to suggest that the holographic reality becomes accessible to a disembodied consciousness. He explains the experience of moving through a dark tunnel as the subjective psychological correlate of consciousness shifting from one domain to the other. In other words, when consciousness shifts gears, Ring's NDErs experience movement through a dark tunnel. This intermediate state, which involves a suspension of time, is experienced as a dark space. Awareness moves into four-dimensional consciousness.

Along with the sense of moving through a dark tunnel, NDErs report a brilliant golden light at the end. It seems plausible that, in becoming sensitive to an entirely new range of frequencies, NDErs tap into a world of extraordinary beauty, brilliance, and light. Both occult literature and popular literature on life after death speak of the "light of the astral plane," which appears to be a different and luminous frequency domain.

Ring (1982) abandons his scientific reserve in advancing a second interpretation of the light. "The golden light is actually a reflection of one's own inherent divine nature and symbolizes the higher self. The light one sees, then, is one's own" (p. 241). The higher self is all-knowing, unconditionally accepting, and so overwhelming and awesome that it is experienced as a brilliant light. It is this self that is sometimes experienced as a "voice," "presence," or "being," and it is this higher self that initiates a life review. In offering this bold speculation, Ring wanders into the land of the mystical disciplines wherein the "higher self" has a decisive and hallowed presence.

How can the last stage of the core experience, the "world of light," be explained in holographic terms? This world, with its preternatural beauty and splendor, is but another frequency domain. At death, the disembodied consciousness continues to function holographically and another reality, the world of light, is constructed out of the higher frequencies to which consciousness now has access. Furthermore, this reality is experienced as real as any other, including the earlier physical world wherein consciousness was connected to a physical body.

The world of light, then, is a consciousness-created world, which may yet have a tenuous link to the thought patterns of the NDEr. Consequently, the paradisiacal imagery of this stage may be tarnished by unpleasant thought patterns at the time of death. This may account for the hellish experiences occasionally described.

METHODOLOGICAL CONSIDERATIONS

A number of methodological problems in near-death research make it difficult to draw firm conclusions on several issues. For example, as Hicks (1995) points out, the majority of the subjects utilized in research are members of the International Association of Near-Death Studies (IANDS), which was formed for the purpose of studying NDEs. Whether that group is representative of a cross-section of NDErs has not been determined. Hicks (1995) also mentions that in several studies, the subjects were mostly white, married, Protestant or Catholic, and almost all of the studies, with rare exceptions (Schwaninger, Eisenberg, Schechtman, & Weiss, 2002; Van Lommel, Van Wees, Meyers, & Elfferich 2001) employed retrospective rather than prospective design. Also, in numerous cases, the subjects were interviewed long after their experiences took place. Lack of adequate description or absence of description of the research instruments and statistical tests and results are also of concern (Hicks, 1995).

Greyson (2000) takes a comprehensive look at the methodological issues in near- death research. He draws attention to a lack of consensus even on a definition of NDE; hence it is problematic to compare results of research of different investigators. "Universally accepted measures of the depth or intensity of the experience" are also missing (p. 342). Small participant samples, the "unrepresentative nature of ... participant populations, the lack of a suitable comparison group, and the lack of a structured interview protocol and standardized, objective scales" are also a source of concern (Greyson, 2000, p. 344). On a positive note, it should be pointed out that the quality of research in this complex field has been improving steadily.

CONCLUDING REMARKS

While there is minimal agreement among the proponents of a plethora of theories concerning NDEs, a consensus is gradually emerging that the real significance of these experiences lies in their transformative effects, and recent NDE research is increasingly focused on these effects. As noted earlier, NDEs often spiritually transform individuals, affecting their self-concept, their relationships, their world view, and their psychological and psychic functioning. The pattern of changes among NDErs "tends to be so highly positive and specific in its effects that it is possible to interpret it as indicative of a *generalized awakening of higher human potential*" (Ring, 1993, p. 248).

The philosopher Teilhard de Chardin (1959) believed that humanity was evolving toward a transhuman state he called "noogenesis," a state characterized by the birth of a planetary mind aware of its destiny. John White referred to this possible emerging form of humanity as *Homo noeticus* (Ring & Valarino, 1998). Ferguson (1980) and Russell (1983) offer evidence of the widespread occurrence of transcendental experiences. Along with NDEs and the kundalini experiences, a family of transformatory experiences seems to be occurring. If these experiences bring about personal transformation, then they may collectively represent an evolutionary thrust toward higher consciousness. If, indeed, the subtle bioenergy known as kundalini underlies these transformations, it may serve as an evolutionary device that "mutates" humankind into loving, compassionate, altruistic, and spiritually inclined beings who have attained a planetary consciousness. Thus kundalini can generate a new kind of human being characterized by a noetic understanding of the universe.

Ring (1984, 1993; Ring & Valarino, 1998) argues that in recent years many such human beings have been and are being created by NDEs and other transcendental experiences, and that a new race that could possibly transform this planet may be coming into existence. Teilhard de Chardin (1959) called the end state of human evolution "the Omega Point." Are we heading toward Omega?

> I think it not improbable that man, like the grub that prepares a chamber for the winged thing it never has been but is to be—that man may have cosmic destinies that he does not understand (Oliver Wendell Homes in Walsh & Shapiro, 1983, p. 273).

REFERENCES

Abanes, R. (1996). *Journey into the light: Exploring near-death experiences*. Grand Rapids, MI: Baker Books.

Abramovitch, H. (1988). An Israeli account of a near-death experience: A case study of cultural dissonanu. *Journal of Near-Death Studies, 6*, 175-184.

Alcock, J. E. (1978). Psychology and near-death experiences. *Skeptical Inquirer, 32*(2), 25-41.

Alvarado, C. (2000). Out-of-body experiences. In E. Cardena, S. J. Lynn, & S. Krippner (Eds.), *Varieties of anamolous experiences: Examining the scientific evidence.* Washington, DC: American Psychological Association.

Atwater, P. (1988). *Coming back to life: The after-effect of near-death experiences.* New York: Dodd and Mead.

Atwater, P. (1992). Is there hell? Surprising observations about the near-death experience. *Journal of Near-Death Studies, 10*(3), 150.

Atwater, P. (1994). *Beyond the light: The mysteries and revelations of near-death experiences.* New York: Avon.

Audain, L. (1999). The near-death experience and the theory of the extraneuronal hyperspace. *Journal of Near-Death Studies, 17*(4), 261-265.

Audette, J. R. (1982). Historical perspectives on near-death experiences and episodes. In C. R. Lundahl (Ed.), *A collection of near-death readings.* Chicago: Nelson Hall.

Badlaw, P., & Badlaw, L. (1982). *Immortality or extinction.* Totowa, NJ: Barnes & Noble.

Bailey, L. W., & Yates, J. (Eds.). (1996). *The near-death experience: A reader.* New York: Routledge.

Balk, D. (1997). The social dimension of the near-death experience. *Death Studies, 21,* 314-317.

Barušs, I. (2003). *Alterations of consciousness: An empirical analysis for social scientists.* Washington, DC: American Psychological Association.

Basford, T. K. (1990). *Near-death experiences: An annotated bibliography.* New York: Garland Publishers.

Bates, B. C., & Stanley, A. (1985). The epidemiology of differential diagnosis of near-death experience. *American Journal of Orthopsychiatry, 4,* 542-549.

Bauer, M. (1985). Near-death experiences and attitude change. *Anabiosis: The Journal of Near-Death Studies, 2,* 102-109.

Becker, C. B. (1982). The failure of Saganomics: Why birth models cannot explain near death phenomena. *Anabiosis: The Journal of Near-Death Studies, 2,* 102-109.

Blackmore, S. (1983). Birth and the OBE: An unhelpful analogy. *Journal of the American Society for Psychical Research, 77,* 224-238.

Blackmore, S. (1986). Out-of-body experience in schizophrenia. *Journal of Nervous and Mental Disease, 10,* 615-619.

Blackmore, S. (1993) *Dying to live: Near-death experiences.* Buffalo, NY: Prometheus Books.

Bremmer, J. N. (2002). *The rise and fall of the afterlife.* New York: Routledge.

Brinkley, D. (1994). *Saved by the light.* New York: Villard.

Brinkley, D. (1995). *At peace in the light.* New York: HarperCollins.

Brumblay, R. J. (2003). Hyperdimensional perspectives in out-of-body and near-death experiences. *Journal of Near-Death Studies, 21*(4), 201-221.

Bush, N. E. (1983). The near-death experience in children: Shades of the prismhouse reopening. *Anabiosis: The Journal of Near-Death Studies, 3,* 177-193.

Bush, N. E. (1991). Is ten years a life review? *Journal of Near-Death Studies, 10,* 5-9.

Callahan, M., & Kelley, P. (1993). *Final gifts: Understanding the special needs, awareness, and communications of the dying.* New York: Posiedon.

Calvin, W. (1990). *The cerebal symphony: Seashore reflections on the structure of consciousness.* New York: Bantam.

Carr, D. (1982). Pathophysiology of stress-induced limbic lobe dysfunction: A hypothesis for NDEs. *Anabiosis: The Journal of Near-Death Studies, 2,* 75-89.

Cobbe, F. P. (1982). *Peak in Darien: With some enquiries touching concerns of the soul and body*. London: Williams & Norgate.
Counts, D. A. (1983). Near-death and out-of-body experiences in a Melanese society. *Anabiosis, 3*, 115-135.
Cressy, J. (1996). Mysticism and the near-death experience. In L. W. Bailey & J. Yates (Eds.), *The near-death experience: A reader*. New York: Routledge.
Crumbaugh, J. C. (1999). A contribution of Tipler's Omega Point Theory to near-death studies. *Journal of Near-Death Studies, 18*(1), 5-11.
DeSpelder, L. A., & Strickland, A. L. (2005). The *last dance: Encountering death and dying*. New York: McGraw-Hill
Ebon, M. (1977). *The evidence for life after death*. New York: Signet.
Ehrenwald, J. (1974). Out-of-the-body experiences and the denial of death. *Journal of Nervous and Mental Disease, 159*, 227-233.
Fenwick, P., & Fenwick, E. (1995). *The truth in the light. An investigation of over 300 near-death experiences*. London: Headline.
Ferguson, M. (1980). *The acquarian conspiracy*. Los Angeles: J. P. Tarcher.
Flynn, C. P. (1986). *After the beyond: Human transformation and the near-death experience*. Englewood Cliffs, NJ: Prentice Hall.
Fox, M. (2003). *Religion, spirituality and the near-death experience*. New York: Routledge.
Freud, S. (1915). Thoughts for the times on war and death. In *Collected Papers* (authorized translation under supervision of Joan Riviere, London, 1959).
Gabbard, G. O., & Twemlow, S. W. (1991). Do "near-death experiences" occur only near death?—Revisited. *Journal of Near-Death Studies, 10*, 41-47.
Gabbard, G. O., & Twemlow, S. W. (1984). *With the eyes of the mind*. New York: Praeger.
Green, C. (1968). *Out-of-the-body experiences*. New York: Ballantine.
Green, J. J. (2001). The near-death experience as a shaman's initiation: A case study. *Journal of Near-Death Studies, 19*(4), 209-225.
Grey, M. (1985). *Return from death: An exploration of near-death experience*. London: Arkana.
Greyson, B. (1981). Toward a psychological explanation of near-death experiences: A response to Dr. Grosso's paper. *Anabiosis: Journal of Near-Death Studies, 1*, 88-103.
Greyson, B. (1985). A typology of near-death experiences. *American Journal of Psychiatry, 142*, 967-969.
Greyson, B. (1991). Near-death experiences precipitated by suicide attempts: Lack of influence of psychopathology, religion, and expectations. *Journal of Near-Death Studies, 9*, 183-188.
Greyson, B. (1992). Reduced death threat in near-death experiences. *Death Studies, 16*, 533-546.
Greyson, B. (1992-1993). Near-death experiences and antisuicidal attitudes. *Omega, 26*, 81-89.
Greyson, B. (1996). The near-death experience as transpersonal crisis. In B. W. Scotton, A. Chinen, & J. R. Battista (Eds.), *Textbook of transpersonal psychiatry and psychology* (pp. 302-315). New York: Basic Books.
Greyson, B. (1997). The near-death experience as a focus of clinical attention. *Journal of Nervous and Mental Disease, 185*, 327-334.

Greyson, B. (2000). Near-death experiences. In E. Cardeña, S. J. Lynn, & S. Krippner (Eds.), *Varieties of anomalous experience: Examining the scientific evidence*. Washington, DC: American Psychological Association.

Greyson, B., & Bush, N. E. (1992). Distressing near-death experiences. *Psychiatry, 55*(1), 95-110.

Greyson, B., & Harris, B. (1987). Clinical approaches to the near-death experience. *Journal of Near-Death Studies, 6,* 41-52.

Greyson, B., & Stevenson, I. (1980). The phenomenology of near-death experiences. *American Journal of Psychiatry, 147,* 1193-1196.

Grof, S. (1975) *Realms of the human unconscious: Observations from LSD psychotherapy.* New York: Viking.

Grosso, M. (1983). Jung, parapsychology, and the near-death experience: Toward a transpersonal paradigm. *Anabiosis: The Journal of Near-Death Studies, 3,* 3-38.

Groth-Marnat, G., & Summers, R. (1998). Altered beliefs, attitudes and behaviors following near-death experiences. *Journal of Humanistic Psychology, 38*(3), 110-125.

Hampe, J. C. (1979). *To die is gain.* Atlanta, GA: John Knox.

Harris, B. (1994). Kundalini and healing in the West. *Journal of Near-Death Studies, 13*(2), 75-79.

Heaney, J. J. (1983). Recent studies of near-death experiences. *Journal of Religion and Health, 22,* 116-130.

Heim, A. v. St. G. (1892). Notezen über den Tod durch absturz [Remarks on fatal falls]. *Jahrbuch des Schweitzer Alpenclub, 27,* 327-337.

Herzog, D. B., & Herrin, J. T. (1985). Near-death experiences in the very young. *Critical Care Medicine, 13,* 1074-1075.

Hicks, B. F. (1995). *The lived experience following a near-death event: A phenomenological study.* Ann Arbor, MI: UMI Dissertation Services.

Hirshfeld-Flores, A. (2002). The spirit molecule: A doctor's revolutionary research into the biology of near-death and mystical experiences. *The American Journal of Psychiatry, 159,* 1448-1449.

Horacek, B. J. (1997). Amazing grace: The effects of near-death experiences on those dying and grieving. *Journal of Near-Death Studies, 16*(2), 149-161.

Insinger, M. (1991). The impact of a near-death experience on family relationships. *Journal of Near-Death Studies, 9,* 141-181.

Irwin, H. J. (1985). *Flight of mind: A psychological study of the out-of-body experience.* Metuchen, NJ: Scarecrow Press.

Irwin, H. J. (1993). The near-death experience as a dissociative phenomenon: An empirical assessment. *Journal of Near-Death Studies, 12,* 95-103.

Irwin, H. J. (1999). *An introduction to parapsychology.* London: McFarland & Company.

Jung, C. G., (1971). *The archetypes of the collective unconscious.* Princeton, NJ: Princeton University Press. (Original work published in 1954.)

Kasan, Y. (1994). Near-death experiences and kundalini awakening. *Journal of Near-Death Studies, 12*(3), 147-157.

Kellehear, A. (1993). Culture, biology, and the near-death experience. *Journal of Nervous and Mental Diseases, 181,* 148-156.

Kellehear, A. (1996). *Experiences near death: Beyond medicine and religion.* New York: Oxford University Press.

Kerr, N. H. (2000). Dreaming, imagery, and perception. In M. H. Kryger, T. Roth, & W. C. Dement (Eds.), *Principles and practice of sleep medicine*. Philadelphia: W. B. Saunders.
Kieffer, G. (1994). Kundalini and the near-death experience. *Journal of Near-Death Studies, 12*(3), 159-176.
Kinnier, R. T., Tribensee, N. E., Rose, C. A., & Vanghan, S. M. (2001). In final analysis: More wisdom from people who have faced death. *Journal of Counseling and Development, 79*(2), 171-177.
Krishna, G. (1970). *Kundalini*. Berkeley, CA: Shambhala.
Krishna, G. (1975). *The awakening of kundalini*. New York: E. P. Dutton.
Krishnan, V. (1995). Near-death experiences and healing. *Journal of Near-Death Studies, 13*(4), 278-281.
Kübler-Ross, E. (1983). *On children and death*. New York: Macmillan.
Lansberry, L. D. (1994). First-person report: A skeptic's near-death experience. *Skeptical Inquirer, 18*, 431-432.
Locke, T. P., & Shontz, F. C. (1983). Personality correlates of the near-death experience: A preliminary study. *Journal of the American Society for Psychical Research, 77*, 311-318.
Loftus, E. (1991). *Witness for the defense*. New York: St. Martin's Press.
Lorimer, D. (1996). The near-death experience and the perenial wisdom. In L. W. Bailey & J. Yates (Eds.), *The near-death experience: A reader*. New York: Routledge.
Lukianowicz, N. (1958). Autoscopic phenomena. *AMA Archives of Neurology and Psychiatry, 80*, 199-220.
Lundahl, C. R. (1993). Lessons of near-death experiences for humanity. *Journal of Near-Death Studies, 12*(1), 5-16.
Lundahl, C. R. (2000). Near-death studies and modern physics. *Journal of Near-Death Studies, 18*(3), 143-179.
Moody, R. (1975). *Life after life*. Atlanta: Mockingbird.
Moody, R. (1977). *Reflections on life after life*. Atlanta: Mockingbird.
Moody, R. A., & Perry, P. (1988). *The light beyond*. New York: Bantam.
Morris, L. L., & Knalf, K. (2003). The nature and meaning of the near-death experience for patients and critical care nurses. *Journal of Near-Death Studies, 21*(3), 139-167.
Morse, M. (1996). Parting visions: A new scientific paradigm. In L. W. Bailey & J. Yates (Eds.), *The near-death experience: A reader*. New York: Routledge.
Morse, M. L. (1994). Near-death experiences and death-related visions in children: Implications for the clinician. *Current Problems in Pediatrics, 24*, 55-83.
Morse, M. L., & Perry, P. (1990). *Closer to the light: Learning from children's near death experiences*. New York: Villard Books.
Morse, M., & Perry, P. (1992). *Transformed by the light: The powerful effect of near death experiences on people's lives*. New York: Villard.
Morse, M. L., Venecia, D., & Milstein, J. (1989). Near-death experiences: A neurophysiological explanatory model. *Journal of Near-Death Studies, 8*, 45-53.
Morse, M. L., Castillo, P., Venecia, D., Milstein, J., & Tyler, D. C. (1986). Childhood near-death experiences. *American Journal of Diseases of Children, 140*, 1110-1114.
Musgrave, C. (1997). The near-death experience: A study of spiritual transformation. *Journal of Near-Death Studies, 15*(3), 187-201.

Neimark, J. (1995). It's magical, it's malleable, it's memory. *Psychology Today*, January/February, 44-49.

Norton, M. C., & Sahlman, J. M. (1995). Describing the light: Attribution theory as an explanation of the near-death experience. *Journal of Near-Death Studies, 13,* 167-184.

Noyes, R. (1972). The experience of dying. *Psychiatry, 35,* 174-184.

Noyes, R. (1979). Near-death experiences: Their interpretation and significance. In R. Kastenbaum (Ed.), *Between life and death.* New York: Springer.

Noyes, R. (1980). Attitude change following near-death experiences. *Psychiatry, 43,* 234-242.

Noyes, R., Hoenk, P. R., Kuperman, S., & Slymen, D. J. (1977). Depersonalization on accident victims and psychiatric patients. *Journal of Nervous and Mental Disease, 164,* 401-407.

Noyes, R., & Kletti, R. (1976). Depersonalization in the face of life threatening danger: An interpretation. *Omega, 7,* 103-114.

Noyes, R., & Kletti, R. (1977). Panoramic memory: A response to the threat of death. *Omega, 8,* 181-194.

Noyes, R., & Slymen, D. (1978-1979). The subjective response to life-threatening danger. *Omega, 9,* 313-321.

Osis, K., & Haraldson, E. (1977). *At the hour of death.* New York: Avon.

Osis, K., & Mitchell, J. L. (1977). Physiological correlates of reported out-of-the-body experiences. *Journal of the Society for Psychical Research, 49,* 525.

Paulson, D. S. (1999). The near-death experience: An integration of cultural, spiritual, and physical perspectives. *Journal of Near-Death Studies, 18*(1), 13-25.

Pastricha, S., & Stevenson, I. (1986). Near-death experiences in India. *Journal of Nervous and Mental Diseases, 174,* 165-170.

Persinger, M. A. (1984). Propensity to report paranormal experiences is correlated with temporal lobe signs. *Perceptual and Motor Skills, 59,* 583-586.

Persinger, M. A. (1989). Modern neuroscience and near-death experiences: Expectancies and implications. Comments on "A neurobiological model for near-death experiences." *Journal of Near-Death Studies, 7,* 223-239.

Pfister, O. (1930). Shockdenken and Shockphantasien bei höchster todesgafahr [Shock thoughts and fantasies in extreme mortal danger]. *Zeitshrift für Psychoanalyse, 16,* 430-455.

Pfister, O. (1981). Shock thoughts and fantasies in extreme mortal danger. Translated by R. Kletti & R. Noyes, Jr. in "Mental states in mortal danger." *Essence, 5,* 5-20.

Pribram, K. H. (1978). What the fuss is all about. *Re-Vision, 1*(¾) 14-18.

Quimby, S. L. (1989). The near-death experience as an event in consciousness. *Journal of Humanistic Psychology, 29,* 87-108.

Rank, O. (1971). *The double: A psychoanalytical study.* Chapel Hill, NC: University of North Carolina Press.

Rawlings, M. (1979). *Beyond death's door.* New York: Bantam Books.

Rawlings, M. (1993). *To hell and back.* Nashville: Thomas Nelson.

Ring, K. (1982). *Life at death: A scientific investigation of the near-death experience.* New York: Quill.

Ring, K. (1984). *Heading toward Omega: In search of the meaning of the near-death experience.* New York: Morrow.

Ring, K. (1992). *The omega project: Near-death experiences, UFO encounters, and mind at large*. New York: William Morrow.

Ring K. (1993). Near-death experiences: Implications for human evolution and planetary transformation. In B. Kane, J. Millay, & D. Brown (Eds.), *Silver threads: 25 years of parapsychology research*.Westport, CT: Praeger.

Ring, K., & Cooper, S. (1997). Near-death and out-of-body experiences in the blind: A study of apparent eyeless vision. *Journal of Near-Death Studies, 16*(2), 101-147.

Ring, K., & Cooper, S. (1999). *Mindsight: Near-death and out-of-body experiences in the blind*. Palo Alto, CA: William James Center for Cousciousness Studies, Institute of Transpersonal Psychology.

Ring, K., & Lawrence, M. (1993). Further evidence for verdical perception during near death experiences. *Journal of Near-Death Studies, 11*, 223-229.

Ring, K., & Valarino, E. (1998). *Lessons from the light: What we can learn from the near-death experience*. Needham, MA: Moment Point Press.

Rinpoche, S. (1996). The near-death experience: A staircase to heaven. In L. W. Bailey & J. Yates (Eds.), *The near-death experience: A reader*. New York: Routledge.

Roberts, G., & Owen, J. (1988). The near-death experience. *British Journal of Psychiatry, 153*, 607-617.

Rodabough, T. (1985). Near-death experiences: An examination of the supporting data and alternative explanations. *Death Studies, 9*, 95-113.

Roe, C. A. (2001). Near-death experiences. In R. Roberts & D. Groom (Eds.), *Parapsychology: The science of unusual experience*. New York: Oxford University Press.

Russell, P. (1983). *The global brain*. Los Angeles, CA: J. P. Tarcher.

Sabom, M. (1982). *Recollections of death: A medical investigation*. New York: Harper and Row.

Sabom, M. (1998). *Light at death: One doctor's fascinating account of near-death experiences*. Grand Rapids, MI: Zondervan.

Sabom, M., & Kreutziger, S. (1977). The experience of near-death. *Death Education, 1*, 195-203.

Sagan, C. (1979). *Broca's brain: Reflections on the romance of silence*. New York: Random House.

Schultz, J. (2004). *Near-death experiences: History, research, and a Christian response*. Unpublished manuscript, Marquette University, Milwaukee, Wisconsin.

Schwaninger, J., Eisenberg, P. R., Schechtman, K. B., & Weiss, A. N. (2002). A prospective analysis of near-death experiences in cardiac arrest patients. *Journal of Near-Death Studies, 20*(4), 215-232.

Schwenk, P. W. (1999). The benefits of working with "dead" patient: Hypnotically facilitated pseudo near-death experiences. *American Journal of Clinical Hypnosis, 42*(1) 36-49.

Serdahely, W. J. (1989). A pediatric near-death experience: Tunnel variants. *Omega, 20*, 55-62.

Serdahely, W. J. (1990). Pediatric near-death experiences. *Journal of Near-Death Studies, 9*, 33-39.

Serdahely, W. J. (1991). A comparison of retrospective accounts of childhood near-death experiences with contemporary pediatric near-death experiences with contemporary pediatric near-death experience accounts. *Journal of Near-Death Studies, 9*, 219-224.

Serdahely, W. J., & Walker, B. A. (1990). A near-death experience at birth. *Death Studies, 14,* 177-183.
Sheikh, A. A., & Sheikh, K. S. (2003). Death imagery: Confronting death brings us to the threshold of life. In A. A. Sheikh & K. S. Sheikh (Eds.), *Healing images: The role of imagination in health.* Amityville, NY: Baywood.
Siegel, R. K. (1980). The psychology of life after death. *American Psychologist, 35,* 911-931.
Siegel, R. (1993). *Fire in the brain: Clinical tales of hallucination.* London: Penguin.
Spraggett, A. (1974). *The case for immortality.* New York: Signet.
Sutherland, C. (1992). *Reborn in the light: Life after near-death experiences.* New York: Bantam.
Sutherland, C. (1995). *Children of the light: The near-death experiences of children.* New South Wales: Transworld.
Tart, C. (1974). Out-of-the-body experience. In E. Mitchell (Ed.), *Psychic exploration.* New York: Putnam's.
Taylor, G. R. (1979). *The natural history of the mind.* London: Penguin Books.
Teilhard de Chardin, P. (1959). *The phenomenon of man.* New York: Harper and Row.
Twemlow, S. W., & Gabbard, G. O. (1984). The influence of demographic/psychological factors and pre-existing conditions on the near-death experience. *Omega, 5,* 223-235.
Vaisrub, S. (1977). Afterthoughts of afterlife. *Archives of Internal Medicine, 137,* 150.
Valarino, E. E. (1997). On *the other side of life: Exploring the phenomenon of the near-death experience.* New York: Insight Books.
Van Lommel, P., Van Wees, R., Meyers, V., & Elfferich, I. (2001). Near-death experiences in survivors of cardiac arrest: A prospective study in the Netherlands. *The Lancet, 358,* 2039-2045.
Van Quekeberghe, R., Goebel, P., & Hertweck, E. (1995). Simulation of near-death and out-of-body experiences under hypnosis. *Imagination, Cognition and Personality, 14*(2), 151-164.
Walker, F. O. (1989). A nowhere near-death experience: Heavenly choirs interrupt myelography. *Journal of the American Medical Association, 261,* 3245-3246.
Walsh, R., & Shapiro, D. H. (1983). *Beyond health and normality.* New York: Van Nostrand Rheinhold.
Wilson, S. C., & Barber, T. X. (1981). Vivid fantasy and hallucinatory abilities in the life histories of excellent hypnotic subjects ("somnambules"): Preliminary report with female subjects. In E. Klinger (Ed.), *Imagery, Vol. 2. Concepts, results, and applications* (pp. 133-149). New York: Plenum.
Wilson, S. C., & Barber, T. X. (1983). The fantasy-prone personality: Implication for understanding imagery, hypnosis, and parapsychological phenomena. In A. A. Sheikh (Ed.), *Imagery: Current theory, research, and application.* New York: Wiley.
Wilson, I. (1997). *Life after death: The evidence.* London: Sidgwick and Jackson.
Yalom, I. D. (1980). *Existential psychotherapy.* New York: Basic Books.
Zaleski, C. (1987). *Otherworld journeys: Accounts of near-death experience in medieval and modern times.* New York: Oxford University Press.

CHAPTER 5

Death Imagery in the Buddhist Tradition

Sundar Ramaswami and Anees A. Sheikh

> It has been said that all the sacred teachings of the world could be summed up in the words: "Let go."
> Richard Boerstler (1982, p. 25)

> Only when you drink from the river of silence shall you indeed sing.
> Kahlil Gibran (1966, p. 81)

Death is perhaps the most important event in life. But most of us are frightened of dying because we don't know what it means to live. To live fully we must confront and transcend death. "If you die to everything you know, including your family, your memory, everything you have felt, then death is a purification, a rejuvenating process.... If you have died to one of your pleasures, the smallest or the greatest, naturally, without enforcement or argument, then you will know what it means to die. To die is to have a mind that is completely empty of itself, empty of its daily longings, pleasures and agonies. Death is a renewal, a mutation . . ." (Krishnamurti, 1969, p. 78). To understand death is to enrich life. This simple truth was well known to the great thinkers of every spiritual tradition. In this chapter, we shall present the concept of death and the use of death imagery in Buddhism. Since Buddhist notions of death and rebirth evolved out of Hindu ideas, we shall begin with an outline of the concept of death in early India. Death is also a source of great anxiety and, consequently, of much psychopathology. Hence, this chapter will conclude with a discussion of the implications of death for psychotherapy.

It is a healthy sign that psychologists have begun to concern themselves increasingly with the problem of dying. That death is a meaningful and integral part of life was readily apparent to Freud. Although he had drawn attention to this problem at the turn of the century, until recently it was ignored by the mainstream of Western psychology. Generally, death as a fact of life has been evaded and even denied.

In his Unpopular Essays, Bertrand Russell captured this mood.

> F.W.H. Myers, whom spiritualism had converted to a belief in a future life, questioned a woman who had lately lost her daughter as to what she supposed had become of her soul. The mother replied: "Oh well, I suppose she is enjoying eternal bliss, but I wish you wouldn't talk about such unpleasant subjects" (1950, p. 141).

But death has always been there, under the surface. Human beings constantly have been preoccupied with death. "If the word death were absent from our vocabulary, our great works of literature would have remained unwritten, pyramids and cathedrals would not exist, nor works of religious art and all art is of religious or magic origin" (Koestler, 1976, p. 239).

Today, death seems to have taken center stage. On the one hand, modern medicine is heroically trying to postpone and even conquer the Grim Reaper, on the other, there is such a

> pervasive preoccupation with the subject of death . . . in contemporary literature, journalism, television and cinema. It is as though modern man had reached a consensus that he might reduce death to a harmless nonentity merely by writing and talking about it to the point of exhaustion (Long, 1975, p. 52).

Our ambivalence toward death is to be expected. No other event evokes such powerful responses as intense anxiety, cataclysmic fears, deep depression, and terrible hopelessness. No wonder then that Rollo May declared, "The price for denying death is undefined anxiety, self alienation. To completely understand himself, man must confront death, become aware of personal death" (May, 1961, p. 65).

Frank (1959) agreed with this view and asserted that death gives meaning to life. Both May and Frankl echo the prevailing view in psychology that in order to live fully, the individual must confront his/her death, and the converse, that only those who have not really lived—who have unresolved problems, unfulfilled hopes and dreams—are afraid to die. This awareness has led to a growing conviction among many psychologists (Kübler-Ross, 1975; Wilcox & Sutton, 1977) that counseling and psychotherapy should embrace not only the art of living but also the art of dying.

The increasing interest in Eastern religions has prompted many psychologists to look to Eastern sources and perspectives on death. In many ways, the concept of death in Eastern religions is in striking contrast to Western notions of death and the afterlife.

CONCEPT OF DEATH IN EARLY INDIAN THOUGHT

When the Aryans—the nomadic tribes of eastern Europe and northwest Asia—entered the Indian subcontinent around 2000 B.C., they brought with them a pastoral culture. The Indo-Aryans, as they were later known, settled the Indus Valley in northwest India. Although their chief occupation was cattle breeding, they later turned to agriculture. Economic and social factors led the Indo-Aryans to develop a fourfold caste system. The highest caste were the priests, the Brahmins, who were the custodians of the Vedas, the sacred books of the Aryans. Next came the Kshatriyas, the warriors whose duty it was to defend the tribe. The Vaisyas, or traders, constituted the third or mercantile caste. The fourth and lowest caste, the Sudras or slaves, were made up of the indigenous population the Aryans had conquered.

The sacred literature of the Indo-Aryans, at first transmitted in an oral tradition, is contained in the Vedas (sacred hymns), the Brahmanas (ritual treatises), and the Upanishads (philosophical works). The Aranyakas (forest treatises) mark the transition from the Brahmanas to the Upanishads (Riepe, 1961). Historical research reveals that the early portions of the Vedas were composed before the Aryan tribes moved to India. The Vedas contain the names of gods found in Greek mythology; for example, Dyaus, a Vedic god, has the same linguistic root as Zeus. Again, the Vedic god Mitra is the Indo-Aryan counterpart of the Iranian Mithra (Hiriyanna, 1964). Studies in comparative mythology and philology show that there are many such names common to the Vedas and to the Iranian and European mythologies (Muller, 1879, 1887).

The hymns of the Rig-Veda reveal that the early Aryans worshipped natural forces.

> They treated the natural forces as divine, offered sacrifices for propitiating them, and prayed for wealth and enjoyment. Theirs was a religion of sacrifices and hymns to varied spirits or "shining" forces. The early Aryans, like the Greeks, were reflective primitive peoples, but not philosophical in the sense of having acquired systems of conceptual and abstract thought. They worshipped the natural forces and beings like the sun, the moon, the wind, the sky, the earth, fire, water and the clouds, as if they were animated beings like men, and made no distinction between body and mind (Raju, 1971, p. 28).

The religion of these Vedic people was organized around the fire sacrifice. Sacrificial offerings of milk, butter, grain, and ghee were bestowed on the gods. "The motive was to secure the objects of ordinary desire—children, cattle, etc., or to get one's enemy out of the way" (Hiriyanna, 1964, p. 35).

The details of the Vedic religion need not detain us. Suffice it to remark that the Vedic religion was life affirming and this-worldly. There is no sign of the ennui that later overtook the Aryans during the period of the Upanishads. The Aryans enjoyed music and dancing, gambling and drinking. The desire for riches is constantly emphasized.

> May the liberal givers, O Agni, attain nourishment, may the rich who bestow gifts [on us] attain to a full span of life. May we win in the battle the booty of him who does not give, obtaining a [rich] share before the gods, that we may win glory (*The Rig-Veda*, Mandala I, Hymn 73, Verse 5, 1897, p. 88).

The Vedas also reveal the more serious concerns of the Vedic poets. The Vedic sages believed in a supreme cosmic principle (Rta) to which they attributed the natural order in the universe. The seasons as well as the fate of a community were due to Rta, whose divine protectors were the deities Varuna and Mitra. The other deities were nature gods and goddesses with specific areas of competence.

There are scanty references to death in the Vedic hymns. The Vedic poets pled for a long and prosperous life while wishing death for their enemies. Certainly, despite the prevailing optimism, there was an awareness of human mortality. There was the recognition that death was inevitable. Nevertheless, death could be postponed by bestowing gifts on the gods. The early parts of the Vedas do not reveal an interest in the afterlife, but the ninth and tenth books of the Rig-Veda do deal with an afterlife (Holck, 1974). When buried or cremated, the body is not to be eaten by insects or animals since the entire person will be restored in the next world. There are two paths: that of the fathers (blessed ancestors now residing in heaven) and that of the gods, by which the dead leave this world. The services for the dead revolve around hymns urging the dead to take the ancestral way (pitryana) to Yama's (the Hindu god of death) realm where

> if he was a liberal giver and had acted in compliance with Rta, he may now join forever the blessed company of Yama, the Fathers, and the gods. This heaven had rather mundane and materialistic features (*The Rig-Veda*, IX, 113, 7-11). Although such pleasures of this world as the drinking of soma, milk, and honey and experiencing love could be enjoyed in Yama's kingdom, the Vedic Aryan was not particularly eager to enter heaven; he was too much this-worldly oriented (Holck, 1974, p. 31).

Yama, the king of death, was himself the first mortal to die and enter that other world. He and his sister Yami also were considered to be the parents of the human race.

There is no mention of postmortem judgment in the Rig-Veda. Yama's world, with its everlasting pleasures, was open to all who had performed good works and the appropriate sacrifices to the Vedic gods. Nevertheless, there are allusions to the punishment that befalls the wicked. There is mention of a deep abyss, which "has been produced [for those who], being sinners, false, untrue, go about like women without brothers, like wicked females hostile to their husbands" (Muir, 1884, p. 312). The Atharva-Veda, in a more explicit reference to hell, describes it as the place for female goblins and sorceresses (Keith, 1925).

On the whole, the Aryans were stoically resigned to death. The belief that Yama had prepared a world of everlasting pleasures, to be enjoyed in the company of one's family and ancestors, made it easier for them to face death. However, these heavenly pleasures did not tempt them to seek an early death. The Vedic people yearned for a long life—100 years was considered the ideal.

Beginning in the tenth century B.C., the gods of the Vedas began to lose their significance. The sacrificial rituals expanded, and commentaries and manuals on the sacrifice proliferated. These manuals, called the Brahmanas, describe with great precision the correct order of the sacrifice. In the Brahmanas, death is "identified with Time, symbolized by the Year, and also identical with divine principle, Prajapati, the Lord of creatures, who created the gods and the mortal beings as well as Death, their consumer" (Holck, 1974, p. 39). Prajapati is said to exist in a symbiotic relationship with his creation. Death is said to consume the creatures for his own sustenance. But, since Prajapati and Death are homologized, it is Prajapati who devours his creatures to quench his hunger and to acquire the energies needed to sustain the world. Thus, Prajapati perpetuates the life cycle, first by devouring his creatures, then by creating them anew. Prajapati is both the creator and the destroyer of the cosmos. The hymns addressed to Prajapati celebrate the fact that life and death are two aspects of a natural cycle. To renew the universe by the procreation of new beings, Prajapati has to destroy existing creatures (Long, 1977).

During the late Vedic period (seventh to sixth centuries B.C.), disenchantment with the sacrifice and the Brahmin priests set in. New movements and schools of thought appeared that questioned the efficacy of sacrificial rites as well as the powers of the embarrassing multitude of gods. The speculations of the philosophers of this period gave rise to the Upanishads, the last branch of Vedic literature. The Upanishads (there are 108 of them), whose authorship and exact age are obscure, are religiophilosophical treatises that use dialogue and parable to explain the nature of reality.

According to the Upanishads, there is a single, eternal, changeless entity underlying the constantly changing forms of existence. In its macrocosmic aspect, it is Brahman, the eternal substrate of the universe. In its microcosmic aspect, it is Atman, the essence of the immortal human soul.

> While the term Atman—originally meaning the breath of life—represents in its development a movement from microcosm to macrocosm, the term Brahman, as the eternal ground of the universe, represents movement in the opposite direction by way of emanation. The two meet in man and become identical when he, in a mystical experience, not in a reasoning thought process, realizes the great oneness with totality (sarvam). Duality is transcended and with it, time and space, moral and social categories, suffering and death (Holck, 1974, p. 43).

This experience is *moksha* or liberation from selfhood, the merger of Atman, the individual self, with Brahman, the universal self. This union with Brahman is immortality; for, in realizing Brahman, the Supreme Self, one is freed from the chain of rebirth.

The individual soul, Atman, is attached to the body and partakes of the pleasures and pains to which the body is subject. Death is no escape; for, although the various components of an individual unite with corresponding elements in nature, karma stays attached to Atman and decides the nature of the next existence.

According to the doctrine of karma, as one acts so one becomes. Human beings, by their actions and behavior, are ultimately responsible for their lives. The law of karma is the moral counterpart of the physical laws of the universe. There is nothing capricious in the moral realm. Individuals reap what they sow. There is salvation not through the gods and sacrifices but through good deeds. People are asked to will the good and do the good (Radhakrishnan, 1951). There is a causal relation between one's actions and the results of those actions not only in this life but over successive lives. Whatever happens to us in this lifetime is largely the result of past actions. Yet, the future is in our hands; for, we can become good through the conscious performance of good deeds.

An understanding of the Upanishadic concept of karma and transmigration of the soul is crucial to an understanding of the later Buddhist view of death. The Upanishads assert that upon death, the fruits of past actions (karma) as well as one's mental tendencies (*vasana*) attach themselves to a *linga sarira*, a "subtle" body, which underlies the gross body in an ethereal form. The subtle body serves as the vehicle for the transport of karma from one life to the next. The Brihadaranyaka Upanishad explains the mechanism of rebirth:

> Then his knowledge and his works and his previous experience take him by the hand. As a caterpillar which has wriggled to the top of a blade of grass draws itself over to a new blade, so does the man after he has put aside his body draw himself over to a new existence (Radhakrishnan, 1951, p. 253).

Thus, death is no escape for the hapless Atman, the individual soul. It not only survives the death of the physical body but also inherits the results of the actions of previous lives. Burdened by its karmic load, the Atman is condemned to *samsara*, the perpetual round of life and death.

> Death can be nothing more than a "way-station" between successive terms of life. A person can expect to escape the sentence of death (lit: "redeath") only by discovering and identifying himself with that deep down essential self which is free from evil, death and all the rest, that Absolute One which is both existence and nonexistence, both birth and death. He who discovers the one, changeless, immortal, unnameable Brahman (= cosmic-self) to be identical with the changeless and immortal atman (= human-self) will be liberated from the sentence of the "Eternal Return," and, on the soul's departure from the world of temporality, birth and death, it will "abide in the world of the Brahman" (Long, 1975, p. 58).

The individual who realizes the essential identity of Atman with Brahman attains to moksha or liberation from the endless cycle of birth and death, time and karma. With the merging of Atman into Brahman, the individual enters the state of *samadhi,* a state of pure consciousness often described as "sleepless sleep." The disengagement of the Atman from the psychophysical complex that thinks, feels, and acts, and its union with Brahman, were the critical problems of Hindu thought in the sixth century B.C. Many were the paths that were purported to lead to liberation. It was into this age of great intellectual ferment that the Buddha was born.

DEATH IN BUDDHIST THOUGHT

The future Buddha was born Gautama Siddhartha, the son of Suddhodhana, king of the Sakya tribe, which made its home along the border with present-day Nepal. The biography of the Buddha is a mixture of history and legend. The details need not detain us. Suffice it to say that on beholding the infant, the sage Asita proclaimed that the boy would attain enlightenment after renouncing the throne. To thwart the prophecy about the renunciation, King Suddhodhana surrounded the young prince with every luxury. At 16, he was married to the lovely Sakya princess Yasodhara.

But the prophecy was not to be thwarted. On several excursions out of the palace, the young prince saw an old man, a sick man, and a corpse. Worldly pleasures lost their charm for the young prince. One more incident was needed to complete Siddhartha's conversion. On the fourth trip out of the palace, he saw an ascetic, begging bowl in hand, at peace with the world. The prince, impressed by the equanimity and self-possession of the itinerant mendicant, resolved to lead such a life.

After bidding farewell to his sleeping son, the prince stealthily left the palace in the dead of night. In his early years as an ascetic, Siddhartha practiced meditation under the tutelage of several yogic teachers. Dissatisfied, he turned to the practice of arduous penances for six long years. At the end of it all, he was nowhere near his goal. He decided to try another way, that of attaining salvation through his mind alone. The decisive moment had arrived, the ascetic was about to become the Enlightened One. Assuming the classic pose of a yogi, Siddhartha vowed not to move until he achieved enlightenment.

On the night of his enlightenment, the Buddha was able to recall, in great detail, more than 500 of his previous lives in animal and human forms. According to legend, he had evolved through these many lives and perfected his qualities such that he was able to come to his last life (Amore, 1974). As he was poised to win final liberation from the endless cycle of rebirth and redeath, the attack by Mara began.

Mara, Death's Advocate

Mara is a powerful god whose kingdom includes the earth, hell, and the spheres of desire. He oversees procreation and replenishes the world. In this aspect, he is the Buddhist counterpart to Prajapati. The various lesser Hindu gods lived in mortal fear of Prajapati lest he end their lives. It was possible to attain immortality by constructing a fire altar exactly according to Prajapati's specifications. This device, however, had potentially disturbing consequences: "If the human mortals should employ the same method, they could share immortality with the gods and thus cheat Death out of his right. Therefore, the gods decided that no living being should enjoy immortality with a body" (Holck, 1974, p. 39). Prajapati in his aspect as Death (*mrtyu*) devoured the body.

When Mara launched his assault on the Buddha, he was merely defending his kingdom. He was both a destructive and a productive agent, Death as well as Love (Kama, hence often called Kama-Mara); and the future Buddha had vowed to destroy this kingdom. In defending his realm, Mara also

> wished to preserve the right of action, of ownership, the right to happiness, the right to love, to marry, to have children, perpetuate the family and so carry on the cycle of earthly life. A frightful cycle of ephemeral joys, illusory happiness, and a perpetual succession of lives furnishing new causes for sorrow and death, contended the monk. Perhaps he in turn was right, but let the whole of humanity become part of the Buddhist Community and in one generation the whole earth will be depopulated. . . . The Buddha's contemporaries did not fail to see this practical result of the Master's doctrine. Soon the people of Magadha were heard to murmur that "Gautama the Ascetic has come to preach the extinction of the families." So Mara was not the only one to protest, and he might well plead not only that he was representing the most legitimate interests of the individual but that he was defending social solidarity (Foucher, 1963, pp. 110-111).

Mara's argument appears persuasive. The future Buddha threatened the world order. Mara had another role to play. He, like Lucifer in Christianity and Iblis in Islam, is the accuser of humankind. He protests that the future Buddha is spiritually unqualified to aspire to enlightenment (Amore, 1974).

Buddhist texts give conflicting accounts of the contest between Mara and the Bodhisattva. On two points all the texts agree: Mara wanted the battle to take place before the Bodhisattva attained enlightenment, since he knew that he could not defeat a Buddha. Further, in this contest the Bodhisattva was completely alone.

> Not only had his five companions abandoned him as a false prophet, but the gods, who had been hovering in the background, prudently left at the approach of the conflict, only to return later for the proclamation of a victory to which they did not contribute (Foucher, 1963, p. 111).

Mara is also the Tempter. The contest represents, in allegorical fashion, Gautama's final temptation, the "dark night of the soul" so familiar to Christian theology. It is safe to assume that all base instincts, evil thoughts, desires, passions, and seeds of sin were cast aside altogether and the mind so prepared for the marvelous flowering of enlightenment.

In the weeks immediately following the enlightenment, Mara again sought to defend his kingdom. If the Buddha could be persuaded to go directly from Enlightenment to Parinirvana (death), Mara's realm would lose only one member and would therefore remain inviolate. Mara approached the Buddha and urged him to enter Parinirvana. The Buddha rejected his plea, declaring that he would enter Parinirvana only after preaching his doctrine.

On the night of his enlightenment, the Buddha is said to have gained insight into the nature of death. In the first watch of the night, he recalled all his previous lives. Thus, he gained knowledge of how humans can spiritually evolve through numerous lives. In the second watch, he saw the death and rebirth of human beings, confirming the doctrine of rebirth. In the third watch, he gained understanding of the impermanence of the universe. It was this insight that he propounded in the Doctrine of Dependent Origination (Conditioned Genesis). We shall briefly outline this doctrine, beginning with the central problem of this volume, namely, death.

Old age and death exist because of birth. They are conditioned by it and could not occur without it. Birth and rebirth are dependent on the process of becoming, which is conditioned by clinging. There are four kinds of clinging: clinging to sensuality, to erroneous views, to rituals, and to belief in the ego/self. Clinging is a developed form of craving and is conditioned by the latter. Craving, in turn, is conditioned by affect (feeling) which is dependent on sense impression. Sense impressions are based on the sensual system inherent in the human body. The sensual system is dependent on the mentality and corporeality of the body. Mentality includes feeling, perception, cognition, and volition. Corporeality refers to the physical elements that make up the body. Mentality and corporeality will not exist in the first place without the karma-laden consciousness, which migrated from one's previous existence. This consciousness is conditioned by the karma formations, which are rebirth-producing volitions. Finally, it is ignorance or lack of insight that prompts the volitions and motivations to be oriented toward rebirth (Amore, 1974). The Doctrine of Conditioned Genesis accounts for birth as well as death.

Viewed from afar, birth and death are normally separated by many years. In reality, though, dying and rebirth occur at successive moments of time. As we have seen, the Buddha denied the existence of a permanent, unchanging, eternal soul or self. The human being is made up of five constituent factors (*skandhas*), physical and mental elements that are continuously changing and succeeding each other. The skandhas are an everchanging bundle from moment to moment and from birth to death. Thus, the human being dies each moment and is reborn at the succeeding moment. This "dying" and "rebirth" at every moment of life is not felt because of *bhava,* the continuity of consciousness over time. "When the Aggregates arise, decay and die, O bhikkhu, every moment you are born, decay and die" (Paramatthajotika I, cited in Rahula, 1962, p. 33). In every instant one is born, and in every succeeding instant one dies.

When what we know as death occurs, the physical organism ceases to function, but the energies that make up the individual do not cease.

> Will, volition, desire, thirst to exist, to continue, to become more and more, is a tremendous force that moves whole lives, whole existences, that even moves the whole world. . . . According to Buddhism, this force does not stop with the nonfunctioning of the body, which is death; but it continues manifesting itself in another form, producing re-existence which is called rebirth (Rahula, 1962, p. 33).

Thus, although there is a complete nonfunctioning of the psychophysical organism, the life energies are not destroyed. They are channeled into another form.

The Doctrine of Rebirth

As mentioned earlier, Buddhism denies the existence of a permanent, unchanging soul or self that endures from moment to moment and from one life to another. The self is but a stream of consciousness, a series of psychophysiological occasions

> changing momentarily and filled with impressions and tendencies created by good and evil actions (karma) which at death is transposed to a new mode of being, while the imagined "self" who thinks in terms of "I" and "mine" does not survive from one moment to the next and hence, does not transmigrate (Long, 1975, p. 66).

What evidence does Buddhism offer in support of the doctrine of rebirth? If there is no permanent substance or soul, what is it that is reborn? Epistemologically, the Buddha was an experientialist, a mystic who claimed a higher, personal knowledge derived from his extrasensory powers of perception. The Buddha, it must be reiterated, was not unique in claiming mystic potency. Thinkers who claimed a final knowledge based on extrasensory perception, the so-called *jnanavadins* (literally, Knowing and Seeing ones), are found in the pre-Buddhist Vedic period as well as in the late Upanishadic period contemporaneous with the Buddha. Although the Buddha classified himself as an experientialist, he asserted that the others had drawn erroneous conclusions—about the soul, Brahman, and so on—from their experiences.

The Buddha is said to have gained his insight into the phenomenon of rebirth on the night of his enlightenment. The Digha-Nikaya describes his insight:

> When his mind is thus composed, clear and cleansed, without blemish, free from adventitious defilements, pliant and flexible, steadfast and unperturbed, he turns and directs his mind to the recollection of his former lives, viz. one life, two lives . . . ten lives . . . a hundred lives . . . through evolving aeons, recalling in what place he was born, his name and title, his social status, his environment, experiences and term of life and dying there in what place he

was next born and so on up to his present existence, he remembers the varied states of his former lives in all their aspects and details. Just as a man who has travelled from his village to another and from that to yet another, when to his former village by the same route, remembers how he came from that village, where he stayed and rested, what he said and what he did; even so, when the mind is composed . . . (*Digha-Nikaya*, 1890-1911, I, p. 81).

At first glance, the Buddhist doctrine of rebirth seems to conform faithfully to the theory propounded by the Upanishadic sages. Nevertheless, there are significant differences between the Upanishadic and Buddhist theories. The Buddha denied the existence of a single, eternal entity—whether it be the microcosmic Atman or the macrocosmic Brahman—underlying phenomenal existence. Therefore, there is no question of the Atman merging with the Brahman upon liberation. For the Upanishadic thinkers, immortality consisted in realizing that one's inner nature is identical with Brahman, the eternal ground substance of the universe. For the Buddha, immortality, or freedom from rebirth, lay in attaining the realization that the self is a causally conditioned illusion. Again, the Upanishadic thinkers propounded the theory that the Atman transmigrated from life to life. It is the Atman that inherits the karmic load of the individual, and this karmic load can be cast aside only though moksha or liberation—the union of Atman with Brahman.

However, the Buddha asserted that karma could end only through attaining Nirvana, the ultimate insight into the nature of existence. Since there was no soul apart from a complex of psychophysical processes, no permanent unchanging substance transmigrated from life to life. The everchanging series of skandhas, the bundle that is perpetually in movement, continues. It is the stream of becoming (*bhava-sota*) or stream of consciousness (*vinnanasota*) that carries karmic volitions.

For the Upanishadic philosophers, identity, in the sense of an individual self, continued unbroken from one life to the next. According to Buddhism, there is continuity without identity. The stream of consciousness moves on like a flame that burns through the night; it is neither the same flame nor is it different. "The corpse and the new baby are causally conditioned and interconnected, but not identical" (Becker, 1981, p. 106).

Despite these differences, the Buddhist notion of karma is similar to the earlier Hindu concept. Both systems assert that human beings cannot escape the effects of their actions. The past produces the present as well as the future. Karma as volitional actions may be good or bad depending on the moral tone of the actions; these ethically good or evil acts give rise to consequences that may be manifested in this life or a future life. The operation of karma is probabilistic, not deterministic. "Karmic laws, therefore, state tendencies rather than inevitable consequences . . . . The general principle is that morally good acts tend to be followed in the long run by pleasant consequences and morally evil acts by unpleasant consequences to the individual" (Jayatilleke, 1975, p. 147).

Karma includes a person's psychological inheritance: unconscious impulses, temperament, character, and so on. This psychological residue is transmitted from one life to the next. Thus, the history of a human being does not commence at birth: it has been ages in the making. Yet, in both Hindu and Buddhist thought, the operation of karma is not inexorable. Human beings are mightier than karma and can ultimately triumph over it. Because they are free, human beings can shape their future; they can forever escape the wheel of karma and achieve immortality through enlightenment.

On the same night when the Buddha gained insight into rebirth, he was able to see, through his powers of clairvoyance, the rebirth of human beings, in various planes of existence. In the Mahasihanada Sutta, the Buddha said,

> There are these five destinies, Sariputta. What five? The lower worlds, the animal kingdom, the spirit-sphere, human existence and the higher worlds. I know these lower worlds, the path which leads to them or the kind of conduct which takes you to that state of existence at death (cited in Jayatilleke, 1975, p. 144).

As we have seen earlier, *The Rig-Veda* (1897) mentioned a heaven with everlasting pleasures and a hell to which the wicked go. The Buddha incorporated this Vedic concept and offered a heaven (the higher or deva world) for the doer of good, a hell for the wicked, and rebirth for the imperfect.

The five planes of existence are classified according to the degree of pleasure or pain experienced in them (McGovern, 1923). In the human world, one experiences more pleasant than unpleasant events. In the spirit sphere, one experiences more unpleasant than pleasant events. The animal world is supposed to be one of unpleasant sensations because animals are motivated by baser instincts. The lower worlds are regarded as wholly unpleasant, in contrast to the deva world, or heaven, which is wholly pleasant. The deva world and the lower worlds correspond to the Vedic heaven and hell.

There is continuity of individuality in all the planes of existence. The human being is regarded as an admixture of both good and evil, and human consciousness is considered as finely attuned to an earthly existence. Consequently, the normal pattern is to return to a human existence upon death.

> But it is possible to regress to animal or subhuman forms of existence by neglecting the development of one's personality or character and becoming a slave to one's passions. It is also exceptionally possible to attain to existence in the deva-worlds (Jayatilleke, 1975, p. 136).

Nevertheless, the various planes of existence are still subject to karma and hence within the cycle of samsara. The individual who is reborn in any of these planes is continuously generating karma and is therefore subject to death and rebirth in a different form. Thus, both heaven and hell are intermediate stations where one enjoyed or suffered, for a short time, the fruits of one's karma before returning to a human existence.

Mechanism of Rebirth

Bhavanga or life continuum, along with intellect, emotion, will, and karma, is transmitted to the next life at the moment of death. This transmission is explained in several ways. The analogy of impressing a seal on muddy ground is often used.

> Our present existence is the seal, our being on an intermediate level the muddy ground. The design carved on the seal is karma. At the moment the seal is impressed on the surface of the ground the design is exactly transposed; in the same way all karma is transmitted to this intermediate state of being at the time of death (Yasutani, 1971, p. 44).

This intermediate being then awaits the opportunity to be conceived and is said to have the capacity to locate its parents-to-be.

Coomaraswamy (1971) used the analogy of billiard balls to explain the transmission of karma. If a moving billiard ball hits a row of stationary balls, the foremost stationary ball will move forward. The moving ball comes to a stop, but it is this ball's momentum, its karma, so to speak, that gives the impetus to the foremost stationary ball. Similarly, rebirth is an unceasing transmission of an impulse. In this transmission, the last thought of a dying person is crucial, since it encapsulates the moral life of the individual. The first thought on rebirth is believed to arise from two causes: the last thought of the previous life and the moral tone of the deeds performed in the previous life. Thus, the last thought of a dying person is potent in determining the destiny of the next life.

The last thought of a dying individual usually reflects a refusal to let go, a clinging to existence. This clinging to existence, known as *upadana*, is the thought force that holds together both karma and the skandhas and makes rebirth possible.

Another view holds that at the moment of death, a psychic force called *vijnana* karmically informs the next life. It is vijnana that migrates endlessly from body to body and life to life; it can be stopped with the attainment of Nirvana, when karma is extinguished and consequently no vijnana is generated that can cause another birth.

The Pudagalavadins, one school of Buddhism, believed that a personal self, the *pudagala,* exists. However, this "self" was not apart from the skandhas nor was it identical to them. By introducing a subtle self that was neither identical to nor apart from the skandhas, the Pudagalavadins avoided being branded as believers in a permanent soul, while at the same time offering an elegant explanation for transmigration. It was the pudagala, they asserted, that transmigrates from life to life, thus providing individual continuity. This Pudagalavadin view is at odds with the orthodox school's (Theravadin) assertion that all five Aggregates, including personal consciousness, are extinguished at death. What passes over into the next life is not a soul or individual consciousness but karma that has not been exhausted and *tanha*, the thirst for existence. Karma and tanha create a new being, a new set of skandhas, as well as a new individual consciousness that descends into the womb. It must be emphasized that Buddhism asserts rebirth but not reincarnation since there is no entity that reincarnates itself.

Buddhaghosa (1976) spoke of a "rebirth-linking" consciousness whose chief function is to link the present state with the immediately following state of existence. This rebirth-linking consciousness is influenced by the last moment of consciousness before death as well as by karma. It is the rebirth-linking consciousness that descends into the womb.

In the *Majjhima Nikaya* (1948-1951), three factors necessary for conception are mentioned: sexual intercourse, the correct phase in the menstrual cycle of the mother-to-be, and the presence of a *gandhabba*. According to Buddhaghosa (1976), the gandhabba is a being ready to descend into the womb. More accurately, the gandhabba is a term for the rebirth-linking consciousness (McDermott, 1980; Piyadassi, 1972).

The Intermediate-State Being

Early Buddhists denied the possibility of disembodied consciousness existing in an intermediate state between death and rebirth. Nevertheless, the concept of *antara-bhava* (intermediate-state being) has intruded into Buddhist tradition. Thus, while Buddhaghosa (1976) denied that the gandhabba is an intermediate being, this Theravadin view is hotly disputed by other schools, such as the Sarastivadins. Arguing the case for an intermediate-state being, Vasabandhu (cited in McDermott, 1980) asserted that the intermediate-state being is found between two destinies. It exists only between the time of death and the time of birth and is made up of five skandhas. Vasabandhu then proceeded to explain the phenomenon of rebirth:

> The Oedipal character of his analysis would do justice to Freud: driven by karma, the intermediate-state being goes to the location where rebirth is to take place. Possessing the divine eye by virtue of its karma, it is able to see the place of its birth, no matter how distant. There it sees its father and its mother to be, united in intercourse. Finding the scene hospitable, its passions are stirred. If male, it is smitten with desire for its mother. If female, it is seized with desire for its father. And inversely, it hates either mother or father, which it comes to regard as rival. Concupiscence and hatred thus arise in the gandharva as its driving passions. Stirred by these wrong thoughts, it attaches itself to the place where the sexual organs of the parents are united, imagining that it is there joined with the object of its passion. Taking pleasure in the impurity of the semen and blood in the womb, the antara bhava establishes itself there. Thus do the skandhas arise in the womb. They harden; and the intermediate-state being perishes, to be replaced immediately by the birth existence (pratisamdhi) (McDermott, 1980, pp. 171-172).

The description of the Bardo (literally, between) state between death and rebirth that is found in the Bardo Thodol, *The Tibetan Book of the Dead* (Evans-Wentz, 1960) is of great interest. The Bardo Thodol—"Salvation by Hearing While in the Intermediate State"—comes from the Mahayana Buddhism of Tibet, which freely borrows from the native Lamaism of Tibet. Probably written in the sixth century A.D., it was meant as a guidebook for the dying. Recited as a breviary to the dying person, the Bardo Thodol outlines the experiences he or she will undergo in the 49 symbolic days of the Bardo, the intermediate state between death and the return to a new birth. Like its counterpart, the *Egyptian Book of the Dead* (1894), the Bardo Thodol is a map through the terrain of the dead and has an initiatory function (Eliade, 1958, 1974). According to Buddhism, the mind is most clear during the process of dying and hence dying offers a unique opportunity to discover one's true nature. Consequently, the Tibetan Book approaches dying as a positive learning experience.

Verses from this book are recited not only at the time of death but immediately following death and during the 49 days intervening between death and rebirth (Beck, 1943). The manner in which the passages are recited is described by Evans-Wentz (1960). Ideally, one's guru should recite the text. If this is not possible, a Buddhist priest should be sought out. If he or she too is unavailable, then a person who can read correctly and distinctly should repeat the verses several times.

> When breathing is about to cease, the guide addresses the dying person thus:
>
> O nobly-born (so and so by name), the time hath now come for thee to seek the path (in reality). Thy breathing is about to cease. Thy guru hath set thee face to face before with the Clear Light; and now thou art about to experience it in its Reality in the Bardo state, wherein all things are like the Void and cloudless sky, and the naked, spotless intellect is like unto a transparent vacuum without circumference or centre. At this moment, know thou thyself; and abide in that state. I, too, at this time, am setting thee face to face (Evans-Wentz, 1960, p. 91).

This verse is repeated many times before breathing ceases. When the person is about to die, he or she is turned over on the right side, to assume what is known as the "lying posture of a lion," the very posture adopted by the Buddha at the moment of his death. If the person appears to slip into a coma or deep sleep, the arteries are pressed firmly—the dying person should die fully aware and conscious. Since the last thought before death is of great importance, the guide attempts to shape it.

> O nobly-born, that which is called death being come to thee now, resolve thus: "O this now is the hour of death. By taking advantage of this death, I will so act, for the good of all sentient beings, peopling the illimitable expanse of the heavens, as to obtain the Perfect Buddhahood, by resolving on love and

compassion towards them, and by directing my entire effort to the Sole Perfection" (Evans-Wentz, 1960, p. 94).

The text describes three stages in the Bardo, and all three are conditioned by karma. The first stage is the Chikai Bardo, which is the state immediately following death. At the approach of death, there is a loss of consciousness. The awareness of objects is lost; this state is often called "the swoon" (Beck, 1943). An intense and blinding light appears, which is the "Radiance of the Clear Light of Pure Reality" (Evans-Wentz, 1960).

> If it is recognized and approached as the void (sunyata), then liberation will be obtained immediately, for this clear light is the Dharma-Kaya, the supreme essence of Buddhahood. If one fails to dwell in the light of the Void, a secondary, lesser clear light appears which can dispel the power of karma. But one's bad karma may cause one to miss this too (Holck, 1974, p. 142).

All dying individuals encounter this dazzling Light and have the opportunity to abandon separate ego/existence and unite with the Light, thus attaining liberation from rebirth. However, the majority of individuals are propelled by ignorance and craving, and are unequal to the task of becoming absorbed in it. They descend progressively into lower states of Bardo existence and eventually find their way back to earthly life. Each Bardo state affords the dying individual an opportunity to overcome karmic propensities; there is an opportunity, at every stage, to arrest one's descent.

In the second or Chonyid Bardo state, the individual recovers from the swoon and partially regains consciousness of objects. He or she asks himself or herself, "Am I dead or not?" without being able to arrive at a conclusion. He or she sees his or her funeral taking place as the guide recites,

> O nobly-born, that which is called death hath now come. Thou art departing from this world, but thou art not the only one; death cometh to all. Do not cling, in fondness and weakness, to this life. Even though thou clingest out of weakness, thou hast not the power to remain here. Thou wilt gain nothing more than wandering in this Sangsara. Be not attached to this world; be not weak. Remember the Precious Trinity (Evans-Wentz, 1960, p. 103).

The guide then recites the verses that interpret the hallucinations that are about to occur. These hallucinations are, in fact, "karmic illusions" woven out of the fabric of one's past thoughts and actions. For seven days, benign deities and Buddhas appear surrounded by bright lights. Another cycle of seven days follows in which terrifying deities appear. Experiences of judgment and punishment in various hells follow. The text reminds the dead individual that these encounters with benign and wrathful deities are fabrications of his or her mind (Hick, 1976).

In the third Bardo state, the Sidpa Bardo, there is intense craving for rebirth. The fierce wind that is karma propels the disincarnate, intermediate being toward rebirth. It is the power of karma that chooses the realm in which rebirth is to take place. Even now, rebirth can be avoided by meditating on the "Clear Light of Pure Reality." If this struggle fails, rebirth is inevitable and is said to occur on the 49th day after death. Beck (1943, p. 202) described the process thus:

> And now, still steadily declining toward earth, the disincarnate one perceives the mating of men and women, and is still drawn downwards to the gateway of the womb. If he is to be born as a male the Knower (the soul) begins to experience the feeling of maleness, to be torn with a feeling of hatred to its future father, of love to its future mother (this is strangely Freudian) and vice versa if it is to be born as a female. Again the swoon takes it, but this time the swoon preceding birth; and it enters the embryonic stage in the womb with its doom pronounced by itself. Future wandering through births and deaths is to be its portion, until the time comes when on seeing the Clear Light it shall recognize it as Itself and its Own, and be one with it by instinctive knowledge and realization.

Heaven and Hell: Postmortem Judgment

Buddhism borrows two concepts from Upanishadic thought: samsara (round of births and deaths) and karma. In both Hinduism and Buddhism, karma acts as a continuous process of judgment. Karma determines not only one's destiny in the next life but also the plane of existence into which one will be reborn.

Buddhist mythology admits heavens and hells that are derived from earlier Hindu notions. The Pali Nikayas classified five realms or destinies in which one may be reborn:

1. *niraya* or hell, commonly referred to as the lower world;
2. *deva* world, or heaven;
3. *tiracchanayoni*, or animal world;
4. *manussa*, or human world; and
5. *pettivisaya*, the world of spirits and ghosts (*Digha-Nikaya*, 1890-1911).

Niraya, the animal world, and the spirit sphere are regarded as unhappy destinies. Heavenly existence and the human world are the only two states of existence considered desirable. The realm into which one is born is determined by one's karma. As we have seen earlier, the Buddha was able to predict, by his clairvoyant knowledge of the individual's karma, the realm into which he or she would be reborn.

While Buddhism denies that there is a Creator behind creation, it recognizes various gods. These devas or gods were former humans, who, through accumulation of merit, had earned the privilege of dwelling temporarily in heaven. With the depletion of their good karma, they too are reborn once again in a lower state of existence. Thus, the gods too are not immune from rebirth. Escape from samsara is possible only through attaining Nirvana. Even the Buddha, who had had many earthly lives and had lived in the heavens as a god, had to be reborn as a human. He was finally freed from the round of birth and death only because of his insight into the nature of Ultimate Reality.

A later development in Buddhist thought, Mahayana (literally, Great Vehicle) Buddhism, created many heavens and populated them with many Buddhas. The most well known of these Buddhas is Amitabha (Unmeasured Light), who is believed to live in a Pure Land to the west. The Pure Land Buddhists believe that devotion to Amitabha will ensure a rebirth in his heaven which is

> adorned with seven terraces, rows of palm trees, strings of bells, and enclosed with four great jewels. There are lotus lakes full of lovely water, lotus-flowers of all colours, heavenly musical instruments always playing, blossoms always raining down, while swans and peacocks sound the remembrance of Buddhist doctrine (Parrinder, 1973, p. 91).

Although there are allusions to postmortem punishment in the Rig-Veda, it is not until one reads the Atharva-Veda that one finds explicit descriptions of hell. The Hindu notion of hell as a terrible pit full of fire and replete with engines of torture and presided over by Yama found its way into Buddhism. The *Anguttara-Nikaya* (1885-1900) described the punishment for wicked deeds. Some deeds, like robbery, are punished in this very life by the laws of the land. Some others may have punitive consequences in a future life. Certain offenses, however, lead to a hellish existence in the very next birth. Also, a heavily demeritorious karma can lead to a hellish rebirth. Buddhist art vividly portrays the tortures of hell. In Buddhist scriptures, there are also references to a Judgment before Yama, the King of the Dead. Yama, it is believed, will hold up in front of the deceased the shining mirror of karma in which all his or her deeds will be reflected. The mirror is the dead individual's memory, and the judgment is also his or her own, the product of his or her past. In reality, there is no Judge of the Dead apart from karmic forces (Conze, 1959).

Beyond Heaven and Hell:
Nirvana as Deathlessness

In the Vedic view, one could "win a heaven" by performing the correct sacrifices. By devotion and sacrifices to a particular god, one could, after death, attain to the heaven ruled by that god. This notion of winning a heaven as a recompense for a lifetime of good works is found in other religious traditions as well (Amore, 1974).

However, in the late Upanishadic period (sixth century B.C.), the concept of winning a heaven was decried. The Upanishads exhorted human beings to strive toward the loftier goal of realizing Brahman. By this period, the concept of reincarnation had become firmly entrenched: heaven and hell were both regarded as temporary, intermediate stations where one enjoyed or suffered, for a short time, the fruits of one's karma. Liberation (moksha) from samsara and karma, the Upanishads asserted, could be had only by realizing Brahman.

The Buddha, too, regarded a heavenly rebirth as a lesser goal than Nirvana, the complete liberation from samsara. Owing to past karma, one may be reborn in various planes of existence, including heaven and hell. But, in all these worlds, one is continuously generating karma. Consequently, one is still subject to death and a rebirth in a different form. Both heavenly pleasures and hellish tortures are temporary since they are subject to time and karma. Death reaches both the lowest hell and the highest heaven (Amore, 1974).

According to the Buddha, death can be overcome by the liberated person who ceases to generate karma and is forever beyond good and evil, death and rebirth. Nirvana is the weapon that annihilates death. Nirvana, which literally means to blow out, refers to the blowing out of the flames of passion. An individual who has attained Nirvana is no longer afire with desire and delusion.

In the sense of extinction or annihilation, Nirvana is the annihilation of all evil in the individual. It signifies the extinction of craving, lust, fear, and the illusion of a separate ego/self. One who has attained Nirvana is no longer dominated by pleasure and sorrow, hope and fear.

Nirvana also means calm and unruffled. Thus, it is described by terms such as the "bliss supreme," the "deathless," "the further shore," "the taintless," "the security" (*Samyutta-Nikaya,* 1884-1904). Nirvana may be described as a lotus flower in a muddy pond.

Understandably, many Western commentators have equated Nirvana with the Christian concept of eternal life or even God. Still others (e.g., Barthelemy Saint-Hilaire, 1962) have declared it to be absolute annihilation. Oldenberg (1882) proclaimed that Nirvana is the domain over which the law of causality has no power. La Vallee Poussin (1912) went so far as to say that Nirvana is synonymous with heaven. Welbon (1968) has summarized the various Western interpretations of Nirvana. Despite the many adventurous attempts at its elucidation, Nirvana remains inexpressible. Parrinder (1973, p. 98) probably had the last word on Nirvana. It is, he said, "beyond all description, definition, location and language."

It must be mentioned that Buddhist thought makes a distinction between the Nirvana that is attainable in life and the final Nirvana at the time of death. The latter is referred to as Parinirvana. The earlier Nirvana that characterizes the *arahat* or enlightened being is "nirvana with the skandhas remaining"; that is, the psychophysical complex that makes up the individual still functions, but without generating karma and in a state of complete egolessness. Parinirvana is the complete extinction of skandha life. There is a dissolution of *namarupa* (individual personality). The arahat ceases to exist and is liberated from rebirth and redeath. The passing of an arahat is likened to a fire that has gone out. The skandhas dissolve without leaving any residue.

DEATH IMAGERY IN BUDDHISM

Buddhaghosa (1976) described in great detail the two meditational contexts in which death is used as a subject. The first of these involves the development of mindfulness of one's death, and the second utilizes corpses as objects of meditation.

Mindfulness of Death

Buddhaghosa (1976) began by describing death as the interruption of the life faculty. Timely death occurs because of exhaustion of good karma, or exhaustion of one's allotted life span, or both. The allotted life span was considered to be 80 years, the age at which the Buddha died. Untimely death occurs as a result of violence or the ability of certain persons to die instantly using psychic powers (Amore, 1974).

One should select a solitary retreat to practice the mindfulness of death. If one imagines the deaths of those whom one loved or hated, either sorrow or joy is bound to arise. This is not mindfulness and should be avoided. The practitioner is exhorted to imagine those already dead but who had been seen enjoying the good things of life, and repeat, "Death will take place."

When a measure of mindfulness has been established using this technique, the individual should recollect death in eight ways:

1. One should imagine facing a murderer and tell oneself, "Just as a murderer appears with a sword thinking, 'I shall cut this person's head off' and applies it to the victim's neck, so death appears." One should reflect on the fact that death is inevitable for that which is born and imagine death appearing like a murderer with poised sword.
2. Death should be imagined as the ruin of success. One should imagine health ending in sickness, prosperity turning to loss, youth yielding to age. One should imagine death as overwhelming an army of elephants, chariots, and infantry.
3. One should imagine the death of others and thus infer one's own mortality. The practitioner is enjoined to imagine the death of seven kinds of persons: those of great fame, those of great merit, those of great strength, those with great understanding, those with supranormal power, arahats, and finally, the Buddha himself. One should imagine the passing away of these persons and remind oneself that even they were not immune to death. Imagining the death of these individuals, one should repeat, "Death will come to me as it did to those distinguished persons."
4. One should remind oneself that one shares this body with "eighty families of worms." These worms live in and depend on the body. One should imagine these worms being born, growing old, excreting, and dying within one's body. One should also reflect that the body is a target for various

diseases as well as for scorpions, snakes, and so forth. Before retiring for the night, the monk should imagine becoming a victim of a snake, a scorpion, and so on.
5. One should reflect on the frailty of the body, its dependence on breathing, temperature, the primary elements, and nourishment. The monk should recollect that disturbances in any of these factors will cause death.
6. One should reflect on the fact that death often attacks without providing prior warning. There are usually no signs to indicate the span of one's life, or the time, place, and manner of one's death.
7. One should reflect on the limited span of life.
8. In the ultimate sense, the life span of an individual is extremely limited, restricted as it is to a single conscious moment. According to Buddhism, the skandhas that make up an individual are dying and being reborn anew every moment. One should imagine this constant dying and rebirth by visualizing the movement of a chariot wheel which, both during rest and motion, rests only on one point, and remind oneself that life actually lasts but a single moment.

There are several benefits associated with the successful practice of mindfulness of death. The practitioner will conquer attachment to life, avarice, and lust. He or she also will realize the impermanence of life and consequently develop serenity. Finally, he or she will be able to face death in a composed and fearless manner.

Meditation on Death

The meditations on corpses serve to overcome fear of death, increase disgust for one's body, lessen attachment to one's body, and remind one of the impermanence of the physical self. The meditations on the corpses take place in a cemetery or cremation area, where one has access to corpses in different stages of decay. These meditations occur under the guidance of an elder monk. The *bhikku* (a male monk) should choose corpses only of his sex. A female body is regarded as unsuitable for a male and vice versa.

The bhikku should choose a bloated corpse and examine it carefully. He should examine its color, shape, location, and delimitation. He should examine its joints, openings, concavities, and convexities. After examining the corpse carefully, the bhikku should close his eyes and imagine the bloated corpse in all its aspects. If he is able to imagine it vividly, he can then return to the seclusion of his room to practice the contemplation. Buddhaghosa (1976) suggested several devices to aid in the visualization of the corpse, if the practitioner is unable to bring it to mind:

> When the sign has vanished the bhikku (monk) should sit down and review the path he took to the cemetery and back noting the directions and markers such as gates, stones, anthills, trees, bushes or creepers. He should then recall,

> "I saw the foulness in such and such a place, I stood there facing in such and such a direction and observed such and such surrounding signs, I apprehended the sign of foulness in this way" (p. 195).

Such a review is said to aid in the vivid visualization of the corpse in all its aspects.

The bhikku should then recall in his imagination the bloated corpse until it is firmly entrenched in his mind's eye. He should cultivate reverence for the imagery, treasure and love it, and anchor the mind on the image. This meditation will lead to the cessation of lust, ill will, worry, agitation, and torpor. The monk will develop tranquility and eventually attain the *jhanas*.

To counteract specific failings, the monk should choose a different type of corpse for meditation. For example, meditation on a livid and discolored corpse is regarded as a corrective to the lust for a beautiful complexion; meditation on a festering corpse with its foul smell leads to disenchantment with bodily scents and perfumes; and visualization of a dismembered body will have a salutary effect on those who lust after a graceful figure.

These visualizations will lead one to the realization that life is impermanent, to the awareness that death is inevitable. It is readily apparent that the death meditations of Buddhism are useful psychotherapeutic tools. Used skillfully and mindfully, death imagery exercises can enhance personal growth and lead to a fuller appreciation of life.

DEATH AND PSYCHOTHERAPY

The fear of death, said Yalom (1980), "plays a major role in our internal experience; it haunts as does nothing else; it rumbles continuously under the surface; it is a dark, unsettling presence at the rim of consciousness" (p. 27). Yalom went on to assert that psychopathology is a consequence of the inability to come to terms with death and that death awareness is vital to effective psychotherapy.

That death is a part of the life cycle has been recognized throughout human history. The Hindus identified Death with Time. Prajapati consumed his own creation in order to generate the energy needed to sustain and replenish the cosmos. Thus, death was necessary for life to take place. "It is only in the face of death," said St. Augustine, "that man's self is born" (Montaigne, 1965, p. 63). And the Stoics declared, "Contemplate death if you would learn how to live" (Montaigne, 1965, p. 65).

Heidegger (1962) stated that the awareness of one's death jolts one into a mindful, authentic state of being. Indeed, it is the possibility of death that makes life interesting. "But suspend judgment for a moment and imagine life without any thought of death. Life loses something of its intensity. Life shrinks when death is denied" (Yalom, 1980, pp. 31-32).

A close encounter with death often precipitates a radical personality change. Koestler, who, during the Spanish Civil War, won a reprieve moments before a firing squad was to shoot him, says that the experience profoundly altered his life (Koestler, 1937). Tolstoy's Ivan Ilyich underwent a tremendous change when he faced imminent death (Tolstoy, 1960). Russell Noyes' (1972) study of 200 individuals who had near-death experiences found that as a result of their experience, a significant number of them developed a greater zest for and appreciation of life.

Death Anxiety

The fear of death plays an important role in human affairs.

> Death transcendence is a major motif in human experience—from the most deeply personal internal phenomena, our defenses, our motivations, our dreams and nightmares, to the most public macrosocietal structures, our monuments, theologies, ideologies, slumber cemeteries, embalmings, our stretch into space, indeed our entire way of life—our filling time, our addiction of diversions, our unfaltering belief in the myth of progress, our drive to "get ahead," our yearning for lasting fame (Yalom, 1980, p. 41).

Choron (1964) asserted that it is the prospect of complete obliteration of the constellation of personality characteristics that constitute the self that is at the core of death anxiety. Thus, it is the prospect of "ceasing to be" that is most dreaded. Garfield (1975), in a study of fear of death among members of five American subcultures, found that the fear of ego dissolution was intimately related to the level of death fear.

According to Yalom (1980), primal death anxiety is rarely seen in clinical practice. The individual uses defenses such as displacement, repression, and sublimation to protect against death anxiety. Skoog (1975) reported that, in a majority of clients with obsessional neurosis, a death experience had occurred immediately prior to the illness. Schwidder (1975), in a study of obsessional/phobic individuals, found frank death anxiety in a substantial number of them. Lazarus and Kostan (1969) stated that death anxiety is present in the hyperventilation syndrome.

The research on death anxiety is instructive. Conscious death anxiety is well correlated with depression in the aged (Templer, 1971). Kastenbaum and Aisenberg (1972) reported that adolescents who reveal symptoms of psychopathology manifest more death anxiety than do controls. Several other studies have reported the presence of significant unconscious death anxiety (Feifel & Branscomb, 1973; Meissner, 1958). Not surprisingly, death anxiety has been found in dreams and nightmares (Cason, 1935; Kramer, Wingel, & Whitman, 1971).

Reviewing the various perspectives discussed so far, Yalom (1980) said that although it is known that death can make life meaningful, promote personality change, and be a source of great anxiety, it has been ignored by psychotherapy.

"Death is overlooked glaringly, in almost all aspects of the mental health field: theory, basic and clinical research, clinical reports, and all forms of clinical practice" (Yalom, 1980, p. 55).

The Child's Concern with Death

Nowhere is this inattention to death more conspicuous than in the literature on child development. There is little doubt that children are aware of and preoccupied with death at a very early age (Anthony, 1972; Rochlin, 1967). According to Yalom (1980), they go through a number of stages not only in their awareness of death but also in the strategies they use—chiefly denial—to cope with their fear of death. Therefore, understanding death is a major developmental task for children. But, sadly enough, Western institutions do little to assist the young in dealing with the vital issue of death. Death education is virtually unknown. Parents, in their eagerness to protect the child from death anxiety, offer information that is often more frightening than reality. An inability to cope with death in early childhood may be an important factor in the development of psychopathology in adulthood.

Psychopathology is almost always the result of inadequate coping with anxiety. Most human beings develop adaptive strategies to cope with death anxiety. However, according to Yalom (1980), when the defensive modes of coping with death anxiety are found wanting, the individual becomes a patient. Searles (1961) suggested that the psychodynamics of schizophrenia can be regarded as strategies to avoid facing the reality of death. The defense mechanisms of schizophrenia, he said, are designed to exclude from the patient's awareness anxiety-inducing phenomena such as death.

Death Awareness

According to Yalom (1980), death awareness may serve as a "boundary situation" (an experience that precipitates a confrontation with one's existential situation) and thus promote personal change. He cited case histories of several individuals who learned to drink deeply from the fountain of life when faced with terminal cancer. A woman riddled with cancer of the esophagus and unable to eat or even drink marveled at the other diners in a restaurant and wondered if they ever realized how fortunate they were to be able to swallow.

> Ordinarily what we do have and what we can do slips out of awareness, diverted by thoughts of what we lack or what we cannot do or dwarfed by petty concerns and threats to our prestige or our pride systems. By keeping death in mind, one passes into a state of rectitude, of appreciation for the countless givens of existence (Yalom, 1980, p. 163).

Given the premise that awareness of one's death can be a catalyst for growth, the task of the therapist, Yalom suggested, is to facilitate the client's awareness of death. The death of a close friend, parent, spouse, or child offers opportunities for us to face our own death. Similarly, the midlife crisis, impending retirement, illness, and the appearance of wrinkles can help foster death awareness.

However, human beings are enormously adept at constructing defenses against death. Hence, props have always been used to bring death to the fore. While the Buddhist visited the burial ground to contemplate on death, the Christian monk kept a skull in his cell as a reminder of death. Montaigne (1991) said that cemeteries were built next to churches to accustom the populace to the sight of death.

Meditation and psychedelic drugs might help us confront death in that they induce ego-dissolution experiences that resemble death. Meditators as well as individuals who use psychedelic drugs like LSD are retraining in ego death, and this training may well be responsible for the reduction in death anxiety in altered-state groups (Garfield, 1975; Kastenbaum & Aisenberg, 1972; McGlothlin, Cohen, & McGlothlin, 1967). Richards, Grof, Goodman, and Kurland (1972), in a study of the psychotherapeutic effects of psychedelics on terminal cancer patients, said that those who experienced ego death claimed that their attitude to death had changed dramatically.

Yalom (1980) has reported on increasing death awareness in psychotherapy clients who had attended meetings of terminally ill patients. He went on to develop the concept of "death desensitization."

> It seems that, with repeated contact, one can get used to anything—even to dying. The therapist may help the patient deal with death terror in ways similar to the techniques he uses to conquer any other form of dread. He exposes the patient over and over to the fear in attenuated doses. He helps the patient handle the dreaded object and to inspect it from all sides (Yalom, 1980, p. 211).

Montaigne (1991) eloquently proclaimed,

> "to begin depriving death of its greatest advantage over us, let us adopt a way clean contrary to that common one; let us deprive death of its strangeness, let us frequent it, let us get used to it; let us have nothing more often in mind than death . . . we do not know where death awaits: so let us wait for it everywhere. To practice death is to practice freedom. A man who has learned how to die has unlearned how to be a slave" (p. 95).

Workshops on death desensitization report success in reducing death anxiety (Kaller, 1975). The Buddhist contemplation on death while in a state of meditation is an optimal behavioral paradigm for death desensitization.

Death Imagery: Psychotherapeutic Aspects

According to Segal (1971), experiencing an event in the imagination comes closest to the actual situation. If so, death imagery is a powerful tool to encounter the experience of one's death. Dying in the imagination can be a relaxing experience. As such, it can be used not only to achieve relaxation but also as a psychotherapeutic tool. Sheikh, Twente, and Turner (1979) described the use of death imagery in relaxation:

> Imagine that you are dead. You have lost all your ability to counter the force of gravity and are completely immobilized and inactive. All your muscles, even all your body cells are pulled down by gravity. You no longer have to struggle, be tense, and spend energy to stay alive.... As your "dead" body is pulled more and more by the force of gravity, you have a feeling that you are shedding off your body. Your thoughts scatter and all the verbal chatter and commotion vanishes into thin air. As you shed your body, you become a weightless, bodiless, pure consciousness. There is stillness and quiet and a benign indifference of nature (p. 154).

The initial anxiety induced by the exercise gives way to feelings of relaxation, peace, and in some individuals, of unity and cosmic consciousness. Sheikh, Twente, Turner, and Frazier (1978) also reported on the use of death imagery in the psychotherapeutic situation. Death imagery has played a crucial role in the meditative tradition of Buddhism. Visualization techniques are used to imagine the body in several stages of decay. The objective is to weaken passionate attachments and sensuality. The practitioner proceeds by stages from disgust to detachment and equanimity (Buddhaghosa, 1976; Nyanaponika, 1962). Death imagery seems to offer the individual a unique opportunity to participate more fully in life by confronting and transcending his or her own death.

CONCLUDING REMARKS

The Dalai Lama (2001) states that death is an inevitable part of samsara or cyclic existence. It is the full acceptance of impermanence and death that enables us to participate more fully in life. By preparing for death, we realize "the great value of human existence, the opportunity and the potential that our brief lives afford us" (p. 39). It appears that death

> acts as a catalyst that can move one from one state of being to a higher one: from a state of wondering about how things are to a state of wonderment that they are. An awareness of death shifts one away from trivial preoccupations and provides life with depth and poignancy and an entirely different perspective (Yalom, 1980, pp. 159-160).

REFERENCES

Amore, R. C. (1974). The heterodox philosophical systems. In F. H. Holck (Ed.), *Death and Eastern thought*. New York: Abingdon Press.

Anguttara-Nikaya (Vols. 1-4). (1885-1900). H. Morris & H. Hardy (Eds). London: Pali Text Society.

Anthony, S. (1972). *The discovery of death in childhood and after.* New York: Basic Books.
Barthelemy Saint-Hilaire, J. (1962). *Le Bouddha et sa religion* (Nouv. ed.). Paris: Didier.
Beck, A. (1943). *The story of Oriental philosophy.* New York: The New Home Library.
Becker, C. B. (1981). *Survival: Death and afterlife in Christianity, Buddhism, and modern science.* Unpublished doctoral dissertation, University of Hawaii.
Boerstler, R. (1982). *Letting go.* Watertown, MA: Associate in Thanatology.
Buddhaghosa, A. (1976). *The path of purification (Visuddhimagga)* (2 vols.) (B. Nyanamoli, Trans). Berkeley, CA: Shambala.
Cason, H. (1935). The nightmare dream. *Psychology Monographs, 209,* 46.
Choron, J. (1964). *Death and modern man.* New York: Collier.
Conze, E. (1959). *Buddhist scriptures.* Baltimore: Penguin Books.
Coomaraswamy, A. (1971). Rebirth. In P. Kapleau (Ed.), *The wheel of death.* New York: Harper & Row.
Dalai Lama. (2001). *An open heart.* N. Vreeland (Ed.). Boston: Little, Brown.
Digha-Nikaya (Vols. 1-3). (1890-1911). T. W. Rhys-Davids & J. E. Carpenter (Eds.). London: Pali Text Society.
The Egyptian book of the dead. (1894). C. H. S. Davis, Ed. and trans.). New York: Putnam.
Eliade, M. (1958). *Yoga: Immortality and freedom.* New York: Pantheon.
Eliade, M. (1974). *Death, afterlife, and eschatology.* New York: Harper & Row.
Evans-Wentz, W. Y. (1960). *The Tibetan book of the dead.* New York: Oxford University Press.
Feifel, H., & Branscomb, A. (1973). Who's afraid of death? *Journal of Abnormal Psychology, 81*(3), 282-288.
Foucher, A. (1963). *The life of the Buddha.* Middletown, CT: Wesleyan University Press.
Frankl, V. (1959). *Man's search for meaning.* New York: Washington Square Press.
Garfield, C. A. (1975). Consciousness alteration and fear of death. *Journal of Transpersonal Psychology, 7*(2), 147-175.
Gibran, K. (1966). *The prophet.* New York: Alfred A. Knopf.
Heidegger, M. (1962). *Being and time.* New York: Harper & Row.
Hick, J. (1976). *Death and eternal life.* New York: Harper & Row.
Hiriyanna, M. (1964). *Outlines of Indian philosophy.* London: George Allen & Unwin.
Holck, F. H. (1974). *Death and eastern thought.* New York: Abingdon Press.
Jayatilleke, K. N. (1975). *The message of the Buddha.* N. Smart (Ed.). New York: The Free Press.
Kaller, D. (1975). An evaluation of a self instructional program designed to reduce anxiety and fear about death and of the relation of that program to sixteen personal history variables. *Dissertation Abstracts International, 35,* 7125A.
Kastenbaum, R., & Aisenberg, R. (1972). *Psychology of death.* New York: Springer.
Keith, A. B. (1925). *The religion and philosophy of the Vedas and Upanishads.* Cambridge: Harvard University Press.
Koestler, A. (1937). *Spanish testament.* London: Victor Gollancz.
Koestler, A. (1976). Whereof one cannot speak . . . ? In A. Toynbee & A. Koestler (Eds.), *Life after death.* London: Weidenfeld & Nicolson.
Kramer, M., Wingel, C., & Whitman, R. (1971). A city dreams: A survey approach to normal dream content. *American Journal of Psychiatry, 127,* 86-92.

Krishnamurti, J. (1969). *Freedom from the known*. M. Lutyens (Eds.). New York: Harper and Row.
Kübler-Ross, E. (1975). *Death: The final stage of growth*. Englewood Cliffs, NJ: Prentice-Hall.
La Vallee Poussin, L. (1912). *Bouddhisme et religions de l'Inde*. Paris: Gabriel Beauchesne et Cie.
Lazarus, H., & Kostan, J. (1969). Psychogenic hyperventilation and death anxiety. *Psychosomatics, 10,* 14-22.
Long, B. (1975). The death that ends death in Hinduism and Buddhism. In E. Kübler-Ross (Ed.), *Death: The final stage of growth*. Englewood Cliffs, NJ: Prentice-Hall.
Long, B. (1977). Death as a necessity and a gift in Hindu mythology. In F. Reynolds & E. Waugh (Eds.), *Religious encounters with death*. University Park: Pennsylvania State University Press.
Majjhima Nikaya (1948-1951). V. Trenkner, R. Chalmers, & C. A. F. Rhys-Davids (Eds.). London: Pali Text Society.
May, R. (Ed.). (1961). *Existential psychology*. New York: Random House.
McDermott, J. P. (1980). Karma and rebirth in early Buddhism. In W. D. O'Flaherty (Ed.), *Karma and rebirth in classical Indian traditions*. Berkeley: University of California Press.
McGlothlin, W., Cohen, S., & McGlothlin, M. (1967). Long-lasting effects of LSD on normals. *Archives of General Psychiatry, 17,* 421-532.
McGovern, W. M. (1923). *A manual of Buddhist philosophy*. London: Kegan Paul, Trench, Trubner & Co., Ltd.
Meissner, W. (1958). Affective response to psychoanalytic death symbols. *Journal of Abnormal and Social Psychology, 56,* 295-299.
Montaigne, M. (1965). *The complete essays of Montaigne*. D. Frame (Trans.). Stanford: Stanford University Press.
Montaigne, M. (1991). *The essays of Michel de Montaigne*. M. A. Screech (Ed.). London: Allen Lane Stanford University Press.
Muir, J. (Trans.). (1884). *Original Sanskrit texts*: Rig Veda, IV. London: Trubner & Co.
Müller, M. (1879). *Origin and growth of religion*. New York: C. Scribner's Sons.
Müller M. (1887). *Science of language*. New York: C. Scribner's Sons.
Noyes, R. (1972). The experience of dying. *Psychiatry, 35,* 174-184.
Nyanaponika, T. (1962). *The heart of Buddhist Meditation*. Rider: London.
Oldenberg, H. (1882). *Buddha*. London: Williams & Norgate.
Parrinder, G. (1973). *The indestructible soul*. London: George Allen & Unwin.
Piyadassi, T. (1972). *The psychological aspect of Buddhism* (Wheel Publication No. 179). Kandy: Buddhist Publication Society.
Radhakrishnan, S. (1951). *Indian philosophy* (Vol. 1). New York: Macmillan.
Rahula, W. (1962). *What the Buddha taught*. New York: Grove Press.
Raju, P. T. (1971). *The philosophical traditions of India*. London: George Allen & Unwin.
Richards, W., Grof, S., Goodman, L., & Kurland, A. (1972). LSD-assisted psychotherapy and the human encounter with death. *Journal of Transpersonal Psychology, 4,* 121-150.
Riepe, D. (1961). *The naturalistic tradition in Indian thought*. Seattle: University of Washington Press.

The Rig-Veda. (1897). Vedic hymns, Part II: Hymns to Agni (H. Oldenberg, Trans.) *Sacred books of the east,* Vol. 46. Oxford: Clarendon Press.

Rochlin, G. (1967). How younger children view death and themselves. In E. Grollman (Ed.), *Explaining death to children.* New York: Beacon Press.

Russell, B. (1950). *Unpopular essays.* New York: Simon & Schuster.

Samyutta Nikaya (Vols. 1-6) (1884-1904). L. Freer (Ed.). London: Pali Text Society.

Schwidder, W. (1975). Cited in J. Meyer, *Death and neurosis.* New York: International Universities Press.

Searles, H. (1961). Schizophrenia and the inevitability of death. *Psychiatric Quarterly, 35,* 631-655.

Segal, S. J. (Ed.). (1971). *Imagery: Current cognitive approaches.* New York: Academic Press.

Sheikh, A. A., Twente, G. E., & Turner, D. (1979). Death imagery: Therapeutic uses. In A. A. Sheikh & J. Shaffer (Eds.), *The potential of fantasy and imagination.* New York: Brandon House.

Sheikh, A. A., Twente, G. E., Turner, D., & Frazier, P. B. (1978, November). *Death imagery: Clinical use for personal growth and awareness.* Paper presented at the meeting of the Second American Conference on the Fantasy and Imaging Process, Chicago.

Skoog, R. (1975). Cited in J. Meyer, *Death and neurosis.* New York: International Universities Press.

Templer, D. (1971). Death anxiety as related to depression and health of retired persons. *Journal of Gerontology, 26,* 521-523.

Tolstoy, L. (1960). *The death of Ivan Ilyich and other stories.* New York: Signet Classics.

Welbon, G. R. (1968). *The Buddhist Nirvana and its Western interpreters.* Chicago, IL: University of Chicago Press.

Wilcox, S. G., & Sutton, M. (1977). *Understanding death and dying.* Port Washington, NY: Alfred Publishing Co.

Yalom, I. (1980). *Existential psychotherapy.* New York: Basic Books.

Yasutani, R. (1971). Rebirth. In P. Kapleau (Ed.), *The wheel of death.* New York: Harper & Row.

CHAPTER 6

The Dynamic, Clinical Use of Imagery to Promote Psychotherapeutic Grieving

James K. Morrison

> I saw a child carrying a light.
> I asked him where he had brought it from.
> He put it out and said:
> "Now you tell the where it is gone."
>
> Hasan of Basra (Arya, 1979, p. 22)

Richard Kalish (1965) has compared the general public's avoidance of the topic of death to their former attitude toward pornography:

> We react to it [death] and its symbols in the same way as we react to any pornography. We protect little children from observing it and dodge their questions about it. We speak of it only in whispers. We consider it horrible, ugly and grotesque (p. 62).

In similar terms, writers such as Gorer (1965), Feifel (1963), and Muggeridge (1970) assert that death has generally been a topic to be avoided in conversation and print.

In recent decades the professional literature on death (e.g., Choron, 1963; Kastenbaum & Aisenberg, 1972; Kübler-Ross, 1969; Shneidman, 1973) has begun to proliferate. However, even though some (Aguilar & Wood, 1976; Melges, 1982; Morrison, 1978, 1981; Ramsay & Noorbergen, 1981;Volkan, 1975) have devoted attention to the use of psychotherapeutic techniques to induce "proper grieving,"[1] and others (e.g., Sheikh, Twente, & Turner, 1979) have written of the therapeutic value of fantasizing one's own death, still there exists a very meager literature on grieving in psychotherapy. Thus, it is possible that psychotherapists too have been avoiding death as an important issue in their work with clients who have lost a loved one (Kastenbaum, 2001).

Related to a theory of grieving, few psychotherapists seem to follow the lead of Freud (1915) in giving death a place of importance in their psychotherapeutic approach.[2] In fact, one is hard pressed to find a clear theoretical delineation of the need of certain clients to more properly grieve the loss of a loved one. Yet, certainly, the death of a loved one can profoundly disturb and disrupt the life of a psychotherapy client. Parkes (1972) concluded from an investigation of widows that women who have lost a husband recently are more likely to die or be physically ill or emotionally disturbed than nonwidowed women. Related to a specific type of death, that is, suicide, Shneidman (1973) maintains that the largest problem in public health is neither the prevention of suicide nor the management of suicide attempts, but the alleviation of the effects of stress among the survivor/victims, whose lives may he forever altered.

The purpose of the present chapter is threefold: first, to present a brief overview of some techniques used to promote proper grieving; second, to briefly suggest a useful theoretical approach to the need for adequate grieving; and third, to outline one specific operational approach (emotive/reconstructive) to grieving in psychotherapy. But first, a definition of some terms would appear to be in order.

NORMAL AND ABNORMAL GRIEF

Although "normal" and "abnormal"[3] grief are quite difficult to define operationally, Engel (1961), and Bowlby (1963, 1973) have outlined a variety of defenses and emotions that occur in normal grieving: shock, protest and anguish, mourning and restitution. The acute stage of grief normally lasts six to eight weeks. During normal grieving, symptoms similar to depression (e.g., insomnia, crying, loss of interest in life, weight loss, etc.) are common and tend to persist for some time after the first eight weeks, but in gradually reduced amounts. It

---

[1] The terms "proper (normal) grieving" and "improper (abnormal) grieving" refer to opposite ends of the continuum of adjustment to the death of a loved one. Whereas "proper grieving" is viewed as adequately processing, both emotionally and intellectually, the dissolution of a relationship, "improper grieving" refers to at least a partial lack of such processing, as exemplified by certain physiological and/or psychological behaviors (e.g., sleep problems, anxiety, depression, inability to speak of the deceased without crying, etc.).

[2] Ironically, Freud (1958) asserted that the normal processes of grieving should not be interfered with.

[3] Generally, the author prefers the terms "proper" and "improper" grieving, since they do not connote "mental illness" as much as the terms "normal" and "abnormal." However, I will use the latter terms when others do so in their discussions of grief.

is sometimes difficult to differentiate normal grief from depressive symptoms (Archer, 1999; Wass, Berando, & Neimeyer, 1995).

Time and intensity may best distinguish abnormal from normal grief (Melges & DeMaso, 1980). In abnormal grieving, the person seems unable to grieve much soon after the loss or grieves too much for too long a period of time after the loss, or both. However, it seems impossible to quantify how much is too little, and too much grieving depends so much on the circumstances of the death (e.g., sudden or expected death, the closeness of the relationship of the survivor to the deceased, the culture in which the death occurs, the personality of the survivor, the support system available, and so on). Perhaps the Texas Inventory of Grief (Faschingbauer, Devaul, & Zisook, 1977) will be a step forward in quantifying grief.

Clinicians have to be aware of the phenomenon of the client who presents a classical picture of depression, but who may be suffering from an unresolved grief reaction to a death which occurred many years ago. I remember one client who presented a picture of classical depression at the age of 48, but was actually still trying to cope with his mother's death when he was four (Morrison, 1981). In the initial interview, the client cried profusely in talking about this death, and so I concluded that the principal cause of the depression may have been the client's inability at such a tender age to cope with his mother's death. The fact that the client experienced a rapid relief from depression immediately after only one session of grieving seemed to confirm this hypothesis (Morrison, 2002).

Melges and DeMaso (1980) list a number of obstacles that have been found to impede normal grieving: (1) persistent yearning for the deceased; (2) over identification with the deceased; (3) the wish to cry or rage about the loss with an inability to express it; (4) misdirected anger and ambivalence toward the deceased; (5) interlocking grief reactions (present grief may combine with grief over another loss); (6) unspoken but powerful contracts with the deceased; (7) unrevealed secrets and unfinished business; (8) lack of a support group and alternative options; (9) secondary gain or reinforcement from others to remain grief-stricken. Thus the presence of many of these defensive reactions may suggest a powerful obstacle to normal grieving which a therapist will need to overcome.

A recent longitudinal study (Parkes & Weiss, 1983) of bereavement among widows and widowers zeroes in on the factors that are involved in successful recovery from the grieving process. The study suggests that some of our assumptions about the bereavement process may be overly simplistic. For example, it is commonly held that the expression of grief following the death of a spouse is an important factor in eventual recovery. However, Parkes and Weiss assert that their data reveal that those whose grief was expressed by an intense yearning for their deceased spouses frequently had problems in recovery. High dependency on the spouse appeared to be the cause of both the intense yearning and the problematic recovery. This dependency factor, according to these researchers, seemed to be one of the most important predictors of poor outcome.

Parkes and Weiss also found that women are more likely than men to express grief and thus have fewer problems arising from repressed grief. Women, however, also seek help in the grieving process more frequently than do men.

Parkes and Weiss identify three major causes of pathological or improper grieving: an unexpected death; ambivalent feelings during the marriage about the spouse; and overdependence on the spouse. Helping clients recover from the grieving process often means helping them to deal with all three of these factors (Neimeyer, 2001).

A BRIEF OVERVIEW OF GRIEVING TECHNIQUES

In this section, the author will briefly delineate some of the more promising techniques described by others related to therapeutic grieving. In a later section, the author will outline his own approach to grieving.

In his interesting book on the important effects of time disorientation on psychological illness, Frederick Melges (1982) describes the approach that he and a colleague (Melges & DeMaso, 1980) developed to assist clients in completing the grieving process. Apparently, this therapeutic approach can be used within the context of other therapies.

Melges and DeMaso use guided imagery as the core of the method. With eyes closed, the patient is encouraged to visualize scenes related to the loved one's death as though they were happening in the present. "Dialogues with the dead" are encouraged. Emotional outbursts are also encouraged in order to increase the client's acceptance that the loss is final.

Melges and DeMaso usually have clients deal separately for about 20 minutes each with the following scenes: awareness of the client's relationship to the deceased shortly before the news of the death; the news of the loved one's death; the happenings at the funeral home; the funeral; saying goodbye to the loved one at the gravesite. According to the authors, this type of grief resolution therapy requires six to ten half-hourly or hourly sessions. Outpatients are usually seen twice a week.

The essence of this guided imagery method involves assisting the client to "progressively relive, revise, and revisit sequences of the loss as though they were taking place in the present" (Melges, 1982, p. 204). The essential steps of this grieving process involve (1) reliving events connected with a death—with eyes closed; (2) revising a scene so as to remove obstacles (e.g., people present at a wake) to full grieving, and (3) revisiting the revised scene in the here and now. In this last phase, the patient is encouraged to engage in dialogues with the deceased in order to acknowledge the finality of the loss, express repressed emotion, and so on. Toward the conclusion of the revisited scenes, the therapist encourages the patient to exchange last words and to ascertain whether the patient is prepared to say goodbye to the deceased.

This type of imagery process is not recommended for acutely manic or schizophrenic patients. It is also not used with patients who are grieving a recent loss. Melges (1982) claims that there have been no lasting "untoward complications" with this treatment process.

Melges (1982) offers a case vignette that illustrates his approach. In this example of imagery-induced grieving, Melges worked with a 43-year-old married mother of three children who came with problems of depression, as exemplified by her suicidal state after being rebuffed by a matronly fellow volunteer worker. Interviews revealed that this client had been severely depressed 10 years previously after the death of her mother. Her father had died 18 months prior to her mother's death. Evidence suggested the client had not adequately grieved either death. After doing some successful clinical grieving of her father's death, the client began to grieve the loss of her mother. She had apparently rejected this vigorously until supportive therapy had helped her to begin the grieving process. The client was amazed how much the guided-imagery process brought back almost total recall of the feelings and circumstances of her mother's death. For example, she could "see" the rose she had placed on her mother's coffin and feel the accompanying resentment that her mother did not deserve the rose. The therapist suggested the client imagine herself alone with her mother's open casket in the funeral home. The client, sounding very insightful, began to release feelings of anger, sadness, and eventually forgiveness.

> Why did you have to drive my father away with your ugly nagging? No wonder he left the family; I forgive him for that. But then, when he died, you had to fight with his wife over his body, his property; yet you had no claim to him. When you couldn't nag him anymore after he left, you took it all out on me. I could never do anything right for you. How I tried to please you, yet I just ended up feeling I had not done enough ever. I hate you, Mother, I hate you. (Much sobbing) No wonder my father's wife didn't want you buried next to him; you are a curse. Now I had to find a place to bury you; you will not like it; it's too grubby. Even in death I cannot please you. But it's your fault; you made your own bed, your own grave. I am going to let you go, Mother, along with all this guilt I will bury you . . . yet even now I feel I am disobeying you, leaving you alone; you needed to cling to me; in a way, I was your mother. Your mother, Grandma, clung to you and made you feel guilty. Maybe that's the only way you knew . . . could you help it? (Much sobbing) MOTHER, I FORGIVE YOU! I forgive you—now I can forgive myself (Relief). I do not owe you anything; I am going to be different from you. I will not drive my husband away; I will be truly loving to my children. Gads, I have almost become like you. . . . Now that you are dead maybe you understand this—I want to be free to be myself (Melges, 1982, p. 211).

After completing this process, the client reported feeling exhilarated and free.

I was surprised to find that I had been developing quite similar operational techniques to those of Melges and DeMaso. And, as Melges (1982) mentions, these techniques are also similar to those of Volkan (1975), although the latter emphasizes more a re-creation of a loss in the past tense, whereas Melges and DeMaso, as well as I, try more to re-create death events in the present tense.

Although Melges (1982) briefly hints at the value of Kelly's (1955) personal construct system as relevant to explaining the change in a patient during the grieving process, the present author has more extensively elaborated Kelly's system in reference to grieving (Morrison & Cometa, 1982). Nonetheless, it is still remarkable how different therapists, in isolation from one another, came to develop such similar grieving techniques.

Another therapist, Ronald Ramsay (Ramsay & Noorbergen, 1981), uses what he terms "Guided Confrontation Therapy" to help people deal with the death of a loved one, as well as with other losses. He usually schedules three 50-minute sessions per week for the grieving patient. The use of tranquilizers and antidepressants is discouraged, since he feels such medications make it more difficult for the patient to breakthrough to an emotional level. Ramsay does not clearly outline his precise style of inducing grieving, but much emphasis is placed on confrontation of the patient to elicit feelings and on active role-playing with the deceased to traverse the various stages of grieving. The process is described as taking a considerable period of time (unlike emotive-reconstructive grieving, discussed later), and the elicitation of screams of pain from the patient seem to be an important goal of the process (also unlike emotive-reconstructive therapy). The authors also do not appear to give imagery a central role in the grieving process.

A case study of a woman who lost her mother and 12-year-old daughter in one tragic accident is offered by Ramsay and Noorbergen (1981), and is perhaps the clearest indication of the active interaction between client and therapist. After the accident, the client's yearning for both became uncontrollable. Losing her mother and daughter within six months after the death of her father was more than she could handle.

The client finally entered Guided Confrontation Therapy. The first session was aimed at getting her to realize the accident really happened and that Beverly, her daughter, would never come back. During this session the client was asked to imagine herself at her daughter's grave and to say goodbye to her. The second therapy session was devoted to her mother. This death seemed easier for the client to handle than that of Beverly. The third session was not as productive as the first two because the emotional upset of the first two sessions had taken its toll.

The fourth session reveals the active, confrontational approach of this style of therapy. The therapist is revealed as constantly pressuring the client to let her mother go in spite of the client's great resistance to doing so. Toward the end of this session, the therapist says, "But you have to send her away first! Then you will get some peace. Tell her to go! She chose to die! Send her away!" (Ramsay & Noorbergen, 1981, p. 116).

It was the last forceful suggestion necessary. Finally the client was able to say goodbye to her mother and to emotionally let her go and accept her death.

On the fifth day of therapy the client finally had to let go of her daughter. Repeated confrontations to do so finally wore down her resistance until she could do so. The client wailed,

> I've got to send you away, Beverly. I've got to send you away. I've got to send you away. I've got to send you away. I've got to send you away. Goodbye, my love. I've got to send you away. I've got to send you away. Goodbye, my love. Goodbye, Beverly. This is how I will always think of you . . . with me. . . . I will always think of you as you are now. Goodbye, my love. I've sent her away! (Ramsay & Noorbergen, 1981, p. 122).

The final session was a test of the successful recovery: the client was able to look at photographs of her mother and daughter for the first time without emotionally breaking down. Furthermore, she could listen to a recording of Beverly's favorite song without an emotional outburst.

The process of Guided Confrontation Therapy seems to differ from the process of grieving recommended by Melges and DeMaso primarily in that the former seems much more active and confrontational, a style which may not suit many therapists, especially those who have a psychoanalytical or nondirective orientation.

A THEORETICAL APPROACH TO THE NEED TO ADEQUATELY GRIEVE

The personal construct theory of George Kelly (1955) provides an excellent general theoretical perspective from which to understand the process of grieving. Although Kelly did not really apply his theory to the grieving process, his theory lends itself nicely to understanding grieving. Thus, in abnormal or *improper* grieving, survivors are confused in the way they construe the deceased. Often some unresolved feelings (e.g., anger, guilt, jealousy) about the deceased are triggered by the death of someone close to them, and such feelings can seem to those grieving to contradict the more conscious feelings (e.g., sadness) they had also maintained about the deceased. If not resolved, such "negative" feelings can cause the survivors some form of anxiety or depression.

In normal or *proper* grieving, the death of someone becomes the occasion for survivors for a better understanding of their relationship with their loved ones. When apparently contradictory feelings about the deceased erupt, rather than dismiss or repress these feelings, survivors examine the meaning of those feelings, and thus elaborate their constructs of the deceased. This process of expanding the conceptual framework in which they understand the deceased further allows them to predict their future feelings about the deceased, thus greatly reducing anxiety.

Kelly (see Mancuso & Adams-Webber, 1982) had a lifelong commitment to applying his theory and his focus was usually psychotherapy. By seeing psychotherapy against the background of current work in developmental psychology (Morrison & Cometa, 1982), one can improve understanding of how persons have organized the experiences that shape their adult constructs of the world. According to Bannister and Fransella (1971)

> the child's construing of his mother's construct system is the jumping-off ground for the development of the child's construing system. He starts out with this and uses it in his dealings with others. Soon he meets others like himself and finds that all the anticipations she makes do not always work out, so he develops new role constructs in relation to others of his age. So he goes on, gradually elaborating his role construing (p. 87).

In clinical terms, if an adult client has lost a parent through death, and if that parent died when the client was younger than 12 (exceptions abound here), it is probable that the child's way of conceptualizing parents, family, and the world in general will suffer a severe rupture. The child may ignore the death event as far as possible and begin to adopt more and more the construct system of the surviving parent, stepparent, or significant other. But what happens to the constructs learned from the deceased parent and all the feelings accompanying this relationship? By relegating these constructs and feelings to a lower level of awareness, the client may only feel the guilt in "giving up" on the deceased parent. Since that is often the only way young children can emotionally survive—by not focusing on that parent—the child is almost condemned to relive the agony in the future. For example, as an adult that person might "fall apart at the seams" when a friend or family member dies. Because the child never construed the death of the parent properly, he or she will be quite unprepared to understand his or her erupting feelings on the occasion of later deaths. Thus, a construct system, or a way of conceptualizing and predicting events, is of absolute necessity to all persons who wish to maintain an emotional equilibrium.

Allow me to offer an example of how therapy can help a client to regain the construct system damaged by a death of the parent. In this case, a female client persisted in using constructions built from the organizing constructs available in early stages of conceptual development. This client had always been the favorite of her now-deceased father, and was troubled by her very negative constructs of her mother, who had come to live with her. The client's negative views of her mother had begun to induce many problems in living with her mother. In grieving her father, the client began to realize that she had built him up to be some kind of god and, conversely, that she had denied information that would have contradicted her excessively harsh view of her mother. As the client became more facile in construing her mother in positive terms, the client's construct system became complex and permeable enough to cope with an aging, lonely mother who needed her support and acceptance.

A child who experiences death then, especially during preoperational or concrete operational stages (see Piaget, 1958), has but limited schemata within which to integrate a great many experiences (fear of death, death of a parent, the wake and funeral, fear of future, loneliness, anger, sadness, guilt, and so on). One begins to realize that the simplistic, structured construct system available to the typical child can never adequately integrate all those data-producing experiences with which a child must try to cope. Since the child does not have useful schemata into which to integrate these episodes, he or she necessarily develops a simplistic and biased view, something that later on causes difficult problems.

In grieving therapy, the use of imagery helps the client to construct more adequately the sensorial and cognitive data about life-changing events such as the death of a loved one. The process, construed in Kellian terms, enables the adult client to use a more adequate construct system to understand the confusion of experiences surrounding the death with which the person could not cope as a child.

At this point, a more specific discussion of some of the tenents of Kellian theory may shed light on the grieving process. Kelly (1955) emphasizes that all persons are similar to scientists attempting to understand what happens around them. When trying to understand our relationship with the deceased, all of us must learn that our comprehension of that relationship may be less than adequate. If we do not accept such limitations to our understanding, our unpredicted emotional reactions (e.g., anger about someone we loved) can throw our construct system into unnerving confusion, causing excessive anxiety. This anxiety is symptomatic of our failure to completely process all of our feelings about the deceased. If we deny this need for further understanding, we might find ourselves depressed.

One can adopt the position that people often foster problem-riddled life patterns because they refuse to elaborate their rigid, simplistic, and unworkable set of constructs (Kelly, 1955). If so, the degree to which people refuse to change their long-cherished constructs of the deceased determines the extent of confusion experienced and thus their need to more properly grieve. Refusing to "loosen" constructs of the deceased—to see the person and our relationship with him or her in a new way—only fosters a "head in the sand" perspective, which does not promote personal growth.

On the contrary, when someone's death causes us "cognitive discomfort," an analysis of how our cognitive system must be stretched to accommodate new information (e.g., I never knew I loved my father so much!) can produce adequate grieving and new constructs of self. Thus, proper grieving can stimulate the type of personal growth that will enable a person to develop a more self-consonant and predictive, albeit implicit, personality theory. Such a perspective will ensure that disappointing cognitive disruptions are minimized in the future. With Antonovsky (1979), one can even assert that a predictive personality theory, or "sense of coherence," is what constitutes a sense of "health." Thus, the more we properly grieve the loss of a loved one, the "healthier" we will feel in the normally depressing circumstances where we lose a loved one.

Furthermore, in cases of proper grieving, even our behavior patterns may change. Thus, a husband who allows himself to properly grieve the death of his mother may, in some cases, discover on her death the extent of his anger toward her. Subsequent construct change may enable him to realize how much he has displaced that repressed anger onto his wife, and such insight may enable him to cease or greatly reduce this unfair displacement.

In brief, in order for the process of grieving to reach a satisfactory conclusion, a client often needs to evolve, in Kellian terms, more workable, superordinate, high-level constructions, which can encompass both the thoughts and feelings of the client about the loved one. Such useful constructs allow the grieving person to experience such thoughts and feelings as integrated, rather than contradictory, systems.

According to Kelly's (1955) fundamental postulate, a person's processes are psychologically channelized by the ways in which he or she anticipated events. In terms of the grieving process, I might apply that postulate to the client who experiences the death of a parent. The client had from time to time thought of the parent dying in the future, but never seemed to feel a great deal of emotion connected with the thought. But then the parent dies, he is overwhelmed with emotion, and feels he is "coming unglued." The client in this case obviously did not have an adequate way of construing his relationship with his parent, or he would have anticipated his reaction. As Kelly also explains, people differ from each other in their construction of events. Not everyone finds inadequacies in how they view a loved one's death. Some, fortunately, have not only thought about the possibility of a loved one's death but have come to some resolution about the meaning of that relationship and are better prepared for the feeling they thus experience.

Although the further theoretical discussion of the usefulness of personal construct theory to understanding the need for grieving would be useful, such a necessarily lengthy discussion will be postponed at this time in favor of elaborating on how construct theory guides the therapist who is helping a client to grieve. Thus, our primary emphasis in this chapter will be clinical, not theoretical.

USING EMOTIVE-RECONSTRUCTIVE IMAGERY TECHNIQUES TO INDUCE GRIEVING

The use of imagery techniques within psychotherapy can greatly assist a therapist in his grief work with a client. A concentration on imagery can re-create so quickly the emotional ambience of the loved one's death that feelings are often easily generated. And with those feelings comes the opportunity to analyze one's constructs about the deceased. Without imagery, a client's defenses against repressed feelings are often stronger. Especially when a client is trying to simply *talk* about the deceased, the opportunity for confronting his or her feelings about that person may be lost. For "events learned in one psychic state can be remembered better when one is put back into the same state one was in during the original experience" (Bower, 1981). And that re-creation of the original experience to elicit clear memories and strong emotional reactions is often best accomplished by having the client concentrate on mental imagery.

The techniques used by the author emerge from a short-term form of psychotherapy called *emotive-reconstructive therapy*. As described in detail elsewhere (Morrison, 1979, 1980; Morrison & Cometa, 1977, 1980), this psychotherapeutic modality is based on the theoretical propositions of Kelly (1955) and Piaget (1972) and uses mental imagery as its primary clinical technique. Ancillary techniques are role-playing and deep-breathing exercises.

The use of this technique to induce proper grieving will become clearer in a discussion of the typical grieving session. After clients are asked to close their eyes, the therapist has them concentrate on imagery, mostly visual, connected with four events: the death, wake, funeral, and burial of the deceased. In some cases, the imagery associated with any one of these events is sufficient to induce powerful expressions of feelings and appropriate insights. In other cases, all four events are sensorially re-created in order to accomplish the same effect. The general principle guiding the therapists that one progresses from the death through the burial, only stopping when the client seems very close to a breakthrough. Often all four events can be covered in a single session. Sometimes two or three sessions are needed before the client will allow certain feelings to be expressed.

When the therapist induces the imagery connected with the *death* of a loved one, the client may react to these stimuli in a variety of ways. Some clients allow this imagery to lead them into strongly repressed feelings (e.g., sadness, anger, guilt, affection, etc.), which often prompt new constructs of self and others. Others breeze through the experience, using every defense available to deny the pain associated with the experience. Usually, the therapist does not choose to immediately fight those defenses, since imagery associated with subsequent events may well weaken such defenses. A death event that is associated with vivid imagery due to certain circumstances (e.g., a parent dies in the presence of a client; a loved one dies, at least partially due to the negligence of the client) is one that seems most capable of inducing a breakthrough in a client's defense system.

If the imagery connected with the death event itself is not sufficient to induce repressed feelings, the therapist may then proceed to the *wake,* if there was one. The more rituals (e.g., saying the rosary) connected with a wake, the better the client seems to be able to sensorially re-create the emotional experience of the wake. Open-casket wakes can be a powerful imagery stimulus, which creates a valuable role-playing opportunity in which the therapist can ask the client to talk to the deceased and to say all the things he or she never had a chance to say before the person died.

In my experience, most *funeral services* do not provoke the kind of imagery or insights that the therapist would value. Most of these services in our culture are quite stiff and unemotional. However, imagery associated with certain services (e.g., an old-time Roman Catholic funeral with black vestments, candles, incense, etc.) can on occasion prompt more useful grieving.

Often more valuable than the funeral service for purposes of grieving is the *burial* of the loved one. One can imagine how emotionally jarring a burial event can be at a military funeral, with images of the flag ceremony, firing of shots, etc. If previous role-playing to express formerly repressed feelings has been unsuccessful to this point, the therapist can use the cemetery scene as the occasion to have the client "say goodbye" to the deceased. Often in such role-playing, clients will discover feelings that lead to new constructs of self and others.

CASE STUDIES ILLUSTRATING PROPER GRIEVING

At this point, four case studies may help to illustrate how I use imagery in grieving sessions to help clients change their dysfunctional constructs.

Case Study 1

Jane was a 32-year-old woman complaining of excessive anxiety and depression. She had recently become obsessed with the fear that she had developed cancer like her parents who had both died of this disease. After just one introductory assessment session, the author contracted with the client to begin attempts to more properly grieve the loss of these parents. The client had long been aware of her need to set in order her feelings about her parents and their deaths.

The first grieving session was purposely abbreviated to test how well the client used imagery, as well as to determine whether the client was emotionally able to cope with such emotionally laden events. The following is a transcript of the emotive or imagery phases of Jane's (C) first and second grieving sessions with her therapist (T), the author. In the first session, the author asked the client to re-create her father's death through imagery.

> T: I want you to close your eyes and first remember what you saw and heard around the time your father died. I want you to remember the circumstances of his death . . . not in an abstract way, but rather I want you to feel as much as possible like you are there again and it is happening right now. I want you to use all of your senses in re-creating the imagery of that death.
>
> C: Dad was disabled for a long time. He had had a stroke on top of the emphysema he had developed. He had hardening of the arteries. He had lost a lot of weight. He looked about 90-years-old. He was in the hospital in Pennsylvania. I saw him two weeks before he died. He was really ill. His skin was cold to touch. He was mad at my sister for something at the time. I felt helpless that he was so ill. Yet, I wished he'd die because he had been so ill for so long.

T: I want you to breathe deeply and relaxingly for awhile. Try to examine what you feel deep down while you are breathing this way. (Client appears to be close to crying after breathing this way for a few seconds.) Talk to your dad and tell him what you are feeling right now.

C: I love you, Dad. I want to tell you that I love you. The words won't come out. Sometimes it doesn't seem to matter anyway. (Client begins to cry.) Oh! I feel hurt. Feels like it hurts all the way inside of me. I don't know what to say to you. You're mad at Lucille (client's sister.) I don't know whether to try to reach you. (Client begins to sob loudly.) Oh! It makes me wish you'd die. I'm so tired of trying to deal with you and reach you. It just doesn't seem to matter. (Client sobs even more noticeably.) (Briefly, speaking to the therapist): I'm angry; he's so unreachable. (Now speaking again to her father): I want to know before you die that you care about me. I'm angry you can't see that. You've always been so wound up in yourself. How awful life was for you! (She says these words sarcastically.) You can't see others care. All you can see is what we *don't* do for you. It makes me angry you're so selfish. What a martyr you are!

T: I want you to begin thinking about the present again and, whenever you feel comfortable doing so, you can just open your eyes and we'll talk about what you just experienced.

Although substantial construct change did not seem to emerge from this brief session, the client felt relieved to express a great deal of repressed anger, frustration, affection, and sadness. In the very next session, the author attempted to elaborate on her simplistic constructs of her father, urging her to image her father's wake.

T: Close your eyes and sensorially immerse yourself in the imagery of your father's wake. Try to see the faces of the people who were there.

C: My brother was there. My husband. My relatives. It was a long wake.

T: Look at the face and body of your father in the open casket.

C: (Client suddenly begins to breathe rapidly as if she is hyperventilating.) I feel confused. "Well, now you're dead," I thought to myself. It's very difficult to think about what he meant to me. I'm so relieved to be able to start dealing with him. I felt really unsettled there. That's how I feel right now. In some ways I always knew he was there. He'd know how to fix anything. He was there to take care of things. I start thinking about having wanted to please him and never having done it. (Client begins to cry.) He was difficult to please. There was never any way he showed me he was pleased with me. He was very negative. He ignored the good I did. He treated others the same. He was emotionally cold. I felt some relief when he died. It used to be a real chore to see him. And how often I would go home to visit him and I would want to get out of there. He didn't want to hear about what I did. He'd talk about the weather and how we hardly ever came to see him. He told others he was proud of us, but he'd never tell any of us. (After a pause) I felt angry at the wake. Angry he hadn't ever let me get to know him.

At this point, the therapist asked the client to briefly image her father's funeral service. The service was brief, and she remembered little about it. She did not go to the cemetery for the burial. So, because I still did not feel the client had significantly changed her constructs of father or self, I asked her to continue to keep her eyes closed and to express more feelings toward him. After asking the client to form a vivid image of her father, I allowed her to continue.

C: He was a terrible father. He was mean to me and Mom. He wouldn't even let us talk to Mom about the cancer she developed. And he wouldn't let Mom go anywhere. I was afraid to go against him. When he'd visit her at the hospital—when she was dying of cancer—he'd only stay ten minutes . . . ten lousy minutes . . . even though we had driven three hours to get to the hospital! She'd beg him to stay longer. But he'd leave and make me leave with him. I feel guilty I didn't stand up to him. I wouldn't talk to him all the way back. I didn't have the guts to confront him.

T: Tell him now what you couldn't say to him then. Tell him what you really feel about how he treated your mother.

C: How could you be so cruel? She *needed* you and you walked out on her! I don't think I can ever forgive you for that. (Client begins to sob loudly.) It was the cruelest thing I've ever seen done. Mom was so scared.

After I allowed the client to cry alone for a few minutes, I asked her to open her eyes and, during the reconstructive phase of therapy, connect her feeling of hopelessness related to her mother's illness to her recent fear that she had breast cancer. She was really afraid that she might be abandoned and left alone as her father had abandoned her mother. This feeling of "aloneness" seemed to form the core feeling of pain that she had been trying to escape since childhood. The client was now able to begin the work of changing constructs of herself and her father due to this new informational breakthrough. She could now understand that her long-felt anger toward her father only masked her long-repressed need for a father who would care for her and protect her from all danger. Now that she could put her finger on what she was really afraid of—being alone—her fear of cancer no longer was a useful construct.

After those two sessions, the client reported feeling significantly less depressed and anxious. She felt much less guilt related to her father now that she could admit her true feelings toward him. She began to sleep better, her stomach problems began to subside, and she reported fewer headaches. The client continued to use the insights into her feelings about her father through several other sessions of emotive-reconstructive therapy in which she was even more successfully able to resolve her conflicted feelings about her father and her boss who, incidentally, she discovered reminded her of her father. The two grieving sessions were so successful that those who knew the client continually commented on how much positive change was evident in the client.

After four more sessions concerned with other topics, the author asked the client to attempt grieving the loss of her mother. Although the client cried a great deal toward the end of the session, it did not appear to the author that the client had any conflicted feelings toward her mother, and that this part of the grieving process could be terminated in just one session. Only some minor elaborations of constructs of self and mother took place. The client eventually finished therapy after 16 sessions of emotive-reconstructive therapy (only three of which were grieving sessions). Evaluation after therapy as well as in a 10-month followup clearly indicated that the client no longer had problems with depression or anxiety.

It is important to note at this point that the dynamics of the above sessions could be explained within many other theoretical frameworks (e.g., psychoanalytic, Gestalt, etc.). However, the clear and ever-constant focus on changing the constructs of a client seems, at least to the author, to provide more consistent guideposts along the way to an ultimate rearrangement of the client's view of the world.

Case Study 2

This case may help to further illustrate how the grieving process can be facilitated by the use of imagery in such a way as to induce construct change. Lucy, a 34-year-old married housewife, initially presented herself as a severely depressed woman who had frequently considered and attempted suicide. She reported feeling depressed about her wife/mother role and appeared to have little hope that life would change in the future. Lucy spent a great deal of time reminiscing about the past, and much of her thinking can be described as morose.

After four sessions of emotive-reconstructive therapy on various life events, it became apparent that the client needed to properly grieve the death of her grandfather who had died when she was eight. It seemed to me that a great deal of emotion was tied up in her comments about her grandfather, and I wondered if he had been a substitute father for Lucy. (She never knew her own father, who had abandoned her shortly after birth. According to Kübler-Ross (1969), children younger than 9 or 10 can have a great deal of difficulty understanding the death of someone close to them. When that happens, it is my experience that children tend to block out the experience and sometimes even the person connected with it.)

The following transcript of Lucy's fifth session illustrates how the therapist (T) can use vivid imagery to induce proper grieving in a client (C):

T: Close your eyes and focus on your grandfather's face. I want you to see him as he looked when you were eight years of age. I want you to get the feeling that you are looking up at him, as you would if you were really eight right now. Try to see him and hear his voice. Maybe there was even a distinctive odor about him. Let all your senses operate to image your grandfather. Eventually I want you to try to remember what happened around the time he died.

C: He's in a special bed, a hospital bed. He looks very, very skinny. He always called me his "Little Pollack" (Her voice begins to sound like a little girl's.) He was always giving me quarters. Grandfather had tubes in him. Now I remember being at home. I'm going upstairs. I go into the bedroom. Daddy's (her stepfather) holding both of Grandpa's wrists. Grandpa's very sick. An ambulance came and took Grandpa downstairs. I went into my room. I'm all alone. My Daddy comes in. He tells me Grandpa has to stay at the hospital. Daddy says he'll be back soon. Then I lie down on my bed. I can see all of this so clearly. Just Mom and Dad, Uncle Jimmy and Aunt Marion around. I sleep on the couch all night. I'm the first one up in the morning. I know Grandpa was sick. He looked terrible! I answer the phone again. It's my Aunt Marion. Grandpa wants to speak to his "Little Pollack." Then Grandpa died. Mommy said that he looked awful, awful sick. But Grandpa still needed to give his quarter to me. Before he died he put on his shoes. Just like the cowboys who put their boots on. Grandpa and I always used to play Cowboys and Indians. (After a short pause) I see a lot of people crying. Mommy had Peggy take me to the wake. Daddy took me up to say goodbye. Grandpa was always so nice. He was always good to me. He played with me. We'd talk all the time.

T: Talk to him now as you see him in the open casket.

C: I love you and you've gone (client begins to cry.) You're dead and can't come back. I loved you. (Now talking to the therapist): I loved him so much.

T: Can you cry for him?

C: He shouldn't have died.

T: He was like a daddy to you?

C: Yes. Yes. He loved me. He really loved me and always had time for me! Always. I think I was his favorite. "Such a pretty Pollack," he'd say. At Christmas he read me stories. He just shouldn't have died. He died of cancer. I don't know why.

T: What do you think your grandfather would say to you today?

C: He'd idolize my kids. He really didn't spoil me. I could talk to him. I could trust him. He'd just talk to me. I wish he were here. He'd listen to me. His advice would be good. He'd never let me down. He'd be proud of me. He'd forget the mistakes. "You're still my beautiful little Pollack," he'd say. I never knew I missed him so much! I never thought that much about him since he died . . . until today.

T: Can you say goodbye to your grandfather?

C: Oh, you were always just so great. I love you so much. I'm happy you don't hurt anymore. I'm going to miss you. Goodbye. Bye. (Client puts her hands over her eyes and begins crying again.) I'd kiss him goodbye, if I had the chance. No one let me do that at the time.

Until this session, the client had completely forgotten what her grandfather looked like. She had no photographs of him to help her recall his appearance. Until this session, she never realized the strong, powerful, positive feelings she had for her grandfather. In reality, he was more of a father to her than her real father.

Up until this point in therapy, the client had been recalling only unpleasant events from her childhood. Perhaps because of her focus on her grandfather's death, and the pleasant memories of him which death imagery evoked, the client was able in her next session to get in touch with repressed pleasant memories of her mother. These memories in turn convinced the client that she had been stereotyping her mother as "bad" and she subsequently concluded, because of the pleasant memories associated with her mother when the client was very young, that her mother had indeed loved her. These positive constructs of her mother substantially changed for the better the client's interaction with her mother.

Beginning after that fifth session, the client reported a substantial lessening of her depression. After 10 imagery sessions, the client was able to terminate therapy with satisfaction that her life had substantially changed for the better. Her original complaints were no longer in evidence and she reported new meaning in her life.

This case illustration demonstrates how persons often need to grieve the loss of a loved one before they can get in touch with the kind of feelings that produce new constructs about self and others. It was almost as if the client had to open herself up to the immense pain of grieving before she could truly live a meaningful life. She had to give up cherished simplistic constructs (e.g., no one loves me), typical of a child, before she could fully understand what her life meant. I have frequently discovered that quite often it is the grieving of a relative or friend that opens up a new way of construing others. As in this case illustration, I have often found that the grieving process can be completed in one 45-minute session.

During a session such as this, the therapist uses vivid imagery to induce powerful feelings, the kind of feelings that provide the necessary input to induce a client to readjust the way she construes other people. For the client to construe her grandfather as someone who loved her flexed her construct system so that she was able to entertain and use a whole new set of constructs about others (e.g., people can love me), thus inducing other valuable constructs (e.g., I am lovable).

Case Study 3

This case study concerns a 41-year-old, never-married executive with a large organization. Being highly intelligent (I.Q. of 165), Robert was able to use intellectualization to partially mask the terrible pain that he felt at the age of 10 when his mother died of cancer. Not being able at such a tender age to properly cope with such a devastating separation from a mother to whom he was so emotionally close, Robert chose to not let himself experience real feelings again. Seldom in later life would he allow himself to get too close to anyone. When women would fall in love with him, he would typically overfocus on their faults until he could pull away from them and eventually drift on to another relationship.

Despite Robert's neurotic attempts to disguise his real pain of separation from his mother, that pain would pierce the armor of his defenses periodically, and he would feel the usual concomitant physiological symptoms of depression and anxiety. Finally he could take it no longer and entered psychotherapy with the author in a highly motivated state. The following is the full text of Robert's third session of emotive-reconstructive therapy, a session that focused entirely on the death of his mother.

> T: Close your eyes, and I want you to slowly go back into the past . . . back to your mother's death at the age of 10. I want you to form vivid images of where you were when you first heard about or witnessed her death.
> C: I was in school. It was a dark, cloudy day. I was in a classroom. The teacher was an Italian. Someone came in and gave her a note. I went through the rest of the day without knowing for sure what had happened. Then I was sent to a children's home along with my siblings. It was a Baptist home. A man was with my father. Dad was crying. I knew then that Mom was dead. But I wanted to feel it by myself and not hear it from a stranger. We were all sitting in chairs and this man, who was the director of this home, talked about the Lord needing an angel. I thought to myself, "He's full of shit, God, I hate his fuckin' guts." I didn't need a fairy story. I looked at Dad with tears in his eyes. I didn't cry. I couldn't feel what was going on. I felt alone. I remember walking downstairs. The light was gleaming on the marble floor. I can see the windows and French doors. I laid my head against the glass. I didn't know what was happening to me. I could see the rain coming down the glass. I began to cry. I remember thinking, "Even God is ashamed today." I let the tears flow. Then I went downstairs—I was still in a daze—to the boy's bathroom and looked out the window. I cried again. I felt a terrible anger toward the director because of the way he told us about Mom's death. (Long pause)

T: I want you now to picture yourself at your mother's wake. I want you to see the room, the coffin, and most of all your mother laid out in the coffin.

C: The funeral parlor was downtown. Mom was laid out to the right of the door. The first time I went to the wake I said to myself: "She's asleep. It's all a joke." I wasn't allowing myself to believe she was dead. There was no sense of pain. I didn't cry. The second time I went to the wake I went to the casket. I remember touching her forehead. Nothing happened when I touched her and I almost collapsed. I felt rubbery-legged. Two guys saw me and brought me into the bathroom. They tried to give me a glass of water, but my hands were too weak. This weak feeling lasted ten or fifteen minutes. It was all because I tried to touch her. It was like she was asleep.

T: Talk to her as if she can hear you right now. Talk to her as you see her in the casket.

C: Mom, why are you doing this to me? Why don't you come back? Don't leave me. I'm angry! How could you make me hurt this way? What have I done to deserve this? Come back to me. I need you. (Client begins to cry.)

T: Tell her about your life after she died.

C: Life was not the same after you died. My feelings stopped and I began to hate. It was all so confusing. I was all full of hate and anger. I couldn't think straight. Maybe I thought you'd come back. We'd keep a place between us at the table. Louise (Robert's stepmother) was not the mom you were. I always wondered if Dad really cared about you. Things are getting better now. I have hope now. I want, Mom, to accept what happened to you . . . to make a life for myself . . . to be able to let go of you so I can grow. But I don't want to forget you.

T: Tell her what she meant to you.

C: You were everything that made me feel good. You screamed a lot, but still you made a home for me. You took care of me. I just feel so sorry for what happened to you. If I did anything to hurt you, I'm sorry. Sorry no one ever told me how sick you were. I lived a big lie. Maybe if we had been told the truth it would have been worse. I'll never forget the look on your face the last time I saw you alive. (Pause) Everyone told me I'd write letters to you begging you not to die. They knew I was affected. I loved you. You were my world! But I couldn't save you from death.

T: Now I want you to place yourself at your mom's funeral. Try to see the images as vividly as you can. Try to let yourself feel what you felt then.

C: The funeral was in a church. An open-casket service. All the adults were in front of us. We were behind them. The adults went up and kissed Mom in the casket. I was afraid they'd make me kiss her too! A man took me to kiss her. I said, "NO!" I couldn't. Total feeling of fear . . . of anxiety . . . of having to kiss a dead person. They allowed me to kiss the icon and put it in her casket. It was like she wasn't really dead. They

took the casket. I wanted to scream, "NO!" It was like she'd been hurt. (Client begins to cry and then to sob loudly.) I didn't want her head to hurt. I didn't want them to hurt my mother.
T: Just let all the tears come. Don't say anything for a little while. Just feel the pain of it all, and then go to the burial.
C: (After a pause) They wouldn't let me go to the cemetery. I knew once the casket was put in the hearse, it'd be the last time I'd see her—then the adults went away with her.
T: I want you to go to the cemetery now and say goodbye to your mother.
C: I guess I imagined what happened there. The casket was lowered and roses were thrown on top before dirt was put on. I felt bad that I had never given her a rose. There was only a stone that said "464." No gravestone then. Dad couldn't afford it. Sometime later my brother and I put twenty-five roses on the grave. I stuck a 26th rose in the ground. "That's mine," I said. It was a chance to give her *my* rose. I wanted to throw that piece of me in with her. "Goodbye, Mom. Goodbye."
T: Take your time now. Let those images fade away slowly. . . . Begin to think about the present and, when you are ready, begin to open your eyes.

This one 45-minute session is an excellent example of the internal pain that a child experiences on the occasion of a parent's death. Robert reexperienced a wide range of feelings (anger, fear, guilt, love, sadness, rage) during this session. After the emotive phase of the session (described above), Robert began to make connections between his mother's death and events of his later life. He realized that since his beloved mother died, he was afraid to let other women get so close to him. He would let no one ever hurt him like that again.

Whenever the subject of having a child would come up in a relationship, Robert would panic. He didn't want a child of his to be anything like him . . . with all that pain. He also realized that most of his real creative abilities seemed to have died with his mother. A voracious reader at the age of 10, he stopped reading after his mother's death, as if to stop new ideas. It was as if he closed off the right hemisphere of the brain from consciousness after his mother's death.

In Robert's case, he needed to reexperience images related to his mother's death before he could change destructive self-constructions (e.g., to feel is always to hurt; no one can take Mom's place; I will always feel dead inside; etc.). To see the death-related images for him meant intense pain. But the pain enabled him to feel again, for he began to construe himself and others in new ways (e.g., not everyone is out to hurt me; I am lovable to others besides my mother).

Although Robert required other emotive-reconstructive sessions on a wide variety of topics, he felt that this third session was a key session, and he reported that life seemed different now that he was letting himself experience feelings again.

Case Study 4

A 39-year-old married artist came for individual psychotherapy because of severe, prolonged depressions, which periodically led him to seriously consider suicide. His depressions frequently affected his work productivity and self-image. One of his goals in therapy was to work on his feelings toward his deceased father, a former policeman, with whom he had always had a strained relationship. The father's death at the age of 64 had left the client confused about his feelings for his father because the client had just begun to get close to him before he died, thus leaving a lot unsaid.

In his fourth imagery session, the client agreed to begin the process of more completely grieving his father's death. The following is a transcript of that session:

> T: I want you to go back to the moment when you first heard about your father's death. I believe you told me that you heard about his death by means of a telephone call. Now close your eyes and imagine you are called to the phone. Try to imagine yourself there by the phone, seeing the room you are standing in, feeling the telephone in your hand, and so on. Take a few deep breaths and try to feel what you felt then.
>
> C: (After a long pause, client begins to sob and, with mouth wide open, actually begins to wail loudly. Tears fall down his cheeks.) Oh, oh, oh! (Client continues to sob loudly.) Oh, oh! Oh, it hurts so much to think about it! (Client opens eyes briefly and then closes them again.) My stepmother (client's father divorced his mother and later remarried) called. She described how she woke up and found Dad dead. He was grey. There was a thin morning light. The death was sudden. He was on vacation in Florida with friends. He had a pacemaker. His wife was very emotional over the phone and couldn't stop crying. I cried for a couple of hours after the call. I had cut off the relationship with Dad when everything was going well between the two of us. We went down to his place as a family: Mom, my wife, and I. My emotions were like steel then. We all tried to avoid crying. My sister was close to cracking, however. All the old friends were there from the old neighborhood. Seeing all those people in this room . . . a sterile room with plastic flowers . . . all the cops there he knew . . . really got to me. The cops were crying. Everyone seemed to be crying. Finally, I cried too. Everyone liked him. We got him this lavish casket. Fortunately for my composure the casket was closed. Thank God! The casket was burgundy enamelled. Very rich. The room where the casket was placed was institutional looking. A few flowers. My eyes filled with tears. I looked at the people and found myself to be screaming and crying more than the rest. Dad's new wife was broken up too. Mom did not go to the wake. She didn't want to face his second wife. She also didn't go to the funeral.
>
> T: Tell me about the images that surround the funeral.

C: The police were all there. There was a Rabbi there. Eulogies were given by different people in the service room of a Jewish funeral home. I don't remember that much about the service. I didn't like the Rabbi. He "fished" for souls. Used guilt.

T: (After a short pause) Did you go to the cemetery?

C: Yes. I was bawling the whole time. I cried from when I saw the casket until they buried him.

T: Talk to your father at the gravesite. Tell him what you've left unsaid all these years.

C: Oh! (Client begins to cry loudly again.) Oh Dad, I couldn't ... I wish when I was growing up we could've been closer to each other. I felt you hated me and wanted to hurt me at times. I couldn't ... (client cries more loudly) I couldn't live up to what you wanted me to be. Only the last few years, when it was too late, could we talk to each other as human beings. Then you just disappeared. I couldn't ever tell you these things. I couldn't tell you how disturbed I was that you and Mom couldn't be together ... that you were having an affair. (Client cries loudly.)

T: Tell your dad the way you really wanted it.

C: I wish we could've done more and talked some together ... talked heart to heart instead of playing roles. Those few times we could embrace each other in the last few years meant so much to me because you accepted me. Now I've got to accept myself. Oh, oh, there were times when I hated him and couldn't express it.

T: But you didn't really want to leave it that way.

C: I didn't. I wanted to be close to him. I'm as much of a man as he was and I wanted him to feel that.

T: What didn't he accept about you?

C: (At this point the client just opened his eyes and left them open for the remainder of the session.) It's hard to put my finger on it. He felt I was self-centered. Only thinking of myself. I wanted him not to feel that way. But I was self-focused. I never really knew him. Like he had a secret life. One face he showed me. I never felt I really knew him. I felt he was cold to me at times. He was more congenial to others my own age. There was a sense that he couldn't forgive me. I was unforgiven for something ... maybe my close relationship with Mom (during the Second World War when his father was away for years in the Army). Part of the agony was being caught between Mom and Dad. His desire for me to be exemplary at the camp he and Mom ran in the summer. Like when he tried to force me to box that other kid and I wouldn't. He wanted me to have great physical powers. He wanted me to be a good competitor. Mom always shielded me and my sister from any strong emotions. Dad wasn't afraid to traumatize me. It was vengeance. I wanted to bury the hatchet these last years. It hurt me so.

T: He sure got to you. It's like he cursed you with always having to question yourself about everything. He never knew how much he got through to you. You never really let him know.

The client explained that this session was an important one in his therapeutic process because he had reexamined his many feelings about his father. He realized he really wanted to make peace with him, and that he had previously not really understood this. The next week the client reported that after he left this grieving session he had a feeling of hope for the first time about the whole process of therapy. He felt all week like he was gradually coming out of a fog. His suicidal thoughts began to decrease significantly, the greatest reduction in a long time. The client had discovered that he had a pattern of developing self-destructive constructs (I should kill myself) whenever he felt guilt about something. Thus, relieving his guilt about his father in the grieving process had reduced his self-destructive constructs.

The client finished eleven more imagery sessions (all but one related to non-grieving issues) before he finished therapy with almost all of his goals achieved. In his fifteenth session, we focused on his own death sometime in the future. He realized how much his family and friends would miss him, and he concluded that he could never take his own life because that would really hurt those he loved, and he loved people too much to do that.

A FEW RECOMMENDATIONS OF CAUTION

Imagery techniques may not be appropriate for those therapists who have not carefully analyzed their own imagery. Especially when therapists suspect that they themselves have not yet properly grieved the loss of a significant person, they must proceed with caution in assisting another to grieve. Otherwise, such therapists may find they are using client time to process their own feelings.

Secondly, therapists should be aware that directed imagery can occasionally provoke traumatic emotional reactions in clients, and they must be ready for them. Although I have never experienced a client becoming psychotic when attempting to face the death of a loved one, I have witnessed a rare client who became psychotic while using imagery to re-create other very traumatic events (e.g., the loss of a childhood friend when the family moved).

RESEARCH

To the author's knowledge, research has yet to be done to determine the effectiveness of imagery techniques in inducing proper grieving. One of the difficulties of doing such research is that most clients come for therapy for multiple reasons, only one of which may be to properly grieve the death of a loved one. In fact, my experience as a psychotherapist in private practice indicates that it is actually very rare for a client to come for therapy with the express purpose of completing the grieving process. Usually they enter therapy because of depression, excessive anxiety, or relationship problems without realizing that in some instances improper grieving may be an important factor impinging on these problems. Thus, a crucial problem in doing research is how to isolate the effect of grieving sessions from the effect of other sessions dealing with other important issues and problems.

One way of proceeding would be to administer dependent measures (e.g., self-report checklists regarding self-image, behavior and symptom change, behavioral indices, etc.) immediately before and after grieving sessions, which would be scheduled consecutively. In this way, the use of imagery or other techniques to deal with other life events (e.g., a father's anger, early sickness, rejection by a girlfriend, divorce, etc.) may be separated from the use of imagery focusing on the grieving process. But this suggestion implies that in one, two, or perhaps as many as three sessions of grieving, the effect of those sessions will show up on various standardized dependent measures. I have found in researching the effect of five imagery sessions (emotive-reconstructive therapy related to relevant life events, sometimes including a grieving session), that a significant effect will show up on dependent measures (e.g., symptom checklists; see Morrison & Cometa, 1979). However, this study was limited in scope and did not include control groups.

Perhaps the ideal research would be conducted on randomly selected family members of hospital patients who have died. Since these family members would, in most cases, not be asking for therapy, perhaps their cooperation in this small-scale project (three sessions on grieving) could isolate the effect, on various dependent measures, of only techniques aimed at inducing grieving. A control group of matched family members, who did not undergo the therapy-structured grieving process, would of course be necessary in such a research design.

THE ROLE OF THEORY

I believe that for several decades psychologists have been caught up so much in empirical research that they have neglected the role of theory. Related to the grieving process and the kind of valuable tool imagery techniques provide therapists, a great deal of theoretical work needs to be done. Although I have suggested in this chapter that personal construct theory may provide a useful theoretical framework in which the need for grieving and imagery techniques can illuminate each other, still the task of elaborating such a framework in greater depth remains to be done. It is my hope that someone will take time and effort to continue this work.

REFERENCES

Aguilar, I., & Wood, V. N. (1976). Therapy through death ritual. *Social Work, January*, 49-54.
Antonovsky, A. (1979). *Health, stress and coping.* San Francisco, CA: Jossey-Bass.

Archer, J. (1999). *The nature of grief: The evolution and psychology of reactions to grief.* New York: Routledge.

Arya. (1979). *Meditation and the art of dying.* Honesdale, PA: Himalayan International Institute.

Bannister, D., & Fransella, F. (1971). *Inquiring man: The theory of personal constructs.* Harmondsworth, Middlesex: Penguin.

Bower, G. H. (1981). Mood and memory. *American Psychologist, 36,* 129-148.

Bowlby, J. (1963). Pathological mourning and childhood mourning. *Journal of the American Psychoanalytic Association, 11,* 500-541.

Bowlby, J. (1973). *Attachment and loss.* New York: Basic Books.

Choron, J. (1963). *Death and Western thought.* New York: Collier Books.

Engel, G. (1961). Is grief a disease? *Psychosomatic Medicine, 23,* 18-22.

Faschingbauer, T. R., Devaul, R. A., & Zisook, S. (1977). Development of the Texas Inventory of Grief. *American Journal of Psychiatry, 134,* 696-698.

Feifel, H. (1963). Death. In N. L. Farberow (Ed.), *Taboo topics.* New York: Atherton Press.

Freud, S. (1915). Thoughts for the times on war and death. In S. Freud (Ed.), *The complete works of Freud.* London: Hogarth Press.

Freud, S. (1958). *Mourning and melancholia* (Standard ed., Vol. 14). London: Hogarth Press. (Original work published in 1917.)

Gorer, G. (1965). *Death, grief, and mourning.* Garden City, NY: Doubleday.

Kalish, R. (1965). Some variables in death attitudes. In R. Fulton (Ed.), *Death and identity.* New York: Wiley.

Kastenbaum, R. J. (2001). *Death, society, human experience.* Boston, MA: Allyn and Bacon.

Kastenbaum, R. J., & Aisenberg, R. (1972). *The psychology of death.* New York: Springer.

Kelly, G. (1955). *The psychology of personal constructs* (Vols. 1-2). New York: Norton.

Kübler-Ross, E. (1969). *On death and dying.* New York: Macmillan.

Mancuso, J. C., & Adams-Webber, J. R. (1982). *The construing person.* New York: Praeger.

Melges, F. T. (1982). *Time and the inner future: A temporal approach to psychiatric disorders.* New York: Wiley.

Melges, F. T., & DeMaso, D. R. (1980). Grief resolution therapy: Reliving, revising, and revisiting. *American Journal of Psychotherapy, xxxiv,* 51-61.

Morrison, J. K. (1978). Successful grieving: Changing personal constructs through mental imagery. *Journal of Mental Imagery, 2,* 63-68.

Morrison, J. K. (1979). Emotive-reconstructive therapy: Changing constructs by means of mental imagery. In A. A. Sheikh & J. T. Shaffer (Eds.), *The potential of fantasy and imagination.* New York: Brandon House.

Morrison, J. K. (1980). Emotive-reconstructive therapy: A short-term, psychotherapeutic use of mental imagery. In J. E. Shorr, G. E. Sobel, P. Robin, & J. A. Connella (Eds.), *Imagery: Its many dimensions and applications.* New York: Plenum.

Morrison, J. K. (1981). Using death imagery to induce proper grieving: An emotive-constructive approach. In E. Klinger (Ed.), *Imagery: Concepts, results, and applications* (Vol. 2). New York: Plenum.

Morrison, J. K. (2002). Imagery techniques in emotive-reconstructive therapy In A. A. Sheikh (Ed.), *Handbook of therapeutic imagery techniques.* Amityville, NY: Baywood.

Morrison, J. K., & Cometa, M. C. (1977). Emotive-reconstructive psychotherapy: A short-term cognitive approach. *American Journal of Psychotherapy, 31,* 294-301.

Morrison, J. K., & Cometa, M. C. (1979). Emotive-reconstructive therapy and client problem resolution: Periodic accountability to the consumer. In J. K. Morrison (Ed.), *A consumer approach to community psychology.* Chicago, IL: Nelson-Hall.

Morrison, J. K., & Cometa, M. C. (1980). A cognitive, reconstructive approach to the psychotherapeutic use of imagery. *Journal of Mental Imagery, 4,* 35-42.

Morrison, J. K., & Cometa, M. C. (1982). Variations in developing construct systems: The experience corollary. In J. C. Mancuso & J. R. Adams-Webber (Eds.), *The construing person.* New York: Praeger.

Muggeridge, M. (1970). *The Observer,* February 20.

Neimeyer, R. A. (2001). *Meaning reconstruction and the experience of loss.* Washington, DC: American Psychological Association.

Parkes, C. M. (1972). *Bereavement.* New York: International Universities Press.

Parkes, C. M., & Weiss, R. S. (1983). *Bereavement: Is there an optimal path to recovery?* New York: Basic Books.

Piaget, J. (1958). *The child's construction of reality.* London: Routledge and Kegan Paul.

Piaget, J. (1972). *Judgement and reasoning in the child.* Totowa, NJ: Littlefield, Adams & Co.

Ramsay, R. W., & Noorbergen, R. (1981). *Living with loss.* New York: William Morrow.

Sheikh, A. A., Twente, G. E., & Turner, D. (1979). Death imagery: Therapeutic uses. In A. A. Sheikh & J. T. Shaffer (Eds.), *The potential of fantasy and imagination.* New York: Brandon House.

Shneidman, E. S. (1973). *Deaths of man.* Baltimore, MD: Penguin.

Volkan, V. D. (1975). "Regrief" therapy. In B. Schoenberg (Ed.), *Bereavement: Its psychological aspects.* New York: Columbia University Press.

Wass, H., Berando, F., & Neimeyer, R (Eds.). (1995). *Dying, facing the facts* (3rd ed.). Washington: Hemisphere.

CHAPTER 7

Hypnotic Death and Suicide Rehearsal

Alexander A. Levitan

> To sue to live, I find I seek to die,
> And seeking death, find life.
> William Shakespeare (*Measure for Measure,* iii I, p. 42)

Hypnotic death rehearsal is a technique initially developed to help patients imminently facing death (Levitan, 1985). It has since been utilized to help many individuals who have particular concerns relative to death and the dying process. The basic rationale of the technique is that humans characteristically and sometimes appropriately have a significant fear of the unknown. Once something has been experienced, however, either through hypnosis or imagery, it becomes more familiar and thus less fear-provoking.

Similar techniques have been described by others (Grof, 2000; Sheikh & Sheikh, 2003; Sheikh, Twente, & Turner, 1979) in which patients are asked to visualize their own death including leave-taking of significant individuals in their lives and thereby resolving conflicts in that relationship. Subjects are then encouraged to describe their individual visualization of the death process.

Subjects usually describe a distancing from their physical self and an integration into a more universal whole. The therapist encourages full involvement and utilization of the visualized experience without offering any psychotherapeutic interpretation or interventions. Subjects are described as experiencing a sensation of tranquility and resolution of conflicts as a consequence of this procedure.

Hypnotic death rehearsal differs from the above in that the therapist is continually involved in reframing and interpreting the visualized images reported by the subject. The principal objective of the hypnotic death rehearsal is to demystify the death experience and allow the patient to approach it with equanimity and confidence. The purpose of the constant reframing that occurs during hypnotic death rehearsal is to support the subject emotionally and allow him/her to perceive alternative positive interpretations of visualized events.

An alternative hypnotic death imagery technique designed to introduce a more critical reality into erroneous preconceptions of the death process and its consequence on significant others is a variant called hypnotic suicide rehearsal. The objective of this technique is to force subjects to critically evaluate the consequences of death by suicide and hopefully eliminate magical thinking in this regard.

Hypnotic suicide rehearsal also involves constant reframing of visualized images, but in a fashion that reintroduces the true reality of the situation at hand and hopefully acts as a deterrent to the proposed, often impulsive, course of action. As opposed to hypnotic death rehearsal, hypnotic suicide rehearsal is designed to cause the subject to evaluate whether suicide is the most optimal approach to accomplishing the objectives of the subject. Not infrequently after having experienced a hypnotic suicide rehearsal, the previously suicidal subject will no longer feel the need to commit suicide, having already performed the act through imagery.

THE TECHNIQUE OF HYPNOTIC DEATH REHEARSAL

This author has principally used the hypnotic death rehearsal for patients with terminal illnesses who have manifested considerable anxiety about their forthcoming death experience. The subject is usually introduced by asking, "Are you afraid to die?" When the response is, "Yes" or an equivalent but less direct response, the next question posed is, "Would you like to know what it feels like to die?" or "Would you like to know more about the death experience?"

If an affirmative response is obtained, then a preinduction discussion is initiated to familiarize the client with hypnosis and with the concept of death rehearsal. In order to achieve a suitable depth of trance, it is necessary to dispel any preconceptions relative to hypnosis that might predispose to resistance.

Clients are advised that all hypnosis is self-hypnosis and that they are totally in control at all times. Hypnosis is likened to attending a movie where one is seated among many other patrons, but after the movie begins, one forgets for the moment that one is in a theater and becomes involved in the action portrayed on the screen.

Nevertheless, one is able to stop watching at any time should one wish to go out for candy or to the bathroom. Similarly, one can be involved in the movie and still have an occasional extraneous thought such as, "Did I mail the letter?" or "What will I have for dinner after leaving the theater?" Thus clients are given permission to allow their thoughts to wander while under hypnosis, therefore defusing concern as to whether they had truly experienced "hypnosis."

The analogy between hypnosis and watching a movie is extended further by pointing out that should the film break, the viewers are not forced to continue to gaze upon a blank screen until the projectionist repairs the problem. Similarly, should the operator die while inducing hypnosis in a client, the client is advised that he/she would come out of hypnosis, say something like, "Too bad about the doctor!" and go home.

Clients usually smile at the above thought while experiencing dissipation of some of their anxiety relative to the forthcoming experience. They are then given the opportunity to ask any questions they might wish. After this they are asked, "If you were to visualize a scene or activity that you would characteristically associate with relaxation, what might that be?"

Frequent responses are visualizing a tropical beach or a scene of natural beauty. Hypnosis is then induced using the desired imagery, and the client is told to experience the scene vividly by involving all the senses, including awareness of color, movement, sound, smell, touch, and taste.

When appropriate, the hypnotic state is deepened with any one of a variety of techniques including descending a staircase, escalator, or elevator. After an appropriate level of trance is achieved, the client is taught how to speak while remaining under hypnosis. The suggestion is then given that he/she will go deeper into trance with each word spoken, thus reversing the tendency for trance to lighten with speaking.

The client is then asked to visualize the circumstances where his/her death is imminent. Often a hospital setting is described with the client surrounded by concerned relatives. Care is taken to point out to the client that he/she is comfortable and free of pain by virtue of nursing and medical care.

The client is then asked to describe the emotions of each relative in attendance and the client's response to those emotions. The client is encouraged to interact fully with loved ones and to resolve any "unfinished business" that might exist. Expressions of sadness are acknowledged and reframed by reminding the client of the many moments of happiness that can never be lost even through death.

After leave-taking has been completed, the client is asked to describe the actual death process. Most clients describe a peaceful transition into another plane in which they feel welcomed and detached from their former physical existence. Not infrequently, clients describe a progression toward a bright light through which they pass, knowing that a warm welcome awaits them on the other side.

Others have described a not unpleasant distancing from their physical selves in which they look on with a detached curiosity at what is occurring, usually from an overhead vantage point. These descriptions are remarkably similar to those described by persons who have experienced a near-death episode, such as cardiac arrest or drowning, from which they were eventually resuscitated (Moody, 1977).

Throughout the client's description of the dying process, emphasis is placed upon how natural and comfortable the process is. The client is asked to note that there is no pain, struggle, or effort involved in the process.

The client is then asked to describe how it feels to be dead. The usual description is that of blending with a universal whole yet returning awareness of what is occurring in the previous plane of existence. The client is then asked to describe in detail the reactions of his/her friends, relatives, doctors, and nurses to his/her death. If grief or anguish is noted on the part of one or all of the above, this observation is reframed to confirm the bonds between the client and family and friends.

The client is reminded that through foresight and planning, he/she can continue to play an active part in the lives of those left behind. This can be accomplished through letters, journals, or audio and video tapes. The client is encouraged to plan ahead to play an active part in future graduations, weddings, births, and similar occasions, via messages recorded or written previously.

The period of time around the actual death is closely scrutinized in order to intensify the reality of the experience. The client is asked to read his/her obituary as it appears in the local newspapers. He/she also is asked to describe those in attendance and what is said at the funeral and at any memorial service.

The client also is asked to note what gives particular comfort to loved ones and enables them to deal with their grief. He/she is reminded of the wonderful shared memories that remain as well as the tangibility of love that once created is never lost.

He/she is then asked to allow time to progress further into the future. He/she is asked how he/she has been remembered and who visits his/her grave. The client is asked to visualize the response to such questions as, "What was Grandma like?" from yet unborn grandchildren.

After exploring as much of the death process and the subsequent impact on their loved ones as is deemed appropriate, the client is asked whether there are any other issues that should be explored. If the response is "No," then, when appropriate, the posthypnotic suggestion can be given that "from now on, your concerns about death and the dying process will be much less bothersome and will occupy far less of your conscious thoughts. Death will seem as natural a process as eating or breathing."

Subjects are then invited to "feel refreshed, energized, and to return to the here and now." Reorientation usually takes a few moments and is often accompanied by a wistful reluctance to return.

On rare occasions, an abreaction is encountered during the death rehearsal process. This is usually manifested by expressions of emotion or by crying on the part of the client. The appropriate response on the part of the therapist is to inquire, "What's happening?" at which point the client usually describes the aspect of the current visualization that is distressing. This can usually be reframed or altered through suggestion to circumstances that are less disturbing or even supporting.

After the client has reoriented, it is important to conduct a posthypnotic interview to process the experience appropriately and to remove any misconceptions that may have occurred. It is also useful to confirm that the client has fully reoriented from the hypnotic state.

Most clients find the experience enlightening. As a consequence of being encouraged and guided to reflect on all the ramifications of dying, they frequently engage in more adequate planning for their demise. Specific attention is directed to each loved one and friend. Letters are written, audio and video tapes are made. Instructions are left relative to specific wishes in regard to disposition of personal property, and so on.

Clients also accept their approaching death with greater equanimity rather than attempting to avoid the inevitable. It is almost as if they had allowed themselves to accelerate through several steps of the dying process as described by Kübler-Ross (1969). They rapidly dispense with denial and bargaining. Preparatory grief is also accelerated since the process is no longer as foreign as it once was. A good portion of the fear that accompanies impending death has been removed as well as the customary associated anxiety.

Perhaps it would be helpful at this point to review an actual transcript of a death rehearsal to acquaint the reader with the specifics of the process.

I.W. is a 68-year-old woman who developed metastatic ovarian cancer eight years ago. The principal manifestation of her disease was a very distended abdomen consequent to marked ascites caused by her malignancy. She has periodically undergone paracentesis with removal of six liters of fluid at a time.

Because of the increasing frequency with which it was necessary to remove the ascitic fluid from her abdomen, along with the associated protein loss and malnutrition, it was decided to admit her to the hospital for surgical insertion of a catheter, which would permit the administration of intraperitoneal chemotherapy. Concomitant with her hospitalization, it was necessary to discuss the topic of possible resuscitation should that become necessary.

The patient expressed a desire to be resuscitated despite the rather advanced state of her disease. Although she remained outwardly calm, it was apparent that the prospect of dying in the relatively near future was very upsetting to her.

An opportune time was arranged to visit her in her hospital room and the topic was raised by the therapist.

"I noticed that you seemed a little upset when I asked you about the question of resuscitation earlier."

"Yes, I was a little," replied I.W.

"Why?"

"I guess I don't like to think about dying."

"Why?"

"It scares me."

"What is it about death that frightens you?"

"I don't know ... I guess I don't know what's going to happen and that's scary!"

"Would you like to know a little more about what it feels like to die?"

"Sure! But how's that possible."

"There's a technique we call Hypnotic Death Rehearsal, which allows you to project yourself forward in time and gain insight into the death experience. Would you like to try it?"

"Sounds weird. Are you sure I can do it? I don't know anything about hypnosis except what I've seen on the tapes at your office."

"I think you'll do very well. Would you like to try?"

"OK, as long as I can stop if I want to."

"That's fine. But first let's talk a little about hypnosis and what it is and isn't." (At this point the therapist went through the conventional preinduction discussion.)

"What would you like to think about that would be particularly relaxing for you?"

"How about sitting on the dock at my son's lake place?"

"Sounds fine. Get yourself good and comfortable in your chair and let's get started." (At this point a standard induction was done with the patient focusing on her son's lake cottage.)

"I think you'll enjoy noticing that while you're relaxing on that lovely dock and noticing all the colors, movements, sounds, smell, and even the textures of the place you've chosen, that you'll be able to speak comfortably and naturally. With each word you say, you'll find that you'll be deeper and deeper relaxed!"

"Just let yourself sink comfortably deeper and deeper into that chair and let your mind go forward in time to when you know that your death is just about to occur. When you're there, just let me know by raising your index finger."

(The patient slowly raises her right index finger.)

"Where are you and what's happening?"

"I'm at home. My family and the hospice nurse are there."

"How do you feel?"

"Comfortable, calm, kind of resigned."

"Do you have any discomfort?"

"No; it's funny, but my back pain is gone."

"What are your relatives doing?"

"My daughter is crying!"

"Why?"

"She's sad to see me go."

"But you're not taking your love for her with you, are you?"

"No . . ."

"Reach out and hug her and tell her that. Tell her also that all the wonderful memories will remain with her forever."

"She understands, but she's still sad about me leaving."

"That's natural, isn't it?"

(The patient nods her head slowly.)

"Who else is there?"

"Her husband and my son and his wife."

"What are they doing?"

"My daughter's husband has his arm around her shoulders. My son looks tired."

"Do you have anything that you want to say to them?"

"Yes, I want them to know that I love them and that everything is O.K."

"What's O.K.?"

"I'm O.K., I'm tired too, and I don't mind going."

"Why not tell them that?"

"O.K. . . ."

"Anything else?"

"Yes, I'd like to tell Kathy that I'm sorry . . ."

"Kathy?"

"My daughter-in-law."

"Sorry?"

"Yes. I'm sorry for the things I said about her before my son married her. I thought she wouldn't make a very good wife or mother. I was wrong. She really loves him and the children . . ."

"Why not hug her and tell her so?"

"O.K. . . . I feel much better now. Like a weight has been lifted off me."

"Does she forgive you?"

(Patient nods.)

"What happens next?"

"I kinda feel myself floating loose from my body. It's like I was being drawn toward something."

"Toward what?"

"Something different, something else. Almost like sunshine. It feels warm."

"And welcome?"

"Yes, yes, that's it . . . welcome."

"Anyone else there?"

"Not exactly, but I feel as if there are people I know here. I feel as if I belong, as if I were part of it all."

"What about your body?"

"Oh, it's there. But I'm here. I don't need it anymore."

"What happens next?"

"They all kiss me and touch my hand but I'm not there; I'm over here."

"How does it feel?"

"Strange. Peaceful. Kind of natural."

"Natural?"

"Yes. . . . Seems to be the right place for me now."

"In what way?"

"Well . . . I'm there and I'm not. Almost like being on the other side of a mirror. I see them but they don't know I'm there. It's nice to know that it goes on. That it's not the end."

"Is there anything else that you want to do?"

"No. I feel kind of tired."

"Well, take a moment to enjoy all the beauty and serenity and peace. Gather your strength and energy. Feel refreshed as if you'd had a lovely long nap, and when you're ready to . . . feeling good all over . . . let yourself come back." (Patient slowly reorients.)

"What was that like for you?"

"Strange. I had forgotten those things I had said about Kathy. I'm sure she has, too."

"How do you feel now?"

"Better. Relaxed. A little tired. My arms still feel heavy."

"That'll pass. I think you'll feel much better from now on."

The patient discussed some of the experience with the hypnotherapist the next day. She said she felt less frightened as a consequence of the experience and had had a dream the previous night of walking through her grandmother's garden while holding hands with her grandmother, whom she loved very much.

HYPNOTIC SUICIDE REHEARSAL

Just as Hypnotic Death Rehearsal can be used to demystify the dying process, so too Hypnotic Suicide Rehearsal can be used to introduce an element of reality into the speculations of patients contemplating suicide. Frequently suicide is an impulsive, hostile act with regard to which few of the eventual consequences are seriously considered.

In the technique of Hypnotic Suicide Rehearsal, the client is directed to seriously consider all the eventual ramifications of the contemplated action. Rather than constantly reframing the visualized experience in order to reduce anxiety as in the case of Hypnotic Death Rehearsal, Hypnotic Suicide Rehearsal attempts to direct the client to consider the often harsh reality of the situation.

It is important to point out that Hypnotic Suicide Rehearsal is not suitable for all patients contemplating suicide. In particular, it would seem inadvisable for use with patients who are merely posturing and not seriously contemplating the act. Neither is it intended for use as a method for instruction in how to successfully suicide or to dispel anxiety so that the contemplated action can proceed.

It has proven most effective for clients who are ruminating about suicide and are developing a preliminary course of action with regard to implementing their plan. These individuals have often given little consideration to the ultimate consequences of their action on their loved ones and friends, and focus only on expressing their hostility toward the party who will "be sorry" as a consequence of their death.

Of those individuals who believe suicide will be an appropriate solution to their current difficulties, few have accurately evaluated alternative outcome scenarios of their considered action.

A representative Hypnotic Suicide Rehearsal follows. The client in question, R.S., was a 47-year-old male who had been under treatment for hypertension. He was divorced and had remarried 2 years previously, but had retained custody of his 16-year-old son. He had a history of chemical dependency (alcohol type), but had been abstinent for 14 months. He arrived at the therapist's office appearing depressed and contemplative. The conversation occurred as follows:

"Hello, Ralph, how are you feeling?"
"Not too good, Doc."
"What's the matter?"
"I've got some problems at home."
"What kind of problems?"
"My wife is down on me since I got laid off."
"When did this happen?"
"Couple of weeks ago. The company is moving out of town and most of the local guys got laid off. I've been looking for something else, but no luck yet. The only thing I've found is minimum wage stuff, and I can't live on that."
"You've still got your unemployment, don't you?"
"Yeah, but that won't last forever. And to make things worse, I'm having troubles with my kid."
"What kinds of troubles?"
"He's into drugs. He won't listen to me. He's been staying away nights and skipping school. I'm worried something bad will happen to him. It's made me real depressed."
"How depressed? Have you thought of killing yourself?"
"Yeah, I have."
"Have you figured out how to do it?"
"Sort of. I've thought about jumping into the river. Or driving my car into a tree or something."
"Would that solve your problems?"
"At least it would get me out of here."
"When will you do it?"
"I dunno . . . sometime soon, I guess. I haven't figured out when."
"Are you sure that's the right answer to the problems?"
"It's the best I can come up with right now."
"Would you like to know what it's like to commit suicide?"
"What do you mean?"
"It's possible to use hypnosis to see and feel what it's like without actually having to do it. Would you like to try?"
"Do you think it will help anything?"
"It might. Would you like to try?"
"Maybe . . . what do I have to do?"
"First it will help if you understood a few things about hypnosis."

(At this point a standard preinduction discussion ensued.)

"Now that you know what hypnosis is and isn't, would you like to see what it feels like?"

"Why not?"

(A standard eye fixation and reversed levitation was employed with the client choosing to focus on a tranquil fishing scene.)

"While you're enjoying fishing in that lovely spot with the beautiful colors, movement, sounds, smell, tastes, and textures, I invite you to let your mind imagine what it would be like for you to commit suicide."

"Where are you?"

"I'm in my car."

"What are you planning to do?"

"I'm going to drive off the bridge into the river."

"Have you written a note?"

"Note?"

"Yes, you want people to understand why you've killed yourself, don't you?"

"I guess so."

"Write a note now. What does it say?"

"It says, I can't take it anymore. This is the best way. I love you. Don't hate me for doing this.'"

"Who is the note for?"

"For my wife and son."

"Where are you putting it?"

"In my pocket, I guess."

"Well, if you're crashing into the river, you might get smashed up and the water will damage the note."

"O.K. I'll put it in a plastic bag and stick it in my wallet."

"That's better. What's happening now?"

"I'm waiting for a time when there's no traffic . . . then I'll get a running start and smash through the guard rail and go into the river. Here I go."

"What does it feel like?"

"I don't know . . . It hurts a little."

"A little? Did the windshield shatter when you went through the guard rail or when the car went into the water?"

"I guess I'm cut up but I don't feel much . . . Maybe I'm knocked out . . ."

"Where are you?"

"Under the water."

"What's it like?"

"Dark, cold, kind of scary."

"What's it feel like to drown?"

"Kinda like suffocating . . . or smothering."

"Do you try to hold your breath?"

"Yeah, but then I can't any more."

"Do you struggle much before you die?"
"Some."
"O.K. Who discovers the accident?"
"I don't know. Somebody else on the road."
"What happens next?"
"The police come. They fish me out."
"How do you look?"
"Peaceful, I guess."
"Not blue in the face?"
"Well, yeah."
"How about your eyes and tongue, are they bulging out?"
"Maybe . . ."
"What do the people who find you say?"
"I don't know, maybe, 'Too bad' or something like that."
"Do you think they understand or respect you?"
"Maybe not."
"Do you think they're happy having to fish you and the car out?"
"It's their job."
"Have they found the note yet? What do they say when they find the note?"
"Just 'Too bad.'"
"Do they approve?"
"No."
"What's happening now?"
"The cops are visiting my wife."
"What does she say? What is her reaction?"
"She's crying. They just gave her the note."
"Where is your son?"
"He's there. Trying to comfort her."
"How does your wife feel about what you've done?"
"She's sad . . . and sorry . . ."
"Does she feel that you've let her down?"
"Yeah, I guess so."
"How about your boy?"
"Him, too, I guess."
"What does your wife tell the relatives?"
"That I had an accident."
"Do you think they'll find out the truth?"
"Could be."
"How about your boy? What does he tell his friends?"
"He just tells them I died."
"Does he tell any of them the truth?"
"Maybe Fred, his best friend."
"Why is that? Is he ashamed?"

"I guess so."
"And angry?"
"Yeah, maybe."
"Any obituary in the newspaper?"
"Just an article about the accident."
"Does it say anything about the cause of the accident?"
"The usual bull: 'Police are investigating.'"
"Go to the funeral home now, and tell me what's happening there."
"Nothing much."
"Who's there?"
"My wife and kid."
"Anyone else?"
"Some of the relatives. My wife's sister."
"What do they say about you?"
"That it's a shame. They're worried about how my wife will manage."
"What does she say to that?"
"She'll manage somehow. Maybe go back to work."
"Do you think she'll go on welfare?"
"Maybe, if she can't find work."
"How do you think that will make her feel?"
"Not too good, I suppose. She never did like the idea of going to others for help."
"Where do they bury you?"
"I don't know. Wherever it's cheapest, I guess."
"What did they put on the headstone?"
"My name and date of birth and death, I guess."
"Anything else?"
"No."
"What would you like them to put on there?"
"Maybe something about being a good man and a good father."
"Do you think that they feel that way about you considering the way you died?"
"Probably not."
"What happens over the next few years to them?"
"I guess my son will leave home as soon as he's old enough to manage."
"How about your wife?"
"She might get married again. She doesn't like being alone."
"How does she feel about you?"
"Kind of angry, I suppose."
"What about?"
"About my leaving her and the kid. About my not being there."
"How about your son? How does he feel?"
"Probably the same as my wife."
"Does he miss you?"

"Some, I suppose. We never were too close."
"What does he tell his children about you?"
"The truth, I guess."
"What do they think about their grandfather?"
"Not too much, I guess."
"Okay. Take a moment now to let yourself see and feel the effect that your committing suicide has on your family and others. And when you're ready to, let yourself come back to the here and now."
(Patient reorients and opens eyes.)
"Well, what do you think of the experience?"
"Well, I never really thought about all the aftereffects."
"Are you ready to go out and do it?"
"I guess not. At least not right away. I kind of feel as if I've done it once. I don't need to do it again."

As is evident, the object of a hypnotic suicide rehearsal is to force the client to face the harsh realities involved in an attempted or completed suicide and the impact it would have not only on the client but on his or her family, friends, and acquaintances as well.

Hypnotic suicide rehearsal differs markedly from death rehearsal as negative reframing is constantly being employed to force consideration of all the ramifications of what customarily is an impulsive and ill-considered act.

CONCLUDING REMARKS

Imagery education and hypnosis have been effectively employed to deal with death anxiety, grieving for the loss of a loved one, and resolution of "unfinished business."

Heterohypnosis and self-hypnosis have been described as being of significant therapeutic benefit in resolving grief relating to the death of a loved one (Fromm & Eisen, 1982). Techniques employed include visualization of progressive distancing from the loved one to the point where existence in the absence of the loved one can be accepted as reality.

Studies have established that education relative to the exact nature of the death experience can appreciably reduce death anxiety as measured by a variety of psychological instruments (McDonald & Hilgendorf, 1986).

Hypnotic imagery can also be employed to allow the completion of "unfinished business" (Lamb, 1982). This technique involves hypnoplasty, in which bereaved individuals are encouraged to visualize conversations and actions on their part, which resolve conflict or anxiety with regard to the deceased.

Hypnosis has also been demonstrated to be of benefit in allowing terminally ill patients to accept the inevitability of death and to reduce their anxiety in this regard (Gross, 1979; LaBaw, 1969; Levitan, 1985; Zelling, 1984). The techniques described in this chapter are two specific applications in this regard. It is not recommended that they be applied to all terminally ill patients nor to all patients contemplating suicide. Nevertheless, in certain selected cases they have been highly effective and have significantly expedited the psychotherapeutic process.

REFERENCES

Fromm, E., & Eisen, M. (1982). Self hypnosis as a therapeutic aid in the mourning process. *American Journal of Clinical Hypnosis, 25*(1), 3-14.
Grof, S. (2000). *Psychology of the future.* Albany, NY: State University of New York Press.
Gross, H. J. (1979). Hypnotherapy in the management of terminally ill cancer patients. *Journal of the Indiana State Medical Association, 72*(2), 126-129.
Kübler-Ross, E. (1969). *On death and dying.* New York: Macmillan.
LaBaw, W. L. (1969). Terminal hypnosis in lieu of terminal hospitalization. *Gerontologia Clinica, 11*(5), 312-320.
Lamb, C. S. (1982). Negative hypnotic imagery/fantasy: Application to two cases of "unfinished business." *American Journal of Clinical Hypnosis, 24*(4), 266-271.
Levitan, A. A. (1985). Hypnotic death rehearsal. *American Journal of Clinical Hypnosis, 27*(4), 211-215.
McDonald, R. T., & Hilgendorf, W. A. (1986). Death imagery and death anxiety. *Journal of Clinical Psychology, 42*(1), 87-91.
Moody, R. A. (1977). *Reflections on life after life* (pp. 23-28). Atlanta: Mockingbird Books.
Shakespeare, W. (1988). *The complete works.* Oxford: Clarendon Press.
Sheikh, A. A., & Sheikh, K. S. (2003). Death imagery: Confronting death brings us to the threshold of life. In A. Sheikh (Ed.), *Healing images: The role of imagination in health.* Amityville, NY: Baywood.
Sheikh, A. A., Twente, G. E., & Turner, D. (1979). Death imagery: Therapeutic uses. In A. A. Sheikh & J. T. Shaffer (Eds.), *The potential of fantasy and imagination.* New York: Brandon House.
Zelling, D. A. (1984). Acceptance of death and dying. *Medical Hypnoanalysis,* April, 66-69.

CHAPTER 8

Death Imagery and Death Anxiety

Rita T. McDonald and Carolyn J. Salyards

> The less the life satisfaction, the greater the death anxiety.
> Irvin Yalom (1980, p. 208)

> Fear not that thy life shall come to an end, but rather fear that it shall never have a beginning.
> John Henry Newman (in Adams, Otto, & Cowley, 1984, p. 145)

Among the various human phenomena studied in the field of psychology, mental imagery has come to be seen as a subject worthy of serious exploration for the increased understanding of its diverse functions in human beings, and also (perhaps especially), for its potential clinical and educational applications. Among the various types of imagery that have been investigated, death imagery in particular presents a useful approach to psychotherapy and to personal growth and development.

Death anxiety has been the subject of an even greater volume of literature. Its development has proceeded through the conceptual stages of (a) initial discovery and labeling, (b) definition of the concept and classification of its subcategories, (c) refinement of measurements designed to quantify its occurrence in individuals and groups, (d) identification of its demographic and personality correlates, and finally, (e) attention to the question of its functional or behavioral consequences.

During the development of research in both of the areas of death anxiety and death imagery, relatively less interest has been shown in the possible relationship and interaction between the two. The studies to have done so, for example, Lonetto (1982), McDonald and Hilgendorf (1986), Parson (1987), and Smith (2000), have found consistent and strong relationships that have generated several hypotheses regarding the possible impact of one upon the other. In order to consider the potential therapeutic usefulness of the death anxiety/ death imagery relationship, it is necessary to review the relevant work that has been done in each area.

DEATH IMAGERY

For the most part, death imagery has been seen in two ways: the imagination of the circumstances of one's own death or that of another; and the personification or reification of death. The first of these has its historical roots in religious meditation. The contemplation of one's own mortality has been an aspect of varying importance in Hindu, Buddhist, Muslim, and Christian mysticism. In the Christian tradition, for example, religious and secular groups set aside specific periods of time, called retreats, days of recollection, or spiritual renewals, in which meditation on death is often the central, or at least a prominent feature. The purpose of such contemplation is seen to be the enhancement of the quality of life through the realization of its transience, and the strengthening of an individual's spiritual life and sense of purpose.

This kind of focused attention to one's mortality has been credited with other positive, as well as some negative, features. Becker (1973), in his Pulitzer Prize winning thesis on the role of death in life, states that innate human fear of death is a principal source of human activity. He subscribes to what he calls the "morbidly-minded argument" for the fear of death, which is graphically summarized by William James (1902) when he refers to death as "the worm at the core" of human beings' pretensions to happiness. Becker then goes on to demonstrate how individuals attempt to transcend death in culturally standardized ways—through heroism, narcissism, charisma, religion, and neurosis.

A similar theme is present in the work of Lifton and Olson (1974), which is a psychohistorical examination of the phenomenon of death. They offer another view of humanity's struggle with death and suggest a solution that utilizes the symbolization of life and death—a symbolization that has both individual and global ramifications. They state:

> We would stress not only the finality of death, but also the human need for a sense of historical connection beyond individual life. We . . . [see] the need to develop concepts, imagery, and symbols adequate to give a sense of significance to experience. This psychological process of creating meaningful images is at the heart of what we . . . call symbolic immortality (p. 75).

They describe a sense of immortality that may be expressed in five general modes: (a) the biological mode, in which individuals achieve a sense of immortality by living on through their children, grandchildren, and so on, through an endless line of generations; (b) the theological mode, or the belief in existence on a higher plane, which provides the opportunity to transcend death through spiritual achievement; (c) the creative mode, in which immortality comes through achievements, such as writing, teaching, and artistic works, that are seen to have an enduring impact; (d) the theme of eternal nature, a participation in immortality by the survival of nature itself; and (e) the state of experiential transcendence, characterized by extraordinary psychic unity and perceptual intensity, not unlike the experience of ecstasy that occurs in religious or secular mysticism, which yields a feeling of the continuous present as in mythical times.

It is interesting to note the parallels between Lifton and Olson's (1974) formulation and Toynbee's (1968) earlier discussion of ways in which human beings have historically sought to reconcile themselves to the fact of death. Toynbee includes not only means of denial or acceptance of death, but also ways in which death can be embraced. He thus proposes hedonism as the most obvious way of reconciling oneself to death: one can make sure of enjoying life to its fullest before death snatches it away. The clear alternative to the illusory solace of hedonism is pessimism, the belief that life is so difficult and hopeless that death is the lesser evil. In this context, Toynbee makes the following interesting assertion:

> One index of pessimism is suicide. In a society in which life is rated at so low a value that death is held to be the lesser of evil, suicide will be held to be one of the basic human rights, and the practice of it will be considered respectable and in some cases meritorious or even morally obligatory (p. 72).

According to Toynbee, human beings have also attempted to circumvent death by physical countermeasures. Historical practices such as mummification; providing corpses with food, drink, and wealth; and searching for the elixir of immortality are cases in point. Another way to circumvent death is to win fame. This is analogous to Lifton and Olson's creative mode of immortality, with perhaps some variation in the size of the audience to whom one offers one's enduring gifts.

Toynbee suggests that reconciliation with the fact of death can be further attempted through liberation from self-centeredness. He proposes that this can occur in two ways: by putting one's treasure in future generations of one's fellow human beings (not unlike Lifton and Olson's biological mode of immortality); and by merging oneself in ultimate reality (the theme of eternal nature).

Finally, the beliefs in the personal immortality of human souls, the resurrection of human bodies, and the reward of heaven and the punishment of hell represent Toynbee is theological approach to the question of death and immortality.

The question of the denial of death and the need for a sense of immortality was still earlier addressed in psychoanalytical literature, which provides another useful perspective. Freud, for example, believed that personal death could not be imagined:

> It is indeed impossible to imagine our own death: and whenever we attempt to do so we can perceive that we are in fact still present as spectators. Hence the psychoanalytic school could venture on the assertion that at bottom no one believes in his own death, or, to put the same thing in another way, that

in the unconscious every one of us is convinced of his own immortality (p. 289).

This statement calls to mind the phenomenon often observed when speaking of some distant future age; that is, that each person in a group is willing to imagine that everyone else has already died, but that he or she is somehow present.

Freud (1957) also proposed a solution to the problem of the denial of death. In the context of the widespread loss of life during World War I, he wrote:

> Should we not confess that in our civilized attitude towards death we are once again living psychologically beyond our means, and should we not rather turn back and recognize the truth? Would it not be better to give death a place in reality and in our thoughts which is its due, and to give a little more prominence to the unconscious attitude towards death which we have hitherto so carefully suppressed? . . . We recall the old saying: . . . If you want to preserve peace, arm for war. It would be in keeping with the times, to alter it: . . . If you want to endure life, prepare yourself for death (pp. 299-300).

Carl Jung (1963), from the very different perspective of his "hygienic" viewpoint, advocated a hopeful imagery of life after death as a way of dealing with the fact of death.

> Yet death is an important interest, especially to an aging person. A categorical question is being put to him, and he is under an obligation to answer it. To this end he ought to have a myth about death, for reason shows him nothing but the dark pit into which he is descending. Myth, however, can conjure up other images for him, helpful and enriching pictures of life in the land of the dead. If he believes in them, or greets them with some measure of credence, he is being just as right or just as wrong as someone who does not believe in them. But while the man who despairs marches toward nothingness, the one who has placed his faith in the archetype follows the tracks of life and lives right into his death. Both, to be sure, remain in uncertainty. But the one lives against his instincts, the other with them. Mythological and religious imagery of life beyond death, that is, constitutes an "archetype," a primordial, inherited, instinctual structure that is worthy of one's "faith" (p. 15).

It may be that all of these philosophical, theological, psychological, and historical perspectives are rich in psychotherapeutic significance and potential, and learning to die may be a prerequisite to living meaningfully. A few specific therapeutic techniques have been developed, which look directly to an individual's confrontation with death and to the positive life outcomes that might ensue from them. Sheikh, Twente, and Turner (1979) outlined just such a technique, which consists of relaxation, confrontation of death, and receptivity to the experience of unity. In representative case histories, the authors described both the process and the outcomes of their death-imagery work. They suggested broader applications of their technique to death-related problems such as grieving and bereavement. In a recent review of death-imagery approaches, Sheikh and Sheikh

(2003) surveyed the beneficial effects of death imagery, including deep relaxation, finishing unfinished business, out-of-body experience, importance of the moment/here-and-now, death and creativity, death and love, and essence vs. accessory attributes.

Aguilar and Wood (1976) applied a related technique, which they termed a death ritual or ritual drama, in their work with Hispanic patients in a state hospital. The procedure was designed to elicit appropriate fantasies and thus to reexperience the loss of a loved one, in the hope that the ensuing catharsis, occurring in the presence of a supportive group, would be therapeutic. The authors report some remarkable results, with patients making pivotal gains in their mental-health status.

Another line of research deserves mention here. Kastenbaum and Aisenberg (1972) explored the phenomenon of thanatomimesis—behavior that imitates death. Included under the heading of thanatomimetic behaviors are tonic immobility, suspended animation, and the low-level behavioral syndromes that are seen in some psychiatric populations as well as in the extended process of dying. The contemporary questions surrounding the definition of death that have been generated by technological life-assistance mechanisms are relevant here. It is no longer invariably possible to know precisely the moment when life has ended and death has taken place. This being the case, it becomes imperative to understand the physical and psychological dynamics of thanatomimesis in order to provide improved treatment techniques for dying persons, as well as for a better understanding of the life-to-death interim experience and the images that accompany it. These images may be central to the therapeutic applications of death imagery.

A different approach to death imagery is the planned obituary, in which individuals are asked to write their own obituaries, either as they expect them to be or as they would wish them to be, or both. Such written obituaries usually include fairly detailed information on age at the time of death, cause and site of death, survivors, and funeral ceremonies. Studies by Sabatini and Kastenbaum (1973), Simpson (1975), and Shneidman (1972) found that young people have difficulty seeing themselves as dead, and that most subjects prefer to live longer than they expect to live. This latter finding was not supported by the investigation into college students' preferences and expectations with respect to their own deaths by McDonald and Carroll (1981). In this study, women preferred to die at an age almost nine years younger than that at which they could expect to die, given actuarial projections. For men, there was no significant difference between the mean preference and the national average life expectancy. Student preferences with respect to the cause and site of death were substantially different from actuarial projections.

Of perhaps greater relevance to the therapeutic potential of death imagery were the unreported findings of the McDonald and Carroll study. In analyzing the obituaries written by 382 college students, the authors found a striking tendency on the part of these students to describe in detail the accomplishments they had achieved in their lifetimes and the generally altruistic and often heroic lives they had led. In follow-up discussions with these subjects, McDonald found that writing their obituaries had led students to reflect on the value of their lives and to conclude that at least a part of their sense of immortality lay in the fruits of unselfishness. They also reported that writing about their survivors strengthened their realization of the importance of the significant others in their lives and renewed their commitment to nurture these relationships. It can be speculated that these insights probably contributed to the enhancement of the quality of the students' interpersonal relationships. If so, the reflection and imagery required by writing one's own obituary may have positive consequences.

The second major way in which death imagery has been studied is by focusing on the ways in which people have personified or reified death. From the earliest records of humanity to the present, death images have permeated art, literature, music, philosophy, and religion. McClelland (1963) speculated about the psychodynamics of death personification and developed the general theme of death as a dark, mysterious lover. To this theme he assigned the term "Harlequin Complex," reminiscent of the well-known figure in art and literature. Beyond McClelland's supportive data, Greenberger (1965) was the first to engage in a formal test of the Harlequin Complex. She administered the Thematic Apperception Test (TAT) to female cancer patients and women hospitalized for minor illnesses. Analysis of the TAT responses revealed that the women approaching death gave twice as many themes of illicit sex as did the control group, thus supporting McClelland's assertions. Greenberger noted that, from some women, these fantasies were a part of their anxiety about death, while for others, these fantasies provided comfort. On the other hand, it is possible that the increased reference to themes of illicit sexuality may have reflected a surge of sexual interest generated by deprivation in the cancer patients. A related study by Papageorgis (1966), with undergraduate students as subjects and using ratings of metaphors rather than the TAT, failed to provide support for McClelland's Harlequin Complex.

In an attempt to further refine the focus on death personification, Kastenbaum and Aisenberg (1972) used an open-end question and a multiple-choice procedure. From the responses, they were able to develop four images of death: (a) the "Macabre," a vivid, horror-laden, repulsive figure; (b) the "Gentle Comforter," a wise and sympathetic individual; (c) the "Automaton," an objective, unfeeling instrument in human guise; and (d) the "Gay Deceiver," a sophisticated, enticing person, using sly techniques to deliver death. The last of these images, the "Gay Deceiver," bears some resemblance to McClelland's Harlequin Complex.

Subsequent studies of death imagery, for instance by Lonetto, Fleming, Clare, and Gorman (1976) and Lonetto (1982), used the Death Personification Exercise developed by Kastenbaum and Aisenberg or a derivation thereof. Results of a study by Kastenbaum and Herman (1997) showed a divergency by gender in type of death personification selected most frequently. Females most often selected "kind and gentle" imagery; males were more likely to see death as a "cold, remote" person. Grim and terrifying images of death were selected least often. Similarly, Feifel and Nagy (1981) created a Fantasy Level Fear of Death Scale that contained two subscales, Positive Death Metaphors and Negative Death Metaphors. The measure is a tool for investigating aspects of attitudes toward death and dying (McLennan, Bates, Johnson, Lavery, & Horne, 1993). As a result of these investigations, there is an increasing body of information, which has begun to establish more specific characteristics of death images and various correlates of death imagery. One of the strongest relationships to emerge to date is that between death imagery and death anxiety.

DEATH ANXIETY

Research interest in death anxiety has paralleled theoretical interest in death imagery. As was stated earlier in this chapter, the phenomenon of death anxiety has been labeled, classified, defined, measured, and studied for demographic personality correlates. Recent attention has been focused on the important question of possible functional or behavioral consequences of death anxiety.

As a construct, fear of death holds a unique position in psychological literature. Writers have generally agreed that the term *fear* is used when the negative reaction (and fear is considered to be negative experience, consisting of alarm, consternation, dread, and expectation of danger) is to some known cause. *Anxiety*, on the other hand, is a term most often technically reserved to indicate a reaction to some unknown cause. Interestingly, while death anxiety seems to be the preferred term for the phenomenon, thus acknowledging that death is basically an unknown experience, fear of death is a frequent label as well, perhaps suggesting that the fact of death, if not the actual experience, is known. Moreover, as was shown in the foregoing discussion of death imagery, it is possible to imagine the circumstances of one's own death as well as those of another; hence, the appropriateness of both terms.

The measurement of death anxiety has been a longstanding problem. Despite a proliferation of instruments, data on the reliability and validity of many of the scales have been questionable. Moreover, the definition of the construct being measured by each scale has been characterized by imprecision. Consequently, research findings are inconsistent.

Most of the early scales developed by researchers measure death anxiety as a unidimensional concept, yielding global scores. Of these early scales, the Death Anxiety Scale (DAS) by Templer (1970) proved to be a very popular research instrument, perhaps because of its relatively few items and straightforward scoring system. It continues to be used in revised form, often in combination with other, multidimensional measures.

The earliest attempt to identify separate components of the global concept of death anxiety was that by Collett and Lester (1969). On the basis of face validity, they subclassified death anxiety into the fears of death of self, dying of self, death of others, and dying of others. Subsequent factor-analysis studies (Hoelter, 1979; Nelson & Nelson, 1975) supported the viability of those four constructs. A revision of the Collett-Lester Fear of Death Scale eliminated a deviant item that reduced the reliability of the scale. Using a sample of 191 undergraduates, four seven-item subscales were derived, with adequate reliabilities and factorial congruence for two of the subscales: Fear of Death of Self and Fear of Dying of Self (Lester & Abdel-Khalek, 2003). Conte, Weiner, and Plutchik (1982), using a principal-components factor analysis, suggested four different, independent dimensions of death anxiety: Fear of the Unknown, Fear of Suffering, Fear of Loneliness, and Fear of Personal Extinction. The Multidimensional Fear of Death Scale (MFODS) is a more recent assessment tool for measuring multiple facets of death anxiety. Dimensions of the MFODS include Fear of the Dead, Fear of the Dying Process, Fear of the Unknown, Fear of Conscious Death, and Fear for the Body after Death.

Amid these efforts to empirically verify the fear of various aspects of death, some writers have approached the question from an intuitive perspective. Schulz (1978) enumerates seven specific fears, noting that they are often interactive: they are the fears of physical suffering, humiliation, interruption of goals, impact of one's death on survivors, punishment in an afterlife, nonbeing or nothingness, and the death of others. Persons employed in hospices, oncology wards, and nursing homes can report a host of other fears on the part of dying persons, such as the fears of being buried alive or of being powerless, isolated, and abandoned.

Besides these intuitive, observational, and direct empirical approaches to the measurement of death anxiety, there is the question of whether a person's public death anxiety (that which one is willing to report when asked) is the same as the private level of anxiety about death, which one does not easily share. There may also be a nonconscious kind of fear, which is not available to the person's awareness, or only infrequently so. Quantification of the private and nonconscious levels of death anxiety requires the use of indirect measures such as projective techniques and physiological reactions. A measurement that blended psychometric and projective components was used to test the dynamic nature of death anxiety in a sample of 392 adults (aged 18-88 years). Findings supported a two-factor model of overt (conscious) and covert (unconscious) death anxiety (Hayslip, Guarnaccia, Radika, & Servaty, 2001, 2002).

A further important effort of research on death anxiety has been to show its various demographic and personality correlates. Lester (1967), Schulz (1978), and Pollak (1979) are among those who have reviewed the correlational studies and outlined the commonalities in findings. Relevant demographic investigations have shown death anxiety differences based on age, sex, occupation, and religiosity. Earlier investigations studied unidimensional correlates, while more recent studies have revealed interactions of multiple factors.

With respect to age, perhaps the most important finding has been that children's views of death proceed through consistent stages of maturation (Nagy, 1959;

Peck, 1966). Death orientation also appears to change across adult development, and there is some evidence of increased comfort with mortality in later life (Neimeyer & Van Brunt, 1995). The relationship between death anxiety (overt and covert) and chronological age has also been explored. Contrary to previous studies, older adults evidenced higher levels of overt fear, while younger adults' covert fears were greater. It is possible that cumulative death and loss experiences over the course of a lifetime could lessen the need to deny fears of one's own death and sensitize older persons to the loss of relationships with others (Galt & Hayslip, 1998). Given the fact that an increasing number of individuals are living to old age, it is apparent that there is a need for further research on death anxiety in older adults. Studies based on sex differences have generally shown women to have a greater fear of death when death anxiety is measured as a unidimensional construct (Iammarino, 1975; McMordie, 1979; Templer, Ruff, & Franks, 1971). The extent to which death anxiety can be attributed to gender differences in emotional expressiveness has also been tested. Results of a study of 59 women and 58 men found that women displayed greater death anxiety than men; but women did not score higher on a death-threat index, suggesting that gender differences may be based on expressiveness (Dattel & Neimeyer, 1990). When death anxiety is subclassified, however, the evidence is not so consistent. For example, males have been found to have a greater fear than females of the effects of their deaths on dependents (Diggory & Rothman, 1961). Men also show more fear of the violent death (Lowrey, 1965). Other researchers (Degner, 1974; Krieger, Epsting, & Leitner, 1974) provide data to suggest that death anxiety in males appears to be cognitive, while death anxiety in females tends to be affective in nature.

Interactions between age and gender have also been examined. For example, in a study using the Revised Death Anxiety Scale (RDAS), the highest death-anxiety scores were obtained by college-age females, followed by college-age males, females over age 55, and males over age 55 (Tomer, Eliason, & Smith, 2000). The relationship between death anxiety and attitudes toward older adults was investigated in a study of 197 men and women (mean age 69.4 years), who completed the Multidimensional Fear of Death Scale (MFODS). Age, ethnicity, and gender were considered. Older women scored higher than men on a dimension called Fear of the Dead. Caucasian participants displayed higher scores on a dimension called Fear of the Dying Process than did older African American participants. Older African American participants reported higher levels of death anxiety on three of the subscales of the MFDOS (Fear of the Unknown, Fear of Conscious Death, and Fear for the Body after Death) when compared with older Caucasian participants, and they also tended to accord less social value to the elderly. These findings were interpreted in terms of patterns of socialization (Depaola, Griffin, Young, & Neimeyer, 2003). A study of 196 adults (aged 18-80 years) indicated that psychosocial maturity was a better predictor of death anxiety than age was. As psychosocial maturity and age increased, death anxiety decreased (Rasmussen & Brems, 1996). Research on the effectiveness of therapeutic interventions for death anxiety in particular populations is especially needed.

There have been a number of studies on occupational correlates of death anxiety. Feifel, Hanson, Jones, and Edwards (1967) were able to substantiate the commonly held belief that physicians have higher than average levels of fear of death. It is interesting to note here that one of the earliest and most significant studies of behavioral consequences of death anxiety, to be reported in detail later, was carried out using a sample of physicians (Schulz & Aderman, 1979). Subsequently, a study of physicians found that, on average, the 40 female participants scored higher in death anxiety than the male participants. Psychiatrists scored higher in death anxiety than surgeons. Furthermore, purpose in life was inversely correlated with death anxiety and external locus of control (Viswanathan, 1996). A longitudinal study of 186 male and 132 female 4th-year medical students found that fear of death decreased over time as physicians became more experienced (Firth-Cozens & Field, 1991).

A final correlational line of research relevant to the link between death anxiety and death imagery is that having to do with religiosity. Early investigations of religious beliefs and death anxiety were clouded by the failure to distinguish between external and internal religiosity. When this difficult but important distinction is made, results may become more consistent and enlightening. Templer (1972) found, in attempting to address this research problem, that in persons who were religiously involved, such as ministers, death-anxiety levels were lower than in the general population. In a study of 389 adults (aged 18-88 years), older respondents scored significantly higher in intrinsic religious motivation and lower in death anxiety. Those who scored higher in religiosity were lower in fear of death. The respondents who were highest in death anxiety were significantly lower in religiosity (Thorsen & Powell, 2000).

Of perhaps greater significance than demographic correlates are the correlates between death anxiety and personality characteristics. While many studies have been done, not all have shown clear, consistent, or significant relationships. Some important indications do emerge, however. Death anxiety appears to be higher in persons lacking a sense of effectiveness, mastery, and power (Nogas, Schweitzer, & Grumet, 1974). It is low in persons who possess high self-esteem and who experience a high degree of meaning and purpose in their lives (Blazer, 1973; Durlak, 1973).

The preponderance of research on death anxiety and personal characteristics has focused on variables that represent the higher levels of human personality development, such as self-actualization, authenticity, integration, and completeness of identity. Many of these kinds of investigations posit that there is an inverse relationship between death anxiety and the ability to confront one's own mortality, and then go on to show that more highly developed individuals are either lower in death anxiety or more nearly able to come to terms with the fact of their own transient existence. For example, a study of 58 residents (ages 52-94 years) of a church-affiliated retirement community found a negative correlation between purpose in life and death anxiety (Rappaport, Fossler, Bross, & Gilden, 1993). A study of 136 students (ages 19-39) found that a sense of purpose of life and symbolic immortality were correlated (Drolet, 1990), and both were significantly stronger in established adults than in young adults. It seems that a sense of symbolic immortality may help individuals to cope with death anxiety. What remains to be discovered is the nature of the relationship between death anxiety, as measured by the numerous instruments now available, and the ability and inclination to encounter the thought and image of the death of the self. Perhaps, as has been postulated by thanatologists, it is not the death of the self that strikes fear into the human heart so much as the dying process, which is fraught with pain, loneliness, and most fearsome of all, the unknown future experiences that may occur before death, such as loss of control over personal decisions, crippling effects of treatment, and uncertain levels of pain, along with questionable possibilities with respect to pain management.

The work that has been done on death fear and levels of human development has, nevertheless, produced some interesting findings. Neimeyer and Chapman (1980) reasoned, according to Sartre, that death would be more threatening to individuals whose projected identities were radically incomplete, since it would finalize the meaning of their lives at a level discrepant with their ideals. In order to test this hypothesis, they studied high- and low-discrepancy groups for their respective levels of death anxiety, as measured by the Templer and Collett-Lester scales. Their prediction was strongly supported; furthermore, they found that the "high split" group, those with discrepant ideals, showed greater concern about the state of death, as opposed to the process of dying. They concluded that the self/ideal discrepancy is a variable that needs to be taken into account in planning strategies for care of the terminally ill.

The psychoanalytic school of thought has approached the notion of facing one's death from another viewpoint. Heuscher (1986) writes: "Death is . . . the ultimate source of anxiety, since it is an ever-present threat to all that we are, own, and cherish" (p. 311), and continues:

> "Death anxiety" refers not only to physical death. As existential anxiety, it refers to any and all situations in which an individual risks or is forced to give up a portion, an aspect of his or her customary ways of seeing himself or herself, or of living, in an environment that is taken for granted. We so identify with externals—with the people we depend on or who depend upon us, with success, position, praise, social expectations, looks, or material possessions—that we tend to forget that behind all these relative values there is our ongoing, genuine, creative identity, namely our Self. We then experience the loss of these externals as "worse than death." Losing his money is worse than death for Scrooge, losing her youth or looks may be worse than death for Hollywood's sex symbol. That losses and changes in fortune

cause pain and sadness is natural and understandable; but why do they cause anxiety? The anxiety seems to derive, first, from the experience of losing the external identity the person has fashioned, at the cost of neglecting and forgetting the true Self. Now we can see existential anxiety as having a second, more profound origin. For existential anxiety reminds us of this neglect; it challenges us to recognize the relativity of the threatened or curtailed external identity and challenges us to give priority to the Self. Just as the anticipation of physical death is experienced as a warning that we may miss the opportunity to become the person we are meant to be, so the anxieties resulting from external losses and changes will remind us of our forgetfulness of the ongoing Self that can rebuild and take responsibility for our world (p. 315).

Beyond the volume of correlational and theoretical information that has been accumulated over the years lies the critical question of whether or not death anxiety, especially at high levels, exerts any influence on human functioning. In other words, are there any consequences of the fear of death? From a theoretical standpoint, Becker (1973), Lifton and Olson (1974), and others have answered affirmatively. Three investigations exemplify this thrust of research efforts.

The first is a work by Schulz and Aderman (1979) already alluded to, who measured the death-anxiety levels of a group of physicians who were treating both terminal and nondying patients. The hypothesis was that terminal patients of physicians with high death-anxiety levels would survive longer during their final hospital stay than would terminal patients of physicians with low death-anxiety levels. This hypothesis was based on the reasoning that physicians high in death anxiety would be less willing to accept their patients' terminality and, therefore, would be more likely to use heroic measures to keep them alive. They might also be likely to admit these patients to the hospital earlier. The findings showed that the length of final hospitalization for patients who died varied directly and significantly as a function of the physicians' level of death anxiety. Terminally ill patients of physicians with high death anxiety were in the hospital significantly longer than were terminally ill patients treated by physicians with low and moderate death anxiety. Similar differences were not found in the hospital stays of nondying patients of these same physicians. A more recent study found that exaggerated death anxiety may influence physicians' professional performance and their ability to provide competent patient care (Neimeyer & Van Brunt, 1995).

A second study demonstrating behavioral consequences of death-related fears looked to the responses of nurses to various work situations (Staller, 1980). Results indicated that death-related fears had little impact on nurses' responses in encounters with the event of death, proximity to a dead body, and provision of care for terminally ill patients. These levels of fear did, however, appear to affect responses to situations requiring interactions with dying patients, such as talking to them, listening to them talking about dying, and finding terminal patients crying.

The third investigation focused on death anxieties and the willingness to donate organs for transplantation after death, an issue of considerable contemporary concern. Hessing and Elffers (1986) showed that it is important to distinguish among several kinds of death anxieties, particularly as they relate to different kinds of behaviors—in this case, donating one's entire body to medical science or donating an organ for transplantation. They tested the following hypotheses: (1) the fear of being declared dead too soon would have stronger influence than the attitude toward death on a person's willingness to donate organs after death; (2) the correlation between death attitudes and the willingness to donate organs would be stronger for persons with low self-esteem than for those with high self-esteem; and (3) the fear of being declared dead too soon and the attitude toward death in general are unrelated death anxieties. Their findings supported all three hypotheses.

There have been a number of studies of death anxiety related to personal health concerns. For example, in a study of 30 cancer patients, there was an inverse relationship between death anxiety and denial over time, lending support to clinical opinions that denial protects against death anxiety (Dougherty, Templer, & Brown, 1986). In a study of gay men with AIDS, perceived positive support from family was more strongly related to lower death anxiety than support received from peers (Catania, Turner, Choi, & Coates, 1992).

An area of widespread speculation, but one that has produced little hard clinical data, has to do with the effect of death anxiety or the expectation of death on actual death or survival following surgery. Fear of death can be distinguished from the conviction of impending death, sometimes referred to in medical literature as predilection to death, although the classic study on predilection to death (Weisman & Hackett, 1961) describes the phenomenon as not only an expectation of impending death, but also a perception that death would be an appropriate outcome. The appropriateness of death within this context stems from the belief that death provides continuity in relationships with those already dead, that it is the consummation of fantasies, and that it is a means of conflict reduction. In the face of this kind of predilection to death, some surgeons refuse to operate and refer such patients to psychiatry, even though the patients in the Weisman and Hackett study were not anxious, depressed, or suicidal. Thus, the more typical fear of death in surgery is different, perhaps both qualitatively and quantitatively, from the expectation of death, which may coexist with fear of death, and predilection to death, which may not. Seeing the distinction may be valuable as a preliminary condition to examining other unexplained deaths, such as anniversary death, voodoo death, and sudden death.

In the study by Weisman and Hackett (1961), patients with intense anxiety before surgery recovered well, and not one died. All of the "predilection" patients, who regarded death resulting from surgery as appropriate, died unexpectedly of difficulties encountered in the postoperative period, usually within days of the surgery. Thus it can be seen that not only death anxiety, but its absence in circumstances in which it is warranted, may have behavioral consequences of substantial significance.

Even this preliminary evidence leads to the consideration of the potentially large number of human situations in which the presence of varying levels of death anxiety might have a significant influence on behavior. Fear of death is also often associated with psychological maladjustment, including anxiety and depression (Neimeyer & Van Brunt, 1995). Obviously, a great deal of research is necessary before the numerous correlates of death anxiety can be separated into those that do and those that do not affect behavior. In the interim, however, it is important, if not yet demonstrably critical, to begin work on the means by which death anxiety levels can be changed. If only a greater individual sense of psychological comfort were to result, the work would still be justified.

THERAPEUTIC IMPLICATIONS

There is growing evidence that death anxiety and death imagery are related. Several studies have addressed the nature of the relationship, with surprisingly consistent results, given the diverse samples of participating subjects and the variety of measures used to assess both death anxiety and death imagery. It would appear that there is a core connection between the two phenomena that transcends the variations of experimental methodology and error of measurement.

Baird (1972) investigated the relationship between death-anxiety scales and ways of thinking about death as revealed in responses to death-related metaphors. The study measured both conscious attitudes and conceptualizations of death and autonomic responses to the metaphors, the latter representing an indirect technique more likely to tap private or nonconscious levels of death anxiety. The main conclusions supported by the data analysis were that people who responded autonomically to human metaphors of death (e.g., the Grim Reaper) thought of death consciously as involving loneliness and sadness, while people who responded autonomically to nature metaphors of death (e.g., winter) did not think of it in those terms. Furthermore, high death anxiety correlated with metaphors of death as ending and finality, rather than with the less final metaphors. Finally, positive thoughts about death were associated with low death anxiety. Baird speculated that the inverse relationship between consciousness of death and reported anxiety about death implied either that denial of anxiety permits the subject of death to be held in awareness, or awareness of death occurs when anxiety is not so great as to require conscious repression of the topic.

Nogas, Schweitzer, and Grumet (1974), using Kastenbaum's personifications of death (the Macabre, the Gentle Comforter, the Automaton, and the Gay Deceiver), found that persons with high death anxiety tended to see death as Macabre, as opposed to persons with moderate or low levels of death anxiety, who saw death as either the Gentle Comforter or the Automaton.

In 1976, Lonetto et al. looked specifically to death anxiety and the perceived sex of death. Their results indicated that subjects, both male and female, who saw death as being sexless showed less anxiety about death than did those who saw death as male or female. Interestingly, however, few subjects saw death as a female figure; those who did were mostly females who demonstrated high levels of death anxiety. In later studies, Lonetto (1982) and Lonetto and Templer (1987, pp. 71-76) found that perceptions of death as a Gay Deceiver were related to the cognitive/affective component of death anxiety; that is, fear of dying, appearing nervous when people discuss death, the frequency of death-related thoughts and their effect, and being troubled by thoughts of life after death and the future. Images of death as the Gentle Comforter or the Macabre were related to an awareness of time; that is, thinking about the rapid passage of time and the shortness of life.

The foregoing studies of the death-anxiety/death-imagery relationships, while using various methods to elicit descriptions of death imagery, all approached the measurement of death anxiety from the unidimensional standpoint. Yet the refinement of measures of the various components of death anxiety would seem to warrant closer scrutiny with respect to death-related images. To this end, McDonald and Hilgendorf (1986), using scales designed to measure death anxiety as both a unidimensional and a multidimensional concept, dealt with five separate measures: the global measure provided by Templer and the four subscales of Collett and Lester's Fear of Death Scale (death of self, dying of self, death of others, dying of others). They also expanded the Kastenbaum and Aisenberg (1972) technique for eliciting descriptions of death images to include specific questions on age, sex, personal characteristics, and the physical appearance of death, in addition to open-ended questions in each area.

Their findings were striking in some ways. For example, of the 179 subjects in the total sample, only 14 imagined death to be young. While no significant differences were found between high and low death-anxiety groups on the young/old death-imagery classification, those who saw death as young had a more positive image of death than those who perceived it as an old person [$t(132) = 2.18$, $p < .05$]. This finding is consistent with those of Lonetto et al. (1976) and Kastenbaum and Aisenberg (1972), and can probably be traced to the fact that contemporary American society values youth over age; hence, a youthful image of death would also tend to be a positive image.

With respect to the sex of death images, they found no difference between high and low death-anxiety groups, but death was imagined to be male by 92% of the male respondents and 74% of the female respondents.

Most significant of all, however, were the results that had to do with the relationship of death anxiety and the positive/negative dimension of death imagery. On all five measures of death anxiety, the subjects with low death-anxiety scores had significantly more positive death images than did those with high scores. Of special importance were the findings on Collett and Lesser's subscales measuring Fear of Death of Self [$t(84) = 4.49$, $p < .001$] and Fear of Dying of Self [$t(84) = 4.68$, $p < .001$]. This is not surprising, in view of the personal nature of imagery. These results support Kastenbaum and Aisenberg's (1972) suggestion that death imagery might be used to assess the nature of death anxiety. For example, in a study by Bassett and Williams (2002), the 300-item Adjective Check List (ACL) was used to describe what death might be like if personified as a human character in a play. Lower death anxiety was associated with more positive ACL descriptions.

These studies raise the important question of the role death imagery could conceivably play in the treatment of death anxiety. Habeck and Sheikh (1984) suggest, for example, that if phobic disorders are rooted in fear of death, therapeutic efforts might well be directed toward the modification of the underlying death anxiety rather than toward the phobic symptoms. They further suggest that the death-imagery technique developed by Sheikh et al. (1979) may be helpful within this context.

Similarly, Morrison (1978), using the framework of George Kelly's personal construct theory, suggested that mental-imagery techniques, especially when used in combination with other psychotherapeutic interventions, could facilitate the grieving process. He urged the use of reconstruction of death-related events, such as the death, the wake, the funeral, and the burial, in order to evoke a variety of strong feelings, which in turn can lead to a successful completion of the grieving process. Reconstruction of positive images of the deceased and enactment of the dying experience that promotes survival is especially important for individuals who witness grotesque deaths or who experience bereavement after a violent or traumatic death of a loved one. For example, survivors of Hiroshima reported preoccupation with death images and death anxiety as fear of dying in a violent or mutilative manner (Rynearson, 1986, Lifton, 1983). Similarly, bereavement after a homicide may trigger fantasied thoughts, feelings, and intrusive images of the victim during his or her last moments (Rynerson, 1993, 1995). Parson (1987) described war-related intrusive symptoms that flood the self with death imagery and death anxiety in Vietnam veterans. Intrusive phenomena include dreams and flashbacks about death, fright, or near-death experiences of war. Death imagery is linked to intense fears that become pervasive in relationships with people, work, and emotional life. The therapist's role is to help the veteran reconstruct the death images of war so that they acquire new meaning. Static death imagery must be changed to vibrant images of life. Pain must be given value so that through the transformation of death images, a special form of knowledge associated with the sense of having "been there and returned" as a changed person is attained (Parson, 1987).

Fear of one's own death can also be addressed through imagery. For example, in one study, Developmental Transformations therapy was used to create a safe, accepting environment for exploring issues of death anxiety in 68 adults, aged 55 to 95. Developmental Transformations uses the encounter between the therapist and clients as well as the embodiment of images and roles as primary modes of healing. Through "play sessions," subjects were able to share and confront their fears and increase their sense of intimacy with their peers (Smith, 2000). Hypnotic techniques using guided imagery have also been used to address fear of dying and have proven especially useful in the management of terminally ill patients (Zahourek, 1990). Research studies are needed to provide empirical evidence of the efficacy of hypnosis and other therapeutic interventions for death anxiety.

These investigations of the use of death imagery in the resolution of psychological distress can only whet the spirit of scientific inquiry. Much remains to be done, as is clear from the long list of correlates and behavioral consequences of death anxiety, as well as from the various theoretical formulations regarding it. Mental-imagery techniques need to be applied in the attempt to modify death anxiety, and in so doing, to reduce the negative effects that are associated with it.

The techniques of imagery, symbolization, and personification need not, however, be merely curative. They can be utilized for integrative purposes, as well. The existentialist contention—understanding and accepting death while in the process of living is more important than confronting death only when it is about to occur—is one argument for the use of death imagery. The assumption underlying this contention is, of course, that life can be appreciated and lived more fully when understood in terms of both being and nonbeing. While arising from a distinct set of premises about human nature and life, this assumption does bear a similarity to the historical religious philosophy concerning the contemplation of death, which was discussed earlier in this chapter.

But the contemplation of nonbeing is not so consonant with human nature that it occurs either frequently or easily. Rather, it seems, it is necessary for an individual to have attained a particular level of understanding of his or her being before the idea of nonbeing can arise, however inchoate that idea might be. Axelrod (1986) makes reference to the innate difficulty with which humans encounter the notion of nonbeing when he points out that, in the Old Testament, God established the fact of death and provided "an abrupt and harsh explanation of its meaning" with the words,

> Until you return to the ground—
> For from it you were taken.
> For dust you are,
> And to dust you shall return.

Axelrod further notes that, despite the fact that Adam and Eve had just received the radical news of their mortality, the Book of Genesis records no reaction. It appears that "Adam does not suffer a single reflection, because death had not yet confronted his imagination" (p. 59).

Not all philosophical and theological writers are in accord, however, on the value of encountering one's mortality through reflection. Epicurus (cited in Bailey, 1926), in a letter to his disciple Menoeceus, advises,

> Become accustomed to the belief that death is nothing for us. For all good and evil consists in sensation, but death is deprivation of sensation. . . . So death, the most terrifying of ills, is nothing to us, since so long as we exist, death is not with us; but when death comes, then we do not exist. It does not then concern either the living or the dead, since for the former it is not, and the latter are no more (3, p. 85).

At the end of the same letter, however, Epicurus appears to contradict himself when he joins Plato, Socrates, and a multitude of religious traditions in exhorting his disciple as follows:

> Meditate therefore on these things and things akin to them night and day by yourself, and with a companion like unto yourself and never shall you be disturbed waking or asleep, but you shall live like a god among men (3, p. 93).

Thus, it can be seen that, even in the midst of the denial of the relevance of reflection on death, it is evaluated as positive and beneficial.

The ability to confront the fact of one's personal mortality does not appear to be evenly distributed among human beings, nor does it seem to be universally possible. Apart from the obvious incapacity for self-reflection in infancy, mental retardation, and certain of the more serious cognitive pathologies, there is probably wide variation in both the intellectual and affective or motivational potential for imagining one's death. Many death-education programs have adopted the reduction of death anxiety as a primary goal. It appears that didactic educational programs may result in cognitive and behavioral changes, but many participants in these programs actually show an increase in discomfort with death. In contrast, experiential programs generally have been found to produce a modest decrease in death anxiety (Durlak & Reisenberg, 1991). Overall, the value of an experiential approach such as imagery in therapy can help individuals to address death anxiety within the context of personal meaning.

It should be noted here that, as with other therapeutic interventions, use of death imagery techniques and the modification of death anxiety levels must be undertaken with caution. Fragile personalities, individuals with highly complex and fixed defensive systems, and those with perhaps an all too suggestive orientation may need certain protective safeguards in the process of confronting the potentially shattering reality of their own deaths. Despite the rather general consensus that it is beneficial to reflect on death, there is also a necessary recognition that the process by which this reflection is generated, the pace at which it progresses, and its effect on the psyche are all factors to be taken into serious consideration. As in other human endeavors, so in death imagery processes, individual differences must be acknowledged and respected.

One investigation has suggested that what is required in order to confront personal mortality is actualized authentic existence. Gamble and Brown (1981) studied two groups of people who were matched on demographic variables. The actualized group was composed of persons in the helping professions; the non-actualized group was composed of patients confined to a state mental institution. The procedure involved relaxation, visualization, and fantasy guided to successively older ages, but with no mention of death or dying. Successful completion of the age-progression procedure required that participants complete the fantasy of dying of natural causes at age 65 or older. Those participants falling toward the actualized and authentic end of the continuum were able to successfully confront the fact of their mortality more often than participants falling at the other end of the continuum. This difference was not affected by the age or sex of the people involved.

It appears, then, that the confrontation of personal death requires a certain level of human development and the absence of a high level of death anxiety. If this is true, the potential of growth deriving from coming to terms with one's mortality may be realized only when death anxiety has been reduced. The alteration of one's images, symbols, and personifications may be a critical phase of the process. Thus it seems that death imagery, having proven its usefulness in the amelioration of negative psychological states, can now embark upon its integrative and growth function. Both the research field and the therapeutic setting have been opened to death imagery. Its role in human actualization and authentic, nonanxiety-ridden existence seems to have just begun.

REFERENCES

Adam, R. S., Otto, H. A., & Cowley, A. S. (1984). *Letting go: Uncomplicating your life.* New York: Science and Behavior Books.

Aguilar, I., & Wood, V. N. (1976). Therapy through a death ritual. *Social Work, 21*(1), 49-54.

Axelrod, C. D. (1986). Reflections on the fear of death. *Omega, 17*(1), 51-54.

Bailey, C. (Ed.). (1926). *Epicurus: The extant remains.* Oxford: Clarendon Press.

Baird, C. F. (1972). Death fantasy in male and female college students. *Dissertation Abstracts, 33,* 1978.

Bassett, J., & Williams, J. E. (2002). Personification of death, as seen in adjective check list descriptions, among funeral service and university students. *Omega, 4*(1), 23-41.

Becker, E. (1973). *The denial of death.* New York: Free Press.

Blazer, J. (1973). The relationship between meaning in life and fear of death. *Psychology, 10,* 33-34.

Catania, J. A., Turner, H. A., Choi, K., & Coates, T. J. (1992). Coping with death anxiety: Help-seeking and social support among gay men with various HIV diagnoses. *AIDS, 6*(9), 999-1005.

Collett, L., & Lester, D. (1969). The fear of death and the fear of dying. *Journal of Psychology, 72,* 179-181.

Conte, H. R., Weiner, M. B., & Plutchik, R. (1982). Measure death anxiety: Conceptual, psychometric, and factor-analytic aspects. *Journal of Personality and Social Psychology, 43*(4), 775-785.

Dattel, A. R., & Neimeyer, R. A. (1990). Sex differences in death anxiety: Testing the emotional expressiveness hypothesis. *Death Studies, 14*(1), 1-11.

Degner, L. (1974). The relationship between some beliefs held by physicians and their life-prolonging decisions. *Omega, 5*, 223.

Depaola, S. J., Griffin, M., Young, J. R., & Neimeyer, R. A. (2003). Death anxiety and attitudes toward the elderly among adults: The role of gender and ethnicity. *Death Studies, 27*(4), 335-354.

Diggory, J. D., & Rothman, D. Z. (1961). Values destroyed by death. *Journal of Abnormal and Social Psychology, 63*, 205-210.

Dougherty, K., Templer, D. I., & Brown, R. (1986). Psychological states in terminal cancer patients as measured over time. *Journal of Counseling Psychology, 33*(3), 357-359.

Drolet, J. L. (1990). Transcending death during early adulthood: Symbolic immortality, death anxiety, and purpose in life. *Journal of Clinical Psychology, 46*(2), 148-160.

Durlak, J. (1973). Relationship between attitudes toward life and death among elderly women. *Developmental Psychology, 8*, 146.

Durlak, J. A., & Reisenberg, L. A. (1991). The impact of death education. *Death Studies, 15*, 39-59.

Feifel, H., Hanson, S., Jones, R., & Edwards, I. (1967). Physicians consider death (Summary). *Proceedings of the 75th Annual Convention, American Psychological Association, 2*, 201-202.

Feifel, H., & Nagy, V. T. (1981). Another look at fear of death. *Journal of Consulting & Clinical Psychology, 49*(2), 278-286.

Firth-Cozens, J., & Field, D. (1991). Fear of death and strategies for coping with patient death among medical trainees. *British Journal of Medical Psychology, 64*(3), 263-271.

Freud, S., (1957). Thoughts for the times on war and death. In *Standard Edition* (Vol. 14, pp. 299-300). London: Hogarth Press.

Galt, C. P., & Hayslip, B., Jr. (1998). Age differences in levels of overt and covert death anxiety. *Omega, 37*(3), 187-202.

Gamble, J. W., & Brown, E. C. (1981). Self-actualization and personal mortality. *Omega, 11*, 341-353.

Greenberger, E. (1965). Fantasies of women confronting death. *Journal of Consulting Psychology, 29*, 252-260.

Habeck, B. K., & Sheikh, A. A. (1984). Imagery and the treatment of phobic disorders. In A. A. Sheikh (Ed.), *Imagination and healing* (pp. 171-196). Amityville, NY: Baywood.

Hayslip, B., Jr., Guarnaccia, C. A., Radika, L. M., & Servaty, H. L. (2001, 2002). Death anxiety: An empirical test of a blended self report and projective measurement model. *Omega, 44*(3), 277-294.

Hessing, D. J., & Elffers, H. (1986). Attitude toward death, fear of being declared dead too soon, and donation of organs after death. *Omega, 17(2)*, 115-126.

Heuscher, J. E. (1986). Death and authenticity. *The American Journal of Psychoanalysis, 46*(4), 310-317.

Hoelter, J. W. (1979). Multidimensional treatment of fear of death. *Journal of Consulting and Clinical Psychology, 47*(5), 996-999.

Iammarino, N. K. (1975). Relationship between death anxiety and demographic variables. *Psychological Reports, 17*, 262.

James, W. (1902). *Varieties of religious experience: A study in human nature.* New York: Mentor Edition, 1958.
Jung, C. (1963). *Memories, dreams and reflections.* New York: Pantheon Books.
Kastenbaum, R., & Aisenberg, R. (1972). *The psychology of death.* New York: Springer.
Kastenbaum, R., & Herman, C. (1997). Death personification in the Kevorkian era. *Death Studies, 21*(2), 115-130.
Krieger, S., Epsting, F., & Leitner, L. M. (1974). Personal constructs, threat and attitudes toward death. *Omega, 5,* 299.
Lester, D. (1967). Experimental and correlational studies of the fear of death. *Psychological Bulletin, 67*(1), 27-36.
Lester, D., & Abdel-Khalek, A. (2003). The Collett-Lester Fear of Death Scale: A correction. *Death Studies, 27*(1), 81-85.
Lifton, R. J. (1983). *The broken connection: On death and the continuity of life.* New York: City University of New York.
Lifton, R. J., & Olson, E. (1974). *Living and dying.* New York: Praeger.
Lonetto, R. (1982). Personification of death and death anxiety. *Journal of Personality Assessment, 46,* 404-408.
Lonetto, R., Fleming, S., Clare, M., & Gorman, M. (1976). The perceived sex of death and concerns about death. *Essence, 1,* 66-84.
Lonetto, R., & Templer, D. I. (1987). *Death anxiety.* Ontario, Canada: Guelph.
Lowrey, R. (1965). *Male-female differences in attitudes toward death.* Unpublished manuscript, Brandeis University.
McClelland, D. (1963). The Harlequin Complex. In R. White (Ed.), *The study of lives.* New York: Atherton Press.
McDonald, R. T., & Carroll, J. D. (1981). Appropriate death: College students' preferences vs. actuarial projections. *Journal of Clinical Psychology, 37*(1), 28-31.
McDonald, R. T., & Hilgendorf, W. A. (1986). Death imagery and death anxiety. *Journal of Clinical Psychology, 42*(1), 87-91.
McLennan, J., Bates, G. W., Johnson, E., Lavery, A. R., & Horne, D. De L. (1993). The Death Fantasy Scale: A measure based on metaphors of one's personal death. *Journal of Psychology, 127*(6), 619-624.
McMordie, W. R. (1979). Improving measurement of death anxiety. *Psychological Reports, 44,* 975-980.
Morrison, J. K. (1978). Successful grieving: Changing personal constructs through mental imagery. *Journal of Mental Imagery, 2,* 63-68.
Nagy, M. (1959). The child's view of death. In H. Feifel (Ed.), *The meaning of death.* New York: McGraw-Hill.
Nelson, L. D., & Nelson, C. C. (1975). A factor analytic inquiry into the multidimensionality of death anxiety. *Omega, 6*(2), 171-178.
Neimeyer, R. A., & Chapman, I. M. (1980). Self/Ideal discrepancy and fear of death: The test of an existential hypothesis. *Omega, 11,* 233-240.
Neimeyer, R. A., & Van Brunt, D. (1995). Death anxiety. In H. Wass & R. A. Neimeyer (Eds.), *Dying: Facing the facts* (pp. 49-82). Washington, DC: Taylor & Francis.
Nogas, C., Schweitzer, I., & Grumet, J. (1974). An investigation of death anxiety, sense of competence, and need for achievement. *Omega, 5,* 245.
Papageorgis, D. (1966). On the ambivalence of death: The case of the missing harlequin. *Psychological Reports, 19,* 325-326.

Parson, E. R. (1987). Life after death: Vietnam veterans' struggle for meaning and recovery. *Death Studies, 10*(1), 11-26.

Peck, S. (1966). The development of the concept of death in male children. *Dissertation Abstracts, 27,* 1294.

Pollak, J. M. (1979). Correlates of death anxiety: A review of empirical studies. *Omega, 10,* 97-121.

Rappaport, H., Fossler, R. J., Bross, L., & Gilden, D. (1993). Future time, death anxiety, and life purpose among older adults. *Death Studies, 17*(4), 369-379.

Rasmussen, C. A., & Brems, C. (1996). The relationship of death anxiety with age and psychosocial maturity. *Journal of Psychology, 130*(2), 141-144.

Rynearson, E. K. (1986). Psychological effects of unnatural dying on bereavement. *Psychiatric Annals, 16*(5), 272-275.

Rynearson, E. K. (1993). Bereavement after homicide: A synergism of trauma and loss. *American Journal of Psychiatry, 150*(2), 258-261.

Rynearson, E. K. (1995). Bereavement after homicide. A comparison of treatment seekers and refusers. *British Journal of Psychiatry, 166*(4), 507-510.

Sabatini, P., & Kastenbaum, R. (1973). The Do-It-Yourself Death Certificate as a research technique. *Life-Threatening Behavior, 3,* 20-32.

Schulz, R. (1978). *The psychology of death, dying, and bereavement.* Reading, MA: Addison-Wesley.

Schulz, R., & Aderman, D. (1979). Physicians' death anxiety and patient outcomes. *Omega, 9,* 327-332.

Sheikh, A. S., & Sheikh, K. S. (2003). Death imagery: Confronting death brings us to the threshold of life. In A. A. Sheikh (Ed.), *Healing images: The role of imagination in health* (Imagery and human development series). Amityville, NY: Baywood.

Sheikh, A. S., Twente, G. E., & Turner, D. (1979). Death imagery: Therapeutic uses. In A. A. Sheikh & J. T. Shaffer (Eds.), *The potential of fantasy and imagination* (pp. 149-169). New York: Brandon House, Inc.

Smith, A. G. (2000). Exploring death anxiety with older adults through developmental transformations. *Arts in Psychotherapy, 27*(5), 321-331.

Shneidman, E. S. (1972). Can a young person write his own obituary? *Life-Threatening Behavior, 2,* 262-267.

Simpson, M. A. (1975). The Do-It Yourself Death Certificate in evoking and estimating student attitudes toward death. *Journal of Medical Education, 50,* 475-478.

Staller, E. (1980). The impact of death related fears on attitudes of nurses in a hospital work setting. *Omega, 11*(1), 85-96.

Templer, D. (1970). The instruction and validation of a death anxiety scale. *Journal of General Psychology, 82,* 165-177.

Templer, D. (1972). Death anxiety in religiously very involved persons. *Psychological Reports, 35,* 530.

Templer, D., Ruff, C., & Franks, C. (1971). Death anxiety: Age, sex, and parental resemblance in diverse populations. *Developmental Psychology, 4,* 108.

Thorsen, J. A., & Powell, F. C. (2000). Developmental aspects of death anxiety and religion. In J. A. Thorson (Ed.), *Perspectives on spiritual well-being and aging* (pp. 142-158). Illinois: Charles C. Thomas Publisher LTD.

Tomer, A., Eliason, G., & Smith, J. (2000). The structure of the Revised Death Anxiety Scale in young and old adults. In A. Tomer (Ed.), *Death attitudes and the older adult: Theories, concepts, and applications* (Series in death, dying, and bereavement) (pp. 109-122).

Toynbee, A. (1968). Various ways in which human beings have sought to reconcile themselves to the fact of death. In A. Toynbee, A. K. Mant, N. Smart, J. Hinton, C. Yudkin, E. Rhode, R. Heywood, & H. H. Price (Eds.), *Man's concern with death.* New York: McGraw-Hill.

Viswanathan, R. (1996). Death anxiety, locus of control, and purpose in life of physicians: Their relationship to patient death notification. *Psychosomatics, 37*(4), 339-345.

Weisman, A., & Hackett, T. (1961). Predilection to death. *Journal of Psychosomatic Medicine, 23,* 232-256.

Yalom, I. (1980). *Existential psychotherapy.* New York: Basic Books.

Zahourek, R. P. (1990). *Clinical hypnosis and therapeutic suggestion in patient care* (pp. 209-221). New York: Brunner-Routledge.

CHAPTER 9

The Use of Guided Imagery in Death Education

Thomas A. Droege

> First I was dying to finish high school and start college. And then I was dying to finish college and start working. And then I was dying to marry and have children. And then I was dying for my children to grow old enough for school so I could return to work. And then I was dying to retire. And now, I am dying . . . and suddenly I realize I forgot to live.
>
> (Anonymous)

People often frown when I tell them that I use death imagery as a tool for learning in the college classroom. Behind the frown is a question that may or may not be made explicit. What is accomplished by engendering fear and anxiety in students through the use of death imagery? That kind of response is not surprising. Death has been regarded with fear by people in every age and every culture. In some periods of history, that has been dramatically expressed, as it was in medieval Europe during the fourteenth and fifteenth centuries. The imagery of death that found expression in art motifs like *The Dance of Death* and *The Triumph of Death*, and in tomb sculptures like the *Transi*, could only have been the product of tortured minds overwhelmed by death on every side. In our modern era we have been successful in distancing ourselves from death in our daily living, but the fear of death remains deeply embedded in our psyches, as Ernest Becker has demonstrated so convincingly in his book *The Denial of Death* (1973).

How then can death imagery be used in a constructive way in death education? The purpose of this chapter is to answer that question—not just theoretically, but with practical suggestions and specific exercises in guided imagery. I have been using guided imagery for the past several years in a college class that I teach on "Understanding Death and Dying." I have found it to be an effective tool for helping students to process the personal thoughts and feelings that are inevitably aroused by a course that is so deeply existential.

The literature on imagery is flooded with commentaries on the therapeutic usages of imagery, but relatively little attention has been given to the many uses of guided imagery for purposes of teaching. That simply reflects the general lack of pedagogical research and training in higher education. Those who teach at the college level get little or no training in instructional methodology. Doctoral programs focus almost exclusively on research methodology within the discipline. Perhaps that is why the lecture method is still so dominant in most college classrooms in spite of the evidence that its effectiveness for teaching is quite low with comparison to other teaching methodologies. The limits of the lecture method are particularly obvious in death education.

I will simply assume the value of death education. It has been included as part of the curriculum in almost every college across the country, and other organizations sponsor lectures, seminars, and workshops for the general public on topics related to death and dying. Even elementary school children are taken on field trips to funeral homes. What was taboo in our culture just thirty years ago, including the academic arena, is now a matter of open inquiry and discussion (DeSpelder & Strickland, 2005).

It is also obvious by now that the academic interest in death-related topics is more than a fad. Thanatology has become a respected field of study that has attracted psychologists, theologians, sociologists, anthropologists, and a wide variety of health-care professionals. All of that is clearly for the good. How much better it is for people to intentionally raise the question of death rather than facing it as a life trauma overladen with grief and feelings of high anxiety (Wass, Miller, & Thorton, 1990).

My experience as a death educator is similar to that of many others. I began by teaching the course on "Understanding Death and Dying" in much the same way that I taught other academic subjects. To understand something in the academic world, particularly at the college level, means using analytical and critical skills that are carefully honed in liberal arts training. Since this was a theology course taught at a university that operates from within the Christian tradition, I engaged the students in a careful and critical study of how Christianity and other religious traditions have understood the meaning of death. We examined the evolution of ideas about death within the biblical narratives with particular emphasis on the accounts of Christ's death and resurrection. This was followed by a study of the history of Western civilization for an understanding of the diversity of different attitudes and ideas about death over time. Finally, we looked at some contemporary studies of death and dying that were written from the perspectives of psychology, sociology, medicine, and other disciplines.

I discovered that students were not able to deal with the subject of death in a purely intellectual way. They complained of mild depression and lack of concentration in reading materials that at one level they found very interesting.

Discussion periods invariably triggered stories of personal encounters with death. Even when not verbally expressed, the strong emotions that the subject evoked could be seen in the faces of students and heard in their voices. The question was not whether the feelings of students would be included as data to be processed in this course, but how that could be done in a constructive and healthy way.

Dealing with death calls for whole-person learning. There is a variety of ways that I have used to facilitate deeper-than-intellectual learning. I invite guest speakers and show videotapes of persons who share personal experiences of bereavement and facing life-threatening illness. I use a variety of exercises that are designed to put students in touch with their personal experience. But what I have found most helpful for heightening personal awareness is guided imagery.

Each person's awareness of death is unique to that person, just as each person's style of living is unique. Guided imagery is a particularly useful tool for exploring the inner world of personal experience because it does not dictate in advance what it is that one will find there. A guide is useful for facilitating the entrance into that inner world and to suggest areas of exploration, but what one finds will be unique to each person.

Another reason for the effectiveness of guided imagery is that it protects the privacy of the person, even when the exercises are done in a group setting. People cannot be expected to express openly personal thoughts and feelings about a subject that is still taboo in our society. Guided imagery is a way of assisting them to explore the meaning of death without the expectation that they will share that experience with anyone else. Sharing experiences can be enormously helpful, as anyone who has participated in a grief group will testify; but a deeply intrapersonal experience in a nonthreatening group setting is the most useful tool I have found to put people in touch with a felt sense of their fear and their faith in relation to death.

Guided imagery is a good learning tool because it fosters the use of the imagination in students who have been taught from early childhood to value their rational powers more highly than their imagination. Guided imagery allows students to structure their experience in a manner that is both realistic and constructive. It can be a creative way to reexperience important events in the past, such as the funeral of a grandparent, and to anticipate events that lie in the future, such as one's own death.

I experimented for a number of years with different types of exercises in guided imagery before settling on a formula that I found most effective. I regularly got feedback from students after each class exercise by asking for both general and specific responses to the method and content of the exercises. This was done anonymously in written form. I continue to get excellent critique and new ideas from students, and I urge all educators to invite regular feedback to their use of imagery.

PRINCIPLES OF GUIDED IMAGERY

I will list the basic principles that inform my use of guided imagery without insisting that they are the only or even the best principles to employ. I will note as well some alternative principles.

The first and most obvious principle is that a deeper level of experience than ordinary consciousness is needed for participants to make effective use of guided imagery. It is for that reason that the beginning portion of each exercise is designed to induce a state of relaxation and readiness for what is to follow. Ira Progoff (1975) calls this a state of "twilight imagery," a spawning ground for images. All methods of guided imagery assume the importance of a trancelike state for exploring the inner world of one's own experience.

Not so obvious is the second principle that guides my use of imagery. I think that the context of a specific faith tradition is a distinct asset for a person who is engaged in the imaging of death. This goes a step beyond those who would argue, as does Progoff, that the nurture of spirituality is an important goal in using imagery. The next section of this chapter will contain an argument in defense of this principle.

A third principle in my use of guided imagery, following directly from the previous one, is that structured exercises work better than unstructured ones for utilizing images that come out of a particular religious tradition. People who are skilled in the practice of meditation and the use of imagery are likely to prefer unstructured exercises, where imagery emerges spontaneously from the person participating in the exercise. They are likely to resist specific directions or modify them to meet their own needs. However, the feedback that I have received from students suggests that most people who have had relatively little experience with the use of guided imagery welcome the suggestion of specific images and the charting of specific journeys (e.g., a mountain-climbing expedition) as long as they are given the liberty to respond to images and events in a manner that is true to their experience and understanding. For example, the death of Christ does not have the same meaning to everyone within the Christian tradition, but the cross provides an image common to all Christians for reflecting on the themes of death and dying. Exercises based on the cross provide ample opportunity for individuals to reflect on that theme with imagery that emerges out of their own inner world of meaning.

A fourth principle (and one of the principles of Progoff's method) that I regard as essential for the process of guided imagery is what he calls "active privacy." He defines it as follows:

> *Active privacy* is the basic means of inner contact available to an individual. It does not mean working alone, nor does it mean holding ourselves aloof from others, for privacy does not involve a physical place or a physical condition. Privacy is primarily an inner place and a quality of being.

> Especially it is the condition of being that is established in a person when his attention is focused toward nurturing the seed and deepening the roots of his life. *Active privacy* is the relation of a person to himself as he works with the inner process of his life (Progoff, 1975, p. 48).

It is always important to protect the privacy of individuals, but it is particularly important in a classroom setting. Exercises in guided imagery are deeply personal, and though sharing after the completion of the exercise may be helpful to some, it is not a necessary part of the process. It will be difficult for some to get any value at all out of a guided imagery exercise if they are not assured of complete privacy.

The fifth principle I propose is that a group setting maximizes the effectiveness of guided imagery. This principle may seem to be in contradiction to the previous principle emphasizing privacy, but it has been my experience that the group environment provides an outer support for the private inner experience. Being in a group need not imply group interaction in either verbal or behavioral ways. One can draw strength from the presence of others while being engaged in an intensely personal experience. Each person in the group works individually on his or her own life, but the nurturing presence of the group is a vital ingredient in facilitating that work. The ritual of a traditional liturgy illustrates the same principle. The ritual behavior (listening, praying, singing, kneeling) has little group interaction, and yet for most people, a religious worship service provides a rich sense of common life.

Is there a danger that the process of guided imagery will weaken the defenses of people with weak egos or overwhelm them with emotions too strong to handle by themselves? I think not. My sixth principle is that participants can assume responsibility for their own journey. I have used guided imagery for years, and I have yet to encounter an instance where it caused someone's pathology to be exacerbated or where the person found it more difficult to cope with life in general or with the particular life issues that were the focus of the exercise. Participants may be deeply affected by the experience, of course, and some will cry. But they will not fall apart. People can be trusted to use an intuitive wisdom in processing their own inner experience, and I have learned to trust that wisdom both as a participant and as a leader of such exercises. There is a big difference between the active privacy of guided imagery and the intrusive probing of an analytical therapist.

The seventh and final principle that informs my use of guided imagery is that some form of writing or journaling will enhance the long-term value of the exercise. Though useful for any form of guided imagery, it is particularly valuable in death imagery. The purpose of the writing is to facilitate spontaneous expression of feelings and reflection on ideas generated by the experience for later reading and meditation. The reflection serves to integrate the experience into the person's evolving perspective on self and world.

THE VALUE OF A RELIGIOUS FRAMEWORK FOR DEATH IMAGERY

As already indicated in the aforementioned principles, I think that there are distinct advantages for using guided imagery within the context of a religious frame of reference. Furthermore, those advantages are enhanced to the degree that the religious tradition that provides the context has rich and powerful images. These images provide reassurance and comfort in facing the death anxiety that can be anticipated in any encounter with death, real or imagined.

By religion I mean simply the broadest and deepest frame of reference used by an individual or group for the understanding of self and world. To be human is to search for meaning, and at no time is the need for meaning likely to be stronger than in facing what have been commonly called "limit experiences"—experiences that force into awareness the realization of the fragility of human existence. Facing one's death, whether real or imagined, is the most absolute form of a limit experience and the measure of all other experiences of lesser loss. Religion supplies the framework of meaning within which one finds the resources for coping with the final limit experience of death.

The questions that people ask in the face of death are ultimate questions calling for religious answers. Our civilization has been moving steadily in the direction of a secular world view, and this loss of a sense of transcendent reality has compounded the burden of finding meaning in life, haunted by the fear of death. More than any other recent cultural analyst, Ernest Becker has exposed the inadequacy of secular solutions to the fear of dying. He notes that many turn to psychotherapy as an aid in understanding their fears and finding a way to cope with them. But psychology cannot provide an ultimate solution to the anxiety that comes with the anticipation of death, because it is not neurotic but existential anxiety, part and parcel of the human condition. As Becker puts it, "There is no way to overcome creature anxiety unless one is a god and not a creature" (1973, p. 261).

Quite apart from ontological questions about the truth of religion, Becker argues along the same lines as Erik Erikson that all people have a psychological need for religion. After citing some other psychological strengths in religion, Becker states:

> Best of all, of course, religion solves the problem of death, which no living individual can solve, no matter how they would support us. Religion, then, gives the possibility of heroic victory in freedom and solves the problem of human dignity at its highest level. . . . Finally, religion alone gives hope, because it holds open the dimension of the unknown and the unknowable, the fantastic mystery of creation that the human mind cannot even begin to approach. . . . Religion takes one's very creatureliness, one's insignificance, and makes it a condition of hope (1973, p. 203).

What I am suggesting on the basis of Becker's analysis is that religious imagery will be much more effective than secular imagery in helping people to face limit situations, and especially death as the ultimate limit situation. One of the most striking indications of the secular age in which we live is the limited number of references to religion in most of the current literature on death and dying. The anthologies that are regularly used as texts for courses in death and dying rarely have an essay written from the perspective of religious studies and contain only isolated references to the role of religion or the clergy in the lives of people who are terminally ill or going through the process of bereavement. I recently did a review of an otherwise excellent anthology of readings on death and dying that had no references at all to ultimate questions of any kind, an omission that would be quite unthinkable in any other than our modern era.

What is true for the authors of the literature on death and dying is true also for most educators who use death imagery as a pedagogical tool. That should not be at all surprising since the vast majority work within state-supported secular institutions. That is as it should be in a pluralistic society that prizes religious freedom, which means both the right to practice my own religion without interference and the right to be protected from anyone who would force his or her religion on me. Political necessity, however, does not make a secular context for using death imagery superior to a religious context. Quite the contrary. I will argue that while a secular use of death imagery is to be highly valued for its humanitarian ideals, only a religious frame of reference can be fully satisfactory in meeting the spiritual needs of people and addressing directly their ultimate questions. In an effort to be clear and concrete in distinguishing between secular and religious contexts, I will refer only to the Christian religion in the next few paragraphs.

The most obvious difference between a secular and a Christian context for using death imagery is that references to a transcendent dimension of reality will be missing from the secular context. Death and dying are strictly natural phenomena within a secular perspective, but they offer to the religiously minded an occasion to experience and reflect on what is believed to be the sacred dimension of life. To understand death as nothing more than an event in nature means that one must face death anxiety, the terror of creatureliness that Becker describes with such painful intensity, without ultimate answers to the questions it raises about human existence. People do find comfort in imagining themselves within the natural flow of life from birth to death, but that view of life receives little support in a society that systematically engages in a rape of nature.

A religious encounter with death can also generate anxiety as well as a feeling of reassurance. For example, St. Paul's interpretation of death in the New Testament is harshly negative. Death came into the world because of sin and is therefore the judgment of God on a fallen humanity. Apart from Christ, death can only bring one face-to-face with an angry God: hardly a source of comfort for the dying and bereaved! Anyone who is even casually familiar with medieval art or Puritan sermons on the theme of death will be aware of just how anxiety producing such imagery can be. However, within the Christian tradition, death imagery yields to the imagery of life and light. It is the emphasis on Easter and the promise of a life after death that makes it possible for Christians to face death unafraid.

This leads to another difference between a secular and a Christian context for death imagery. The difference is whether death is imaged as a wall or as a door. The image of a wall emphasizes finality while the image of a door suggests the continuity of life beyond death. The issue of historical continuity cannot be avoided by anyone using death imagery, as Robert Lifton has suggested throughout his writings (e.g., Lifton & Olson, 1974). To be human is to remember and to anticipate. Throughout our lives we anticipate the future and its hoped-for rewards, often to the detriment of our appreciation of the present and the past; but we woud be less than fully human if we ignored the future altogether. That is as true when we reflect on our dying as it is when we imagine what life will be like after college or after retirement.

One can meet this human need for a sense of historical continuity within a secular perspective. Lifton and Olson (1974) have identified five modes of symbolic immortality, four of which can be utilized within a secular frame of reference: biological or biosocial (living through your children), creativity (being remembered for what you have done), nature (the eternal return of the four seasons), and experiential transcendence (altered state of consciousness). The fifth mode is religious, which by definition cannot be secular, though each of the other four modes can be and have been utilized within a religious framework.

The third major difference between a religious and a Christian frame of reference for death imagery is that the dominant images for secular death imagery are likely to be drawn from within nature and history, while the dominant images of Christian imagery will be drawn from beyond nature and history. While it is true that Christian imagery draws heavily on nature and history, what is seen as significant from this perspective is always the "something more" than nature and history. However one identifies it, it is this deeper dimension to reality that is of the essence in religious death imagery. Death imagery that lacks it might be appreciated as helpful and, within its own limited sphere, as true; but it will lack the meaning and significance that can only come from an encounter with the sacred.

We live in a secular age, and I for one would opt for no other, but we need to recognize that its values are limited and not always appropriate for meeting our basic needs. Most people know that intuitively and live their lives accordingly. A scientist may spend a lifetime in his or her laboratory without even entertaining a hypothesis about transcendent reality, but at the same time draw heavily on religious imagery when contemplating his or her own death. There is no self-contradiction in that unless one assumes that the secular assumptions that undergird the use of the scientific method are the only appropriate assumptions for a total worldview.

Though I have no statistical data to offer as evidence, my hypothesis is that most people, including thoroughly secular people, look to religious imagery when reflecting on their death. What I would cite as evidence, rarely noted in the current literature on death and dying, is that the clergy are the professionals who are most deeply involved in the lives of people who are terminally ill or grieving the loss of another. They are the only members of the helping professions who still have direct access to the homes of people and who make house calls at times of dire need, like a death in the family. The religious ideas and values that are affirmed in and through funeral liturgies undergird individuals and communities in periods of great loss. Even people who have never had formal ties to a religious institution regularly request a religious ritual for burials.

Why is that? One reason, I think, is because Christianity, the dominant religion in the Western world, has made victory over death such a prominent motif in its belief system. And this has been true throughout the period when death denial has been so characteristic of this culture. Death imagery appears again and again in Christian hymnody. The rituals that surround death highlight its importance and offer comfort to survivors. And, above all, death imagery appears at the center of the Christian contemplation of the mystery of the cross. The primary purpose of religion is to provide meaning, and at no time is that function more important than when the secular values that have sustained people throughout their lives appear to be weak and unsatisfying in an encounter with death.

STRUCTURED EXERCISES IN GUIDED IMAGERY FOR DEATH EDUCATION

The use of imagery needs more structure when used for educational purposes than it does in a therapy session. Although I have used structured and unstructured exercises in both therapy and classroom settings, I generally prefer structured exercises in a classroom setting. Each of the examples of guided imagery that follow are replete with an induction and specific directions concerning the content of the exercise, place, and time of pauses, and a commentary on how the exercise shoud be introduced and concluded. What I am assuming is that the instructor has not used guided imagery before and would be helped by careful instructions about how to proceed. Most college teachers have no formal education in teaching methodologies and are often hesitant about trying new techniques. That is even more true if the technique is imagery, due to the fear that repressed death anxiety might overwhelm a vulnerable student.

Students are also well served by exercises that are structured. First, one must assume that at least some of them are neophytes in the use of imagery, and thus explicit directions will alleviate anxiety about what to do and provide the reassurance of being guided through the exercise. Second, a common experience (e.g., a mountain-climbing expedition) facilitates a bonding of the group even though there is no interpersonal sharing in the exercise. Third, the common experience facilitates sharing at the end of the exercise among those who choose to do so. Fourth, a structured exercise permits direct focusing on particular images of faith within a religious tradition. Though the fourth point applies only to groups that share a common faith tradition, it is applicable in a broader sense to any culture that is bound together by common values and beliefs.

Examples of three structured exercises in guided death imagery will be provided: two that assume the Christian faith as the common tradition of the group participating in the exercise and one that would be appropriate for use in any secular setting.

A Life-Threatening Experience

The first exercise, based on Psalms 90 and 121, takes the form of a life-threatening experience while climbing a mountain. It is obviously an imaginary experience since very few people are mountain-climbers. There is an advantage to an experience that is so clearly imaginary. One can surrender fully to the experience because nothing like it has ever happened or is ever likely to happen to the participants in real life. Life-threatening experiences prompt people to reevaluate their lives and to reorder their priorities. A guided imagery exercise is certainly not the same as a real event, but for some it may be an occasion for reflecting more deeply on the course of their lives and for making significant changes if their life-review warrants it.

It is important in this exercise, as well as others, that the pace of speaking by the leader be deliberate. Long pauses are needed only where indicated, but those doing the exercise should never feel rushed. The leader should also tell the participants that they will be doing some writing during the course of the exercise so that pen and paper are ready to use.

Before beginning the exercise, the leader should read Psalms 90 and 121 in a slow, meditative way. The three or four verses of these psalms that are included within the script are from the Revised Standard Version of the Bible. Another translation can be substituted, but the quotations in the script should match the translation that is used when reading the psalms before the beginning of the exercise.

An opportunity for sharing should be provided at the close of the exercise for those who could benefit from that. Of course, nobody should be asked to share their experience if they have not volunteered to do so. Small groups of three to four work well for this purpose. The exercise follows:

Be aware of your body for a moment. Feel places of tension in your body—perhaps in your shoulders or the back of your neck, perhaps in your lower back or in the pit of your stomach, perhaps a tightness you feel in your head. Wherever it is, let the tension flow away. Stretch your arms and legs, and then let them relax. Rotate your head. Take a deep breath and exhale slowly.

Relax in your chair and close your eyes so that you can see what is going on inside of you rather than concentrating on what is happening outside . . . concentrating on the natural rhythm of your breathing . . . breathing in . . . and breathing out... breathing in... breathing out... feeling the rhythm of your inner life... letting the rhythm of your breathing carry you easily and naturally into the realm of your interior life... moving more deeply into the inner recesses of your being, into the quietness of the center of your being... feeling the goodness of being alive at this very moment and preparing yourself for a spiritual journey that will take you to the very brink of death... letting yourself be guided along paths that your imagination will construct with ease.

In your mind's eye, picture a snow-covered mountain. Imagine yourself as part of a mountain climbing party with a common goal to reach the top. Give yourself permission to be as young and physically able as you would need to be to engage in such a mission. You've established a base camp high up on the mountain, and five of you have been selected to make the final ascent to the peak. You feel the exhilaration and challenge of this special moment in your life.

Let yourself feel the majesty and the mystery of the mountain, its permanence and its power. As you reflect on the awesomeness of the natural surroundings, you begin to reflect on the majesty and the mystery, the permanence and the power of the God who formed mountains, the God for whom a thousand years is as a passing night. Suddenly you feel quite small in relation to the majesty and mystery, the permanence and power of this mountain and the God who created it. How fragile your life seems as you carefully chip away one foothold after another into the icy mountainside until you reach a plateau. One slip and the crevasse opens its wide jaws to swallow you up. One false step and your life hangs in the balance. How solid this mountainside is in comparison with your soft flesh. How permanent it is compared with the fleeting hours and days that you have to spend on this earth. Far below you see a field of wild flowers growing on the mountainside, and you sense that your life is as fleeting and as fragile as the grass and flowers in that field—here today, gone tomorrow. So is human life in comparison with the life of a mountain, to the life of God.

Suddenly a snowstorm hits with an intensity known only high up on a mountainside, and you find yourself momentarily separated from the rest of the climbing party. Unable to see two feet in front of you but unwilling to simply stay in the same spot, you stumble and find yourself hurtling over the steep precipice of a narrow crevasse. When you hit the bottom, you breathe a sigh of relief that you are unharmed, but then you realize you are pinned in the narrow crevasse, unable to move. You call out with all your might, but hear only the howling wind in return. You hope and pray that others in the party will find you, but you know your life hangs in the balance, and that it's only a matter of time until the bitter cold claims your life. Feel the cold of that place as it gradually penetrates into a body unable to move. Hear the howling wind of the winter storm. Experience the loneliness and the isolation of being left alone to die. (*Pause for a minute.*)

Unable to do anything but wait, you find your whole life passing before you as if it were projected on a screen. As each passing event appears on the screen, you hear a voice in the background intoning the same word again and again:

"GUILTY, GUILTY, GUILTY." As scene after scene reveals both the flaws and the failures of your past life, you hear in the background the faint strains of a chorus, "We are consumed by your anger, by your wrath we are overwhelmed. You set our iniquities before you, our secret sins in the light of your countenance." You come to the gradual realization that you are in a twilight zone at the border that separates this life and the next, that the scenes of your past life are blending into the scene of the last judgment. And you wish fervently that you could relive some of the past and extend some of your days into the future. If you could be snatched from this pit, then surely you would value every year, every month, every day, every hour. And you would number your days and use each one wisely.

In time the storm passes and you are able to see above you the mighty mountain you had set out to master, only now it seems to be the master, you the vanquished. As the cold penetrates ever more deeply, numbing both body and mind, you turn your eyes one last time to view the majesty of the mountain you had set out to climb, and just over the precipice of the crevasse you see the figure of a climber preparing to descend, and you know in an instant that you will be rescued, and a whole new life opens up before you. The figure that slowly but surely makes its way down the crevasse looks bigger than life, and these words begin to form on your lips: "I will lift up my eyes to the hills. From where does my help come? My help comes from the Lord, who made heaven and earth." As you are carefully lifted from your frozen tomb by expert climbers on each side of you and assisted by them up the steep incline to the top of the crevasse, other words of the psalm come into your mind: "He will not let your foot be moved; he who keeps you will not slumber. The Lord will keep you from all evil; he will keep your life. The Lord will keep your going out and your coming in from this time forth and forevermore."

After you have been brought down to a chateau high up on the mountainside, given a warm bath and some hot broth, you are placed in a warm bed in order to restore your body temperature to its normal level. As you lie in bed, looking out a picture window at a panoramic view of the mountains, still too stimulated by all that has happened to sleep, your thoughts return to the events of the day, and you begin to reflect on the meaning of it all for your life and faith. Imagine yourself alone and reflective at the end of such a day. In what way do you think you are different as a result of what happened? Have your priorities in life been changed? Is God nearer or farther away for you? Has your attitude toward death changed? As you are ready, write whatever comes to your mind as you reflect on your journey up the mountain and the implications of its nearly fatal outcome for your life and faith. Let your writing be as free and spontaneous as if you were dictating it at the close of that awesome day. (*Allow 15 minutes for writing.*)

The purpose of the above exercise is to provide an opportunity for participants to reflect on the finitude of human existence and examine the priorities of their lives in the light of the limited life span of every human being. The exercise could be adapted for use in a secular setting by simply removing all religious references.

It would then be a life-threatening experience with a dramatic rescue and time to reflect on one's values in light of the experience. The exercise is considerably enhanced, however, if it is done within the framework of a particular religious tradition that is shared by all of the participants. That makes it possible to use common symbols and strengthen the bonding of the group. Though the exercise is intrapersonal in that it calls for no sharing, doing the exercise in solidarity with a group that has a common bond deepens the experience considerably.

Before the Judgment Seat of God

The next exercise is based on a passage in the New Testament, Mathew 25:31-46. It is a parable of Jesus about the last judgment that is familiar to almost every Christian. For fully half of the two thousand years of recorded Christian history, the primary image of death has been an image of judgment. It was with fear and trembling that Christians contemplated a coming day of judgment when their souls would be weighed on the scales of justice. Demons tempted the dying and waited anxiously to pounce on the soul as it departed the body. Even if one were fortunate enough to escape the fires of Hell, one's soul would still need to be purged of its remaining evil before dwelling in the presence of a holy God.

People in the modern era no longer live with the same kind of fear of judgment that characterized the medieval period of Christian history, but guilt is still a fundamental dynamic of Christian consciousness and, as any grief counselor knows, at the forefront of awareness for anyone wrestling with loss. The purpose of the following exercise is to give expression to the feelings of guilt and the fear of judgment that are an inevitable part of facing death. For Christians, the experience of judgment, no matter how negative the feelings it evokes, can be faced with the confidence that nothing can separate them from the love of God in Christ.

Though the parable of the last judgment will be familiar to most Christians, it should be read slowly before the beginning of the exercise so that the imagery in the parable is fresh and clear in the minds of the participants. The exercise follows:

Letting the self become still . . . letting the tension fade away . . . letting tranquility flood the mind . . . letting breathing become even and slow . . . sitting in quietness with eyes closed . . . waiting for the muddiness in the water of our lives to settle. As the waters become quiet and clear, as the inner awareness deepens, as the heart yearns for understanding, the moment of revelation is near. Let the breathing come evenly and deeply as you wait in silence. The waters are clear now and quiet . . . transparent as you look into them . . . quiet as a still lake that mirrors the environment around it. Looking into the quiet waters that are you . . . waiting for images to appear that will reveal what is within . . . looking deeply within yourself for a clear picture of yourself as others see you, as God sees you, as you in your most open and vulnerable moments see yourself.

In your mind's eye, imagine yourself seated on a hard-backed chair in the middle of a room. Surrounding you on every side are tiered rows of seats filled with people who have known you, plus some who are strangers. All of those present have needed you in some way. Some are hungry. Some are poor. Some are emotionally starved. Some are very young. Some are very old. The number is great, so many people who have needed so much from you.

As you sit in this room with all eyes focused on you, one of this array of needy people comes forward and sits directly in front of you. It is somebody you know. Let the image of that person form in your mind as he or she approaches. This person looks directly into your eyes and tells you what he or she needed from you that you were never able or willing to give. Listen carefully to what is being said as you look directly into the eyes of the person who is speaking. Do not attempt to defend yourself or offer excuses. Simply listen to what is being said. (*Pause for 1 minute.*) After having listened carefully to what this person has needed but not received, let the image of that person fade away and be replaced by an image of Jesus sitting in front of you. Let the image form spontaneously in any way that seems natural to you. Look closely at the face of Jesus for the expression that you find there. What do you see in his eyes? Disappointment? Judgment? Compassion? Perhaps a mingling of all those expressions and more?

Now let another person come forward, this time someone who is a stranger to you. Let an image of a stranger who may have needed you take shape in your mind. He or she takes the chair directly in front of you. Let the image form spontaneously without forcing it. What does this stranger look like? How old is the person? How is he or she dressed? Don't second-guess your choice of images. Simply let the image take shape in any form that your inner consciousness suggests. As this stranger sits across from you and looks directly into your eyes, listen carefully to what this person tells you about what he or she needed from you that you were not willing or able to give. Listen carefully to what is being said as you look directly into the eyes of the person who is speaking. Do not attempt to defend yourself or offer excuses. Simply listen to what is being said. (*Pause for 1 minute.*) Having listened carefully to what this person has needed but not received, let the image of that person fade away and be replaced by the image of Jesus sitting in front of you. Look closely at the face of Jesus for the expression that you find there. (*Pause for 30 seconds.*)

As you remain seated in the same chair, the room around you is transformed. All the people are gone, and the room is empty. There is no door. There are no windows. The room is brightly lit, but there is no obvious source of the light. The walls, the ceiling, and the floor are all mirrors. No matter where you look, you see a reflection of yourself. You look to the right and then to the left; you look up and then down—only to see images of yourself from different perspectives, images reflected over and over again so that the whole room is filled with images of you. Take a moment to experience what it is like to be in a room where there is no escape from images of yourself. (*Pause for 1 minute.*)

Now recall a time when you were feeling very bad about yourself, but instead of being judged you received an act of kindness from another, an act that you could never deserve or expect much less ask for. Recall the circumstances around that event and with the aid of your imagination reenter the experience. Recall in as much detail as you can what it was that made you feel so badly about yourself. What did the person do that helped you to feel better about yourself? Feel the goodness of being cared for when what you expected was only judgment and criticism. Now let the image of that person fade from your mind and be replaced by an image of a forgiving God. Let yourself feel the full weight of your sinfulness and then let images of God's forgiveness flood your mind. There may be many images—images that come from the Bible, images that come from your experience, images that come from stories you've heard. . . . As those images come to mind, select the one that seems the strongest and let it form fully in your mind. (*Pause for 4-5 minutes.*)

Now let the image shift once more, this time to the scene of the last judgment. You are a part of a vast throng of people surrounding the judgment seat of Christ. Where do you see yourself in this crowd and what do you expect to hear from Jesus? Let that drama unfold of its own accord as you watch it being projected on the screen of your mind's eye. Let it unfold spontaneously without any effort on your part to direct it or change it. (*Pause for 2-3 minutes.*)

As you feel ready, write what you feel and think as you reflect on the experience of being judged and still loved and cared for without reservation or condition. (*Allow 10-15 minutes for writing.*)

This exercise on judgment could also be adapted for secular use, but that would not likely happen, and if it were used, it would lack the framework of meaning that would make the experience positive. I think it woud not be used because most people would regard scenes of judgment as guilt inducing and entirely too negative. The truth is that feelings of guilt are a given for those who grieve. The question is how to deal with those feelings in a constructive manner. The forgiveness of sins is a central motif within the Christian tradition. That assumes both an awareness of guilt and a willingness for confession on the part of the penitent and it assumes also the unconditional love and acceptance of a forgiving God. It is within that framework of meaning that this exercise becomes constructive for Christians.

Care for the Dying

The third exercise has no religious frame of reference, though it could be adapted to include religious symbols shared by those in a common faith tradition. The purpose of the exercise is to facilitate an experience of caring for the dying by identifying resources within the person for that task. I have found this exercise particularly useful for students who are being trained as health-care personnel and know that care for the dying will be part of their professional responsibility. The exercise has the additional value of helping people to reflect on how well they will be able to receive care from others at the time of their own dying.

It is possible to divide the exercise into "Care for the Dying" and "Being Cared for While Dying." One reason for keeping the exercise as a single unit is that a person who has confronted the reality of his or her own dying will be much more sensitive, open, and honest in providing care for those who are dying. I have heard more than one terminally ill person say, "I felt as though I had to take care of her rather than the other way around," or "I felt like he wasn't even here, at least not as a person." One way to retain the unity while dividing the exercise is to invite some sharing in between the divided exercise.

The exercise calls for participants to choose a person to care for who has already died. However, the exercise can be adapted so that they are directed to provide care for someone who is likely to need their care. It is better not to advise them ahead of time that they will be making this choice. That will rob the exercise of its spontaneity. It will be enough to tell them that the exercise is designed to assist them in future tasks of caring for the dying. The exercise follows:

Sitting in the quiet and calm of this protected space with eyes closed, removed from the noise and busyness of the outside world, find a relaxed position for your body . . . become aware of your breathing . . . feel the tensions of the day float away . . . let your body feel more and more relaxed, tensions draining away like water flowing down the side of a hill.

In the quiet and calm of your inner space, so relaxed that your body feels as though it is floating on air, be aware of the goodness of being alive at this very moment, whatever problems you may have. . . . Feel the peace of being alone with yourself and in touch with the deeper part of yourself. . . . Feel the unity with others who share your concern for the dying and who want, like you, to provide gentle care for their human spirit as well as their ravaged bodies. . . .

In the quiet and calm of your inner being, so relaxed that your body feels as though it is floating on air, let your mind drift back over the years in an unhurried, leisurely pace, and remember people you have known who have died. Let the memories come spontaneously. You may be surprised at some of the names and faces that come to your mind. . . . As those names and faces come to you, jot them down, opening your eyes just long enough to put the first name or the initials on the paper and then returning to the region of your inner self. As you write each name, remember the circumstances around the dying and some of the feelings you had at the time. Take a few moments to complete that list. For some of you it will be short, for others longer. (*Pause 3-5 minutes.*)

When you have completed the list, select a person whose dying was gradual rather than sudden, preferably a person with whom you spent some time when he or she was dying. It doesn't have to be the most important person on the list, not even someone that you knew well. If you have had no occasion to be with a person who was dying, imagine being with a person on your list whom you wish you could have been with while he or she was dying. (*Pause for 30 seconds.*)

With your eyes closed, feeling safe in the quiet and calm of this protected space, enter or reenter the experience of being with someone who is dying for whom you have a deep, caring attitude. Picture that person in your mind at different stages of your knowing him or her; first during a time of relatively good health . . . then at the onset of the illness . . . and then at different stages of the process of dying. . . . Be aware of your reaction to the growing awareness of the imminence of his or her dying. . . . As you let that awareness deepen in your heart and mind, focus on your relationship to the person at the end-stage of his or her dying. Imagine yourself being at your present age even if you were much younger when the death occurred. Picture in your mind's eye the place where you and the person are located. You can choose any location you wish and furnish it in a manner that makes it a good place for both of you to be, a place where you would feel comfortable either in giving or in receiving care. Let that scene come clearly in your mind, and let yourself blend slowly into that scene. In your mind's eye, approach the bedside and look into the eyes of the person who is dying. What do you see there? Is it a sense of personal loss? A feeling of inadequacy? A fear of your own dying? Though you will be aware of both physical and emotional needs, focus also on spiritual needs, the needs of the human spirit. What is it that the person needs from you? Is it some form of assurance that you are there and will not leave? Is it reassurance that everything will be O.K.?

How adequate do you feel in meeting those needs? How ready would you be to talk openly and honestly about his or her dying, as well as your own? How do you feel within yourself in this situation? As you are ready, write down some of the feelings and thoughts that come from within the experience of caring for someone who is dying. Let the writing flow spontaneously without analysis or criticism from the rational side of your brain. (*Allow 5-10 minutes for writing.*)

Closing your eyes once again, and feeling safe in the calm and quiet of your inner world, return to the room where you were before, only this time imagine yourself as the one who is dying and being cared for by anyone that you would like to select for that role. Choose someone with whom you would be comfortable. It can be someone who is no longer alive or even someone who doesn't know you but whom you know and respect. (*Pause for 1 minute.*)

Picture your ravaged body close to the time of your death. Imagine yourself lying in bed, looking into the eyes of the person who is caring for you. What do you see there? What are you feeling as you gaze into the eyes of this person who is there to meet your needs? What is the hardest thing for you in being cared for? Is it fear of facing the reality of your dying? Is it fear of rejection? Fear of being abandoned? Is it hard for you to admit your need of others? Hard to ask for what you need? What needs are you aware of in yourself? Though there will be physical and emotional needs, focus also on your spiritual needs, like the need for meaning and purpose. Do you have confidence that the person taking care of you could meet those needs if you could ask for the help you need? Would you be able to speak openly and honestly about your dying? If so, how do you think this person would respond?

Take a moment to let the experience deepen and then, as you are ready, write down some of the feelings and thoughts that come from within the experience of being cared for in your dying. Let the writing flow spontaneously without analysis or criticism from the rational side of your brain. (*Allow 5-10 minutes for writing.*)

At the close of this exercise, the participants are encouraged to share thoughts and feelings without putting pressure on anyone to do so. Dividing into small groups of three or four makes it easier for some to share, though others may feel greater pressure in a smaller group.

Most participants say that they find it easier to provide care for the dying than to receive it. The old adage that it is better to give than to receive is common in our culture. But for everybody who gives care, there has to be somebody who receives it, and by the law of averages, that means that everybody has to be on the receiving end once in a while. Not many people are prepared for that, however, and most cringe at the thought of becoming dependent. Caregiving and care-receiving go hand in hand, and the receiving of care is probably the most necessary and valuable part of the exercise.

LOOK TO THE FUTURE

The greatest need that I see is for research on the effects of using imagery exercises in death education. Psychological studies of death attitudes have multiplied in the past decade. For a good review of those studies, see Robert Neimeyer's review in *Dying, Facing the Facts* (Wass, Berardo, & Neimeyer, 1995). The scales used to test for variables like death anxiety are becoming more sophisticated and reliable, and it would not be difficult to adapt them for measurement of the effects of guided imagery in death education.

There are numerous questions that could be addressed with the aid of psychological testing. What are the psychological effects of using death imagery, especially imagery that is negative? Is there any evidence that the use of death imagery is harmful, for example, engendering a state of depression that is debilitating? Are the feelings that are evoked in the use of death imagery (anxiety, sadness) likely to dissipate fairly soon (within a day), or will they have long-term effects? Does the use of death imagery result in more or less death anxiety? Are there differences in the use of death imagery between men and women? Between young and old? What are the cross-cultural differences in the use of death imagery?

The thesis that I have defended in this chapter, that the context of a specific faith tradition is better for using death imagery than a secular context, also needs to be tested empirically. It may be difficult to obtain a valid statistical measurement since the comparison needs to be made between two different instruments (one using religious imagery and the other secular imagery) in two different settings (religious and secular). The best method for gathering reliable data may be through individual interviews, which might reveal a pattern of response that suggests some definitive differences.

In the future I plan to have students construct their own exercises of guided death imagery as a class project. Part of the project will be for the student to lead others in the exercise, which could be the whole class, a small group, or one other person. The purpose of the project is to demonstrate to students that it does not require professional training to construct and lead exercises in guided imagery. The project should be helpful in moving students from a position of passive receptivity to responsible leadership. In so doing, they will not only be more likely to continue in their use of guided imagery for themselves, but also be more strongly motivated to serve as a guide for others.

Guided imagery is a useful teaching tool for many different subject areas. Within the discipline of theology, it could be used in teaching biblical studies by having students imagine themselves as participants in the stories that are being studied. Guided imagery can be used to make social concerns more relevant; for example, having students identify with people who are disabled or oppressed. Certainly Christian doctrines can be made more existentially relevant with the aid of guided imagery. I once conducted a guided imagery exercise on the meaning of baptism by encouraging members of the group to remember or create in their mind's eye the day of their baptism. Most of the members of this group had been baptized as infants, but the experience was both vivid and compelling. One person who had been born in Germany but had lived in the United States since he was a young child heard the officiant speaking in German. A woman who had been so terrified by water for years that she could shower only with great anxiety completely lost that phobia after the exercise.

The use of guided imagery for death education has value far beyond the confines of a college classroom. As I have argued throughout this chapter, I think it has particular value within the context of a specific faith tradition. I have written a book entitled *Guided Grief Imagery* (Droege, 1987) for use in Christian congregations. The first portion of the book is an exploration of the images of faith that have provided comfort to Christians facing death. The last half of the book contains 26 structured exercises of guided imagery for use in homilies, adult study groups, and pastoral care situations.

There are many other appropriate settings for the use of imagery as a resource for death education. Every wellness program should have a component devoted to death education; imagery is an excellent method for helping people to "live" their dying in a natural, healthy way. The use of death imagery belongs in any program devoted to life-cycle issues in that death imagery is the paradigm for any transition event. It is a mistake to associate death imagery exclusively with terminal illness. At its best, imagery can help people "see" death as a part of life in a way that is enriching, not debilitating.

Death education is here to stay. That presents a challenge for death educators to develop the best possible tools for that task. In my judgment, there is no subject area of education where imagery can be used to better advantage than in death and dying. There are many opportunities for experimentation and research in the use of death imagery. If interest in this subject area during the coming decade matches the interest of the last decade, we should be hearing about many promising developments.

REFERENCES

Becker, A., (1973). *The denial of death.* New York: Free Press.
Droege, T. (1987). *Guided grief imagery: A resource for grief ministry and death education.* New York: Paulist Press.
DeSpelder, L. A., & Strickland, A. L. (2005). *The last dance: Encountering death and dying.* New York: McGraw-Hill.
Lifton, R., & Olson, E. (1974). *Living and dying.* New York: Praeger.
Progoff, I. (1975). *At a journal workshop.* New York: Dialogue House Library.
Wass, H., Berardo, F., & Neimeyer, R. (Eds.). (1995). *Dying, facing the facts* (3rd ed.). Washington: Hemisphere.
Wass, H., Miller, M. D., & Thorton, G. (1990). Death education and grief suicide intervention in the public schools. *Death Studies, 14,* 253-268.

CHAPTER 10

Confronting Death: An Experiential Imagery Exercise

Anees A. Sheikh

> Someone once said, "If stars come out only once in a lifetime, everyone would be out to see them." Not only would we be out to see them but all who saw them would remark about the grandeur of the experience. The media would announce it for weeks in advance and proclaim the beauty of it long after the lights were stilled. We would be prepared and finely tuned to experience the stars if they came out only once, but when they shine every night we go for months without even looking up.
>
> Adams, Otto, and Cowley (1984, pp. 130-131)

As Stephen Levine reminds us in his book, *Who Dies?*, about 200,000 people died today. Some killed themselves, others were murdered. Some died before they were born, others died of old age. Some died thirsty, others were drowned. Some overate, others starved. Some surrendered in peace, others died angry and confused. Lewis Thomas, in *The Lives of a Cell*, points out, "There are 3 billion of us on the earth and all 3 billion must be dead, on a schedule, within this lifetime. . . . Everything that comes alive seems to be in trade for something that dies, cell for cell" (see Levine, 1982, pp. 1-2).

    It is strange that the death of another human being seldom alerts us to the impermanence of all things. As Krishnamurti (1964) says, life is like a river, deep and wide, vital and beautiful, "endlessly moving on, ever seeking, exploring, pushing, overflowing its banks, penetrating every crevice with its water" (p. 156). But Krishnamurti also notes that we human beings have a tendency to dig a little pond for ourselves "away from the swift currents of life," because we want permanence. We barricade ourselves in this pond with our families, ambitions, cultures, fears, guilt, and then we stagnate and die, letting life pass us by (p. 154). In fact, the whole secret of life seems to lie in the acknowledgment of our impermanence, or better still, in our encounter with our impermanence. "An awareness of death shifts one away from trivial preoccupations and provides life with depth and poignancy and an entirely different perspective" (Yalom, 1980, p.160). As Montaigne (1945, p. 65) claimed, "He who would teach men to die, would teach them to live"; or as Santayana asserted, "The dark background that death supplies, brings out the tender colors of life in all their purity" (see Yalom, 1980, p. 163).

Several years ago, Joseph Garai (personal communication, 1982), an art therapist from New York, shared with me the findings of one of his studies. In one group, college students in art therapy were guided through the imagery experience of their rebirth; in another group, subjects first experienced their death in imagery and then their rebirth. Immediately following these experiences, the subjects were encouraged to paint whatever came to them spontaneously. When Garai compared these two sets of paintings, he discovered that the paintings of the second group contained many more vibrant colors, many more flowers and other symbols of joy than the paintings of the first group. Garai's study almost literally bears out Santayana's claim that the dark background that death provides brings into focus the beauties of life.

All major religions and philosophies of the world teach that a purposeful and meaningful life is possible only through the unflinching acceptance of death as an integral constituent of life. Facing death draws us to the threshold of life; it promotes the feeling of joy and intimacy. Paradoxically, we enjoy fully only what we are prepared to relinquish. (Adams et al., 1984). "The acceptance of death as a never-ending process in our life allows to fully enter into the dance of life, the joie de vivre, the child-like astonishment of discovery, of adventure, of pleasure and continuous joyful unfoldment" (Otto, 1973, pp. 100-101).

Following is an example of how a near-fatal automobile accident transformed an individual's life:

> It is hard to describe how "different" I felt about myself and about my whole life after the accident. Somehow, my whole ordering of what was important in life seemed totally wrong. I was more sensitive to how we all waste time—and much less willing to do so myself. I was more aware of the beauties of nature, the common joys, and the fragility of relationships . . . and vowed to live each day so I would be "ready" if it were my last. . . . Why do we have to almost lose life in order to really appreciate it? (Adams et al., 1984, p. 144).

Instead of letting clients wait for a life-threatening event to wake them up, many therapists have developed ways to encourage them to face the fact of death. Over the years, in my imagery workshops, I have routinely employed a death imagery procedure with largely salutary effects. In this exercise, the group first is engaged in a general discussion of death and dying and the life-giving qualities that ensue from an encounter with death. Next, the group works through a couple of brief exercises that tangentially deal with this issue, such as,

On a blank sheet of paper draw a straight line. One end of that line represents your birth; the other end, your death. Draw a cross to represent where you are now. Meditate upon this for five minutes (Yalom, 1980, p. 174).

This simple procedure almost always elicits profound reactions, particularly from adults in their late thirties and older. After a brief sharing of the experiences, the participants are guided to deep relaxation; they are encouraged to feel the natural rhythm of their breathing, to regard each breath as an opportunity to let go, to imagine giving in to gravity, to experience the peace and silence ever present deep within them. While the participants are relaxed and preferably with their eyes closed, they are read an excerpt from the poem *"Keeping Quiet"* by Pablo Neruda, the Nobel laureate from Chile (see Kornfield, 1984, pp. 88-99):

> For once on the face of the earth,
> let's not speak any language;
> let's stop for one second,
> and not move. . . .
> It would be an exotic moment. . . .
>
> If we were not so single-minded
> about keeping our lives moving,
> and for once could do nothing,
> perhaps a huge silence
> might interrupt this sadness
> of never understanding ourselves
> and of threatening ourselves with death.
>
> Perhaps the earth can teach us
> as when everything seems dead in winter
> and later proves to be alive.

After a brief pause, participants slowly are read the following instructions about a detailed death/rebirth imagery,[1] with sufficiently long pauses at appropriate points to conjure up images and to process them. They are informed that they will be led through an imagery of their death and will be brought back through a rebirth imagery. They also are told that if they become concerned or frightened at any time during the guided imagery, they can come out of it. The instructions for the guided imagery follow:

Imagine that you are only days or weeks away from your death, wherever and however it is going to occur. Recall some of the happy moments and some sad moments in your life. Notice what it is that makes you happy or sad. Now think of some important decisions that you made in your life or some decisions that you feel you ought to have made, but did not. Let the images of some of the significant

---

[1] This imagery exercise was in part inspired by the works of a number of individuals (Levine, 1982; Koestenbaum, 1976; Kornfield, 1984; Simonton-Achley, 1981; Yalom, 1980).

individuals in your life emerge. What is it about these individuals that makes them significant to you? If you were to say only one sentence to each of these individuals, what would that be. Say it, if you like.

Now imagine being close to your death. Become aware of the process of dying. Notice any bodily sensations, thoughts, feelings. In this moment close to death, who is with you? What kind of communication is going on between you and these people. At this moment of death, what is it that is most difficult for you to give up, to lose, to let go? What is it?

Now you are even closer to the moment of your death. Who is there? What is being said? You can have anyone that you want to be present. Remember this is your very last chance to say what needs to be said and hear what needs to be heard. This is your last chance to finish any unfinished emotional business. What is still unfinished between you and anyone else present? See how you can achieve resolution. If anyone caused you pain by their words or actions, intentionally or unintentionally, maybe you would like to forgive him/her. Feel that person in your heart center and say, "I forgive you for what you did that caused me pain. I forgive you." Maybe you also need to ask for forgiveness from something that you had done. Remember, this is your last chance to say what needs to be said and to hear what needs to be heard, to say or hear "I love you" or "I am sorry."

Now you see yourself as a corpse. What happens around you? You have the opportunity to watch your own funeral. What kind of service is it? Is it as you always wished? Who is there? What is being said about you? What are the thoughts and feelings of those present? Look at people's faces closely one by one. Can you accept all the good things being said about you? Is there anything you would like to say to them? They won't hear it, but say it anyway, if you like. The service is now finished. Your body is now being laid to rest or cremated. Attend to your thoughts and feelings as this is happening.

Imagine that as your body is buried or cremated, your essence merges with the source of the universe, with the universal energy, which lies beyond the reality that you have known in your earthly life. Worldly objects and events are beginning to recede into the distance. You feel more like a spirit in outer space observing the affairs of the world rather than participating in them as a human being. You are in touch with your universal, eternal consciousness.

Now you have been given an opportunity to be reincarnated. You are in complete control of all the details of this new life. What would you want to create for yourself this time? What kind of models would you follow? What kind of people would you like to surround you? What would have priority in your life? What would be the purpose of your life? What would be your passion? What would stir your soul? What would be your song, your dance in this new life? See, feel, and experience this human being that you want to become in your new life. Let this image sink into the very core of your being. Let yourself become this person.

Now allow yourself to come back to your body, to slowly return to the world. Although you are returning to your body and to this world, you will never be the same again. Now you know exactly how you want to live your life, and you feel deeply motivated to live it that way.

Following this exercise, participants are encouraged to share their experiences, which often leads to a deeply meaningful discussion. Almost always the experiences are profoundly positive and, in many ways, similar to the experiences reported by the near-death experients (Ring & Valarino, 1998), by subjects in psychotherapy under the influence of LSD (Grof, 2000; Grof & Halifax, 1977), or by individuals surviving life-threatening emergencies (Yalom, 1980). As Grof and Halifax (1997) surmise, it is not only that we know we are going to die, but deep down we also have the knowledge of how it feels to die.

The benefits of confronting death are discussed in detail in Chapter 1. Most importantly, these experiences have the power to lead to an enhanced appreciation of one's potentials, of one's relationships with others, and of the countless blessings in one's life. As the poet/mystic and Nobel laureate, Rabindranath Tagore (1962, p. 85), says:

> When I think of this end of my moments, the barrier of the moments breaks and I see by the light of death thy world with its careless treasures.

REFERENCES

Adams, R. S., Otto, H. A., & Cowley, A. S. (1984). *Letting go: Uncomplicating your life.* New York: Science and Behavior Books.

Grof, S. (2000). *Psychology of the future.* Albany, NY: State University of New York Press.

Grof, S., & Halifax, J. (1977). *The human encounter with death.* New York: Dutton.

Koestenbaum, P. (1976). *Is there an answer to death?* Englewood Cliffs, NJ: Prentice-Hall.

Kornfield, J. (1984). The smile of Buddha: Paradigms in perspective. In S. Grof (Ed.), *Ancient wisdom and modern science.* Albany, NY: State University of New York Press.

Krishnamurti, J. (1964). *Think on these things.* New York: Harper and Row.

Levine, S. (1982). *Who dies? An investigation of conscious living and conscious dying.* New York: Anchor Press/Doubleday.

Montaigne, M. (1945). *The complete essays of Montaigne* (D. Frame, Trans.). Stanford: Stanford University Press.

Otto, H. A. (1973). *Group methods to actualize human potential.* Beverly Hills: The Holistic Press.

Ring, K., & Valarino, E. E. (1998). *Lessons from the light: What we can learn from the near-death experiences.* Needham, MA: Moment Point Press.

Simonton-Achley, S. (1981). *Death/Rebirth fantasy and discussion of death.* (Audiocassette). Dallas: Health Training and Research Center.

Tagore, R. (1962). *Gitanjali.* New York: Macmillan.

Yalom, I. (1980). *Existential psychotherapy.* New York: Basic Books.

Contributors

THOMAS A. DROEGE, Ph.D., is Professor Emeritus in the Department of Theology, Valparaiso University, Valparaiso, IN. He was the recipient of the Distinguished Teaching Award from Valparaiso University in 1986. He has published numerous journal articles and book chapters, and his books include *Guided Grief Imagery, Faith Passages and Patterns, Ministry to the Whole Person, Self-Realization and Faith,* and *The Faith Factor in Healing.*

COLLEEN M. HEINKEL, M.A., is a member of the research team at the Center for Health Systems Research and Analysis at the University of Wisconsin–Madison, a group most recently named to serve as a Center of Excellence in Cancer Communication Research by the National Cancer Institute. Ms. Heinkel is currently researching the role of meaning in mitigating treatment distress of patients with breast cancer and is completing her doctoral degree in clinical psychology at Marquette University.

ROBERT G. KUNZENDORF, Ph.D., is Professor of Psychology at the University of Massachusetts Lowell, coeditor of the journal *Imagination, Cognition, and Personality* and past president of the American Association for the Study of Mental Imagery. Dr. Kunzendorf has published four edited books and over 75 articles, which focus on conscious reality testing and various aspects of the mind/body problem.

ALEXANDER A. LEVITAN, M.D., is board certified in medical oncology, internal medicine, and medical hypnosis. He has served as Clinical Associate Professor at the University of Minnesota and teaches at the Minnesota School of Professional Psychology. He is a past president of the American Society of Clinical Hypnosis and the American Board of Hypnosis. He is a Fellow of the American College of Physicians, the American Society of Clinical Hypnosis, and the Society for Clinical and Experimental Hypnosis. He has published and lectured extensively on the topics of hypnosis and oncology, and he is the coauthor of *No Time for Nonsense: Self-Help for the Seriously Ill.*

RITA T. McDONALD, Ph.D., is Associate Professor Emerita of Psychology at Marquette University and a consultant to public and private organizations. She holds a Ph.D. in Clinical Psychology from Loyola University, Chicago, and an Honorary Doctor of Laws from Cardinal Stritch University, Milwaukee. She designed and taught courses in thanatology at Marquette University and at the Medical College of Wisconsin. Her work on the topic of death anxiety has been published in several professional journals.

JAMES K. MORRISON, Ph.D., is Clinical Associate Professor in the Department of Psychiatry at Albany Medical College and is in private practice. Also, he has served as team leader and then as unit chief with the Capitol District Psychiatric Center, Albany, N.Y. Dr. Morrison has published numerous articles on death imagery, psychotherapy, and attitudes toward mental illness, as well as the book, *A Consumer Approach to Community Psychology*.

SUNDAR RAMASWAMI, Ph.D., is a native of Madras, India, where he studied with J. Krishnamurti. He completed his graduate studies at the University of Newcastle, Australia, and at Marquette University. Currently, Dr. Ramaswami is Supervising Clinical Psychologist at Southwestern Connecticut Mental Health System, where he directs the Mobile Crisis Unit and the Forensic Services. Formerly, he was Supervisor at Nova University Clinic.

CAROLYN J. SALYARDS, Ph.D., completed the doctoral program in clinical psychology at Marquette University. She also holds a master's degree in library science (MLS) from the University of Wisconsin–Milwaukee, and a Bachelor's degree in sociology from the University of Minnesota. Her research deals with issues related to complicated grief, focusing and imagery, and imaginal exposure treatment of individuals with posttraumatic stress disorder and non-visual flashbacks.

ANEES A. SHEIKH, Ph.D., is Professor and former chairman of the Department of Psychology at Marquette University and Clinical Professor of Psychiatry and Behavioral Medicine at the Medical College of Wisconsin. He is internationally recognized for his contributions to the field of imagery. A former editor of the *Journal of Mental Imagery*, he now edits the *Imagery and Human Development Series*. Dr. Sheikh has published 14 books on imagery and related topics.

KATHARINA S. SHEIKH, M.A., was formerly on the faculty of Clara Schumann Schule, Bonn, Germany; Cardinal Stritch University; and St. Francis de Sales College in Milwaukee. She is the President of the Institute for Human Enhancement. Educated in Germany, France, Canada, and the United States, she holds graduate degrees from the University of Toronto and Marquette University. She is coeditor of *Imagery in Education* and *Eastern and Western Approaches to Healing*.

Index

Abnormal manifestations of death imagery, 51-53
Acceptance of death bringing one to threshold of living, 2-3
Active privacy, 206-207
Adjective Check List (ACL), 194
African Americans and death anxiety, 187
Age and death anxiety, 186-187
Ambivalence toward death, 110
Ancient approaches to death imagery. *See* Death imagery, overview of ancient/modern approaches to
Anguttara-Nikaya, 126
Annihilation, death as an image of personal
   abnormal manifestations of death imagery, 51-53
   Freud's arguments, 49-50
   Koestenbaum's phenomenological description, 48-50
   overview, 47
   repression of death imagery, 50-53
   See also Artistic expressions of death imagery
Anoxia and NDEs, 88
Antara-bhava (intermediate-state being) in Buddhism, 122-125
Anxiety, death
   authentic existence needed to confront personal mortality, 196-197
   behavioral consequences of, 190-192

[Anxiety, death]
   caution in using therapeutic interventions, 196
   children, 132
   consequences of, functional/behavioral, 185, 190-192
   demographic and personality correlates, 186-188
   dreams/nightmares, 131
   education, death, 177, 196
   fear of death plays important role in human affairs, 131
   hypnosis, 50-51, 177
   identity incompleteness, 189-190
   imagery, relevant work done in field of death, 180-185
   imagery and, studying relationship between death, 179-180
   literature on, 179, 185
   maturity, psychosocial, 187-188
   measuring, 185-186, 190, 193-194
   metaphors of death, 192
   occupational correlates, 188
   older adults, attitudes toward, 187
   organ donation, 191
   personality characteristics, 188-189
   physicians' professional performance, 190
   private and nonconscious levels of, 186
   psychopathology manifested through, 131, 132

[Anxiety, death]
  reflection, encountering one's mortality through, 195-196
  religiosity, 188
  sex of death, perceived, 193
  surgery, 191-192
  therapeutic implications/treating, 192-197
Anxious Journey, The (de Chirico), 58, 59
Appreciation of life, 32, 131
Aranyakas (forest treatises), 111
Archetypes, NDEs as, 94-95
Aronson, Elliot, 12
Artistic expressions of death imagery
  crucifixion, images of Jesus', 54-58
  deathbed theme, 58, 60-61
  insignificance/nothingness, 58-59
  overview, 53-54
  subjectivity of personal annihilation, 61-63
Aryans, 111-115
Atman (individual self), 113-115, 119
Authentic state of being/existence, 130, 196-197
Awareness of one's compassionate nature, 30-31
  See also Mindfulness of death

Bardo Thodol, 4, 123-126
Beauty, appreciation of, 18-19
Becker, Ernest, 208
Belly meditation, soft, 31-32, 35
Benefits of death imagery work
  beauty, appreciation of, 18-19
  creativity, 17
  essence sifted from accessory attributes, 19-20
  here and now: importance of the moment, 16-17
  love, 17-18
  other possible effects, 20
  out-of-body experience, 15-16
  potential, achieving one's, 18
  relaxation, 14-15
  unfinished business, finishing the, 15
Bhikku (male monk), 129-130

Birth experiences, NDEs as recollections of, 94
Blind people and NDEs, 78-79
Boerstler, Richard, 109
Boswell, James, 1
Brahmanas (ritual treatises), 111, 113
Brahman (universal self), 113-115, 119, 126
Brain, NDEs and a damaged, 88-92
Brain, psyche escaping its space-time limitation to the, x-xi
Buddhaghosa, 122
Buddhism
  birth of Buddha, 115
  corpses as objects of meditation, 129-130
  heaven/hell: postmortem judgment, 125-126
  historical beginning, 115
  Indian thought, concept of death in early, 109, 111-115
  intermediate-state being, 122-125
  Levine's (Stephen) introduction into, 28-30
  Mara: death's advocate, 115-118
  meditation on death, 4-5
  mindfulness of death, 4-5, 128-129
  near death experiences, 67
  Nirvana as deathlessness, 126-127
  rebirth, doctrine of, 118-121
  rebirth, mechanism of, 121-122
Byrd, Richard, 69

Children, 75-77, 132
Children of the Light, 77
Christ and the Magdalene (Rodin), 54, 57
Christian contemplation, 180
Christianity and death education, 209-211
Clinging and Buddhism, 117, 121
Closer to the Light: Learning from Children's Near-Death Experience (Morse), 77
Cognitive discomfort and personal construct theory, 147
Collett-Lester Fear of Death Scale, 185-186, 193-194

INDEX / 233

Compassionate Buddha, The (Burt), 28
Conference of Birds, The (Attar), 6
Confrontation therapy, guided, 144-145, 224-227
Consciousness
  holotropic therapy, 11
  Levine, Stephen, 8, 32
  living/dying, conscious, 8, 32
  NDEs and awakening to a higher, 83-86
  NDEs as altered states of, 95-96
  nonlocal model of, x-xi
Construct system/theory, personal, 144, 145-148, 150-156, 194
Contemplation of one's mortality, religion and, 180, 195
Corporeality and Buddhism, 117
Corpses as objects of meditation, 129-130
Craving and Buddhism, 117
Creativity as a benefit of death imagery work, 17
Crucifixion, images of Jesus', 54-58
Crucifixion with the Virgin, Saint John, Saint Jerome and Saint Mary Magdalene (Perugino), 46, 54
Cultural influences and NDEs, 75, 95

Dalai Lama, 134
Dance of Death, The, 203
Davies, Paul, ix
Death 101: Workbook for Educating and Healing (Straub), 7-8
Death Anxiety Scale (DAS), 185
Deathbed theme in death imagery, 58, 60-61
Death Chamber, The (Munch), 58, 60, 61
Death imagery, overview of ancient/ modern approaches to
  Buddhist meditation on death, 4-5
  Freud, Sigmund, 109
  grieving through imagery, 8-9
  holotropic therapy, 11-12
  hypnotic death and suicide rehearsal, 10
  initiation rites, 3-4
  Koestenbaum's (Robert) exercises, 7

[Death imagery, overview of ancient/ modern approaches to]
  Levine's (Stephen) work, 8
  literature on death, increase in professional, 139
  other related techniques, 12-14
  perinatal experiences and LSD, 10-11
  practicing death, 6-7
  Sufi contemplation upon death, 5-6
  summary/conclusions, 20-21
  technique, death imagery, 9-10
  See also Benefits of death imagery work; *individual subject headings*
Death of Ivan Ilyich (Tolstoy), 3
deMello, Anthony, 1
Denial of Death, The, 203
Depersonalization and NDEs, 92-93
Depression, 52-53, 142
Desensitization, death, 133
Developmental Transformations therapy, 194-195
Dimethyltryptamine (DMT) and NDEs, 90
Disidentification, 19
Dissociative coping and NDEs, 75
Doctor Zhivago (Pasternak), 2
Dossey, Larry, ix-xi
Drama, ritual, 183
Dreams/nightmares and death anxiety, 131
Dreyfus, Ann, 12
Drugs and NDEs, 90
Dukha (suffering), 29
Dyaus (Vedic god), 111
Dying, Facing the Facts (Neimeyer), 220

Eastern philosophy, 28-30, 110
  See also Buddhism
Education, death
  anxiety, death, 177, 196
  classroom, settings other than the, 221
  difficulty in dealing with topic, students', 204-205
  faith tradition vs. secular context, 220-221

[Education, death]
   imagination, fostering the use of the, 205
   lecture method, limits of the, 204
   literature on, lack of, 204
   overview, 203-205
   principles of guided imagery, 206-207
   privacy protection, 205-207
   religion, 204, 208-211, 220-221
   research needs, 220
   structured exercises
      care for the dying, 217-220
      judgment, parable of the last, 215-217
      life-threatening experience, 212-215
      overview, 211-212
      students constructing their own exercises, 221
   summary/conclusions, 221-222
   whole-person learning, 205
Ego death, 11, 20
Egyptian Book of the Dead, 123
Electromagnetic forces and NDEs, 86
Emotive-reconstructive imagery techniques to induce grieving, 148-150, 153, 156-158
Encounter-prone personality and NDEs, 76
Endorphins and NDEs, 89-90
Epicurus, 195-196
Erikson, Erik, 208
Essence sifted from accessory attributes, 19-20
Ethnicity and death anxiety, 187
European and Indo-Aryan mythologies, comparing, 111
Experience, mediation and the openness to the fullness of, 8
Experiences Near Death (Kellehear), 95
Experiential imagery exercise: confronting death, 224-227

Fana (annihilation of the ego), 20
Fantasy Level Fear of Death Scale, 185
Fantasy-prone individuals and NDEs, 76, 93

Fear of death, 95, 109, 130, 203
   See also Anxiety, death; Hypnotic listings
Feifel, Herman, 7
Fetishistic fantasies, 51-52
Feynman, Richard, ix
Flash-forwards, NDEs and personal, 87
Forgiveness meditation practice, 35
Formless/spaciousness, one's true nature as, 30
Freud, Sigmund, 49-50, 53, 92, 109, 140, 181-182
Funeral services, 149-150

Garai, Joseph, 224
Gautama Siddhartha, 115
Gender
   anxiety, death, 187
   grieving process, 142
   near death experiences, 74
   widows/widowers, study of bereavement among, 141
Genesis, The Doctrine of Conditioned, 117
Gennep, Arnold van, 3
Genocidal fantasies, 51, 52
Gilbran, Kahlil, 27, 109
Gradual Awakening, A (Levine), 34
Grief Process, The (Levine), 28, 33
Grieving, psychotherapeutic
   case studies, 150-161
   caution, recommendations of, 161
   construct theory, personal, 145-148
   emotive-reconstructive imagery techniques, 148-150, 153, 156-158
   Levine, Stephen, 39-40
   normal and abnormal grief, 140-141
   obstacles impeding normal grieving, 141
   overview, 139-140
   regrieving, 15
   research to determine effectiveness of imagery techniques, 161-162
   successful recovery from grieving process, 141

[Grieving, psychotherapeutic]
techniques, overview of grieving, 8-9, 142-145
theoretical work needs to be done, 162
unfinished emotional business, finishing the, 15
Grist for the Mill (Ram Dass & Levine), 28
Grof, Christina, 11
Grof, Stanislav, 11
Guided Grief Imagery (Droege), 221
Guided imagery. *See* Education, death; individual subject headings
Guided Meditations, Exploration and Healing (Levine), 28, 33, 34

Hanuman Dying Project, 28
Harlequin Complex, 184
Harvey, Andrew, 6
Hawaiians, NDEs and early, 68
Heading Toward Omega (Ring), 83
Healing into Life and Death (Levine), 28, 36
Healing through uncovering the heart, 31-32
Health and death anxiety, 191
Health changes and NDEs, 86
Heart, exploring suffering and uncovering one's, 31-32
Heart of the Buddha's Teaching, The (Thich Nhat Hanh), 30
Heim, Albert, 68-69
Hemingway, Ernest, 69
Hinduism, 111-115, 125, 126
Hiroshima and death anxiety, 194
Holography/holographic theory, 98
Holotropic therapy, 11-12
Homo Faber (Frisch), 2
Hunter, R. C. A., 92
Hygienic viewpoint, 182
Hypercarbia and NDEs, 88
Hypnotic death rehearsal, 10, 50-51, 165-172, 177-178
Hypnotic suicide rehearsal, 10, 172-178

Identity incompleteness and death anxiety, 189-190
Idiot, The (Dostoyevsky), 17
Immortality, symbolic, 180-181
Impermanence, acknowledgment of/ encounter with our, 29, 223-224
India, NDEs in, 74
Indian thought, concept of death in early, 109, 111-115
Indo-Aryans, 111-115
Inevitability of death incorporated into fabric of life experience, xiii
Initiation rites and ancient death imagery, 3-4
Intermediate-state being and Buddhism, 122-125
International Association of Near-Death Studies (IANDS), 99
Interpersonal relationships and NDEs, 85
In the Heart Lies the Deathless (Levine), 34, 38
Iranian and Indo-Aryan mythologies, comparing, 111

James, William, 180
Journal of Near-Death Studies, 69
Journey Into the Light (Abanes), 95
Jung, Carl G., x-xi, 69, 182

Kabir, 21
Kalish, Richard, 139
Karma, 119-122, 125-127
  See also Buddhism
Keeping Quiet (Neruda), 225
Kelly, George, 144-146, 194
Ketamine and NDEs, 90
Koestenbaum, Robert, 7, 48-50, 61
Krishnamurti, Jiddu, 223
Kübler-Ross, Elisabeth, 28
Kundalini experience and NDEs, 96, 100

Levine, Stephen
  appreciation of life, 32
  awareness of one's compassionate nature, 30-31

[Levine, Stephen]
   belly, softening the, 31-32, 35
   conscious living/dying, 8, 32
   death transition meditation, 43-45
   dying, guided meditation on, 41-43
   Eastern philosophy, 28-30
   forgiveness meditation practice, 35
   grief meditation practice, 39-40
   heal to the infinite, the capacity to, 32-33
   heart, healing uncovers the, 31
   life/death as complementary dimensions of a single/integrated process, 8
   love, 18, 33-35
   mindfulness of death, 31-32, 37-38
   overview, 27-28
   pain meditation practice, 40-41
   practice, regular, 33
   summary/conclusions, 45
Life After Life (Moody), 69, 71, 77
Life at Death (Ring), 97
Life cycle, death as part of the, 12, 130
Life/death as complementary dimensions of a single/integrated process, 8
   See also Levine, Stephen
Light/luminosity and NDEs, 75, 85
Light/luminosity and near death experiences, 98-99
Liminal percepts, 53
Line of life exercise, 12
Literature on death, increase in professional, 139
Lives of a Cell (Thomas), 223
Lobe seizures, NDEs and temporal, 88-89
Loss and suffering, 29-31
Love as a benefit of death imagery, 17-18, 33-35
LSD (lysergic acid diethylamide) and perinatal experiences, 10-11

Magic Mountain, The (Mann), 2
Mahayana Buddhism, 126
Majjhima Nikaya, 122
Mann, Thomas, 2
Mara (Indian god), 115-118

Materialism and NDEs, 85
Maturity and death anxiety, psychosocial, 187-188
May, Rollo, 2, 110
Meaning, spiritual path and a search for, xi
Meditation practice in confronting/accepting death, 8, 180
   See also Buddhism; Education, death; Levine, Stephen; *individual subject headings*
Meetings at the Edge (Levine), 28
Melanesians and NDEs, 74
Melges, Frederick, 142-144
Memory syndromes, NDEs and false, 94
Meno (Plato), 6
Mentality and Buddhism, 117
Metaphors of death and death anxiety, 192
Metaphysical theories of NDEs, 96-99
Michelangelo, 2
Mindfulness of death
   authentic state of being/existence, 130, 196-197
   Buddhism, 4-5, 128-129
   depth/poignancy, life filled with, 223-224
   Levine, Stephen, 31-32, 37-38
   overview, 110
   therapist facilitating client's awareness of death, 132-133
Mindsight (eyeless vision), 79
Mithra (Iranian god), 111
Mitra (Vedic god), 111
Mohammed (Prophet), 5
Moment, importance of the: here and now, 16-17
Multidimensional Fear of Death Scale (MFODS), 186, 187
Munch, Edvard, 61
Myers, F. W. H., 110
Mythologies, comparing Indo-Aryan/Iranian/European, 111

National Training Laboratory, 12
Nazis and genocidal fantasies, 52

NDEs. *See* Near death experiences
Near death experiences (NDEs)
   appreciation of life, 131
   in the blind, 78-79
   characteristics of, perceived, 69-75
   in childhood, 75-77
   consequences of
      call to awaken, 83-85
      consciousness, search for a higher, 86
      negative, 81-83
      overview, 80-81
      positive, 83-88
      psychic development, 86-88
      self, the revolution of the, 85-86
   defining terms, 67-68
   demographic factors, 73-74
   distressing, 79-80
   Heim, Albert, 68-69
   history of, 68
   Levine, Stephen, 33
   modern concept of, 69
   psychological profile of individuals with, 75-76
   recent interest in, 69
   sex differences, 74
   social conditioning, 74-75, 95
   summary/conclusions, 100
   theories of
      metaphysical, 96-99
      methodological considerations, 99
      neuropsychological, 88-92
      psychological, 92-96
Neuropsychological theories of NDEs, 88-92
Newman, John H., 179
Nietzsche, Friedrich W., 2
Nirvana as deathlessness, 126-127
Nonbeing, humans inability to accept concept of, 195
Nonlocal model of consciousness, x-xi
Normality in middle of continuum between psychotic repression/existential depression, 53
Nothingness/insignificance in death imagery, 58-59
Noyes, Russell, 92, 131

Obituary, planned, 183-184
Occupational correlates to death anxiety, 188
Older adults, death anxiety and attitudes toward, 187
Omega, 69
Organ donation and death anxiety, 191
Origination, Doctrine of Dependent, 117
Out-of-body experiences (OBEs), 15-16, 71, 97-98
   See also Near death experiences

Pain meditation practice, 40-41
Pantanjali, 28-29
Peak in Darien (Cobbe), 97
Perinatal experiences and LSD, 10-11
Personality characteristics and death anxiety, 188-189
Personal transformation due to brush with death, 2-3, 85-86, 131, 224
Personification, death, 184-185
Pfister, Oscar, 68-69, 92
Phaedo (Plato), 6, 7
Phaedrus (Plato), 6
Physicians' professional performance and death anxiety, 190
Planetary consciousness/vision, 83, 87-88
Plato, 6-7
Pornography, comparing attitudes toward death and, 139
Potential, achieving one's, 18
Practicing death, 6-7
Prajapati (Lord of creatures), 113
"Presence" encountered during NDEs, 84-85
Privacy protection and death education, 205-207
Progoff, Ira, 206
Psychedelic drugs, 90, 133, 227
Psychic development and NDEs, 86-88
Psychic Vision Theory, 97
Psychosocial maturity and death anxiety, 187-188

Psychotherapy and death
  anxiety, death, 131, 132, 194
  awareness of death, facilitating client's, 132-133
  construct theory, personal, 146
  dying individuals in meetings, 13, 133
  Eastern sources and perspectives on death, 110
  ignoring the issue, 131-132
  imagination, dying in the, 133-134
  NDEs, psychological profile of individuals with, 75-76
  NDEs, psychological theories of, 92-96
  psychopathology as consequence of inability to deal with death, 130
  relaxation, death imagery in, 133-134
  See also Grieving, psychotherapeutic
Pudagalavadins (school of Buddhism), 121-122

Ram Dass, 28
Ramsay, Ronald, 144
Rebirth, Buddhism and doctrine of, 118-122
Reflection, encountering one's mortality through, 195-196
Regrieving, 15
Reified/personified death, 184-185
Reincarnation, 126-127
Relaxation as a benefit of death imagery, 14-15, 133-134
Religion
  anxiety, death, 188
  contemplation of one's mortality, 180, 195
  education, death, 204, 208-211, 220-221
  Vedic, 111
  See also Spirituality
Repression of death imagery, 50-53
Republic, The (Plato), 6, 68
Revised Death Anxiety Scale (RDAS), 187
Rig-Veda, 111, 120, 126
Ring, Kenneth, 67, 70-73, 83
Rinpoche, Sogyal, 67

Rites of passage, 3
Ritual drama, 183
Russell, Bertrand, x, 110

Santayana, George, 2, 224
Schizophrenia as defense against recognizing death, 51
Scream, The (Munch), 61, 62
Scrooge, Ebenezer, 3
Self-centeredness, accepting death through liberation from, 181
Self-transformation and NDEs, 85-86
Sex of death, death anxiety and perceived, 193
Shamanic training, 3
Sheikh, Anees A., xiii-xiv
Sheikh, Katharina S., xiii-xiv
Siddhartha, Gautama, 115
Sivananda (Swami), 28, 29
Small Crucifixion, The (Grunewald), 54
Social conditioning and NDEs, 74-76, 95
Soul Travel Theory, 97
Space-time perception, reassessing absolute validity of, x-xi
Spirituality
  loss and, 29-30
  meaning, search for, xi
  near death experiences, 84-85
  See also Religion
St. Augustine, 130
Straub, Sandra, 7-8
Suffering and loss, 29-32
Sufi contemplation upon death, 5-6, 20
Suicide rehearsal, hypnotic, 10, 172-177
Surgery and death anxiety, 191-192
Symbolization of life and death, 180-181

Tagore, Rabindranath, 14, 27, 227
Tanha (thirst for existence), 122
Teaching, guided imagery used in. *See* Education, death
Teilhard de Chardin, Pierre, 83
Thanatology, 204
Thanatomimesis, 183
Theaetetus (Plato), 6

Thematic Apperception Test (TAT), 51, 184
Tibetan Book of the Dead, 4, 123-126
Time-contingent meanings of death, reassessing, ix-x
Tolstoy, Leo, 131
Toynbee, Arnold J., 181
Transformation due to brush with death, personal, 2-3, 85-86, 131, 224
Transi, 203
Transition to another state, more acceptance of death as a, xi
Triumph of Death, The, 203
Truth, search for a deeper, 29-30
Turning Toward the Mystery (Levine), 28, 32
Twilight imagery, 206

Unfinished emotional business, finishing the, 15
Unpleasant reality, Western cultures regarding death as an, 1
Upadana (clinging to existence), 117, 121
Upanishads (philosophical works), 111, 113-115, 119, 125, 126

Valarino, Evelyn E., 67

Vasabandhu, 122
Vedas (sacred hymns), 111-113
Vietnam War and death anxiety, 194
Vijnana (psychic force), 121
Vivekananda (Swami), 28-29

War and Peace (Tolstoy), 2
Watts, Alan, 16
Western cultures' notions of death, 1, 110
Who Dies? (Levine & Levine), xiii, 28, 223
Whole-person learning and death education, 205
Widows/widowers, study of bereavement among, 141
With the Eyes of the Mind (Gabbard & Twemlow), 76
Workshops, death awareness, 12-13
Yalom, Irvin, 2, 179

Yama (Vedic god), 112, 126
Year to Live, A (Levine), 27, 28, 32

Zen Buddhism, ix
    See also Buddhism